Advanced Therapy for Hepatitis C

Advanced Therapy for Hepatitis C

EDITED BY

Geoffrey W. McCaughan MBBS, PhD, FRACP

Head of Liver Immunobiology Program
Centenary Research Institute
A.W. Morrow Professor of Medicine
Director A.W. Morrow GE/Liver Center
Director Australian Liver Transplant Unit
Royal Prince Alfred Hospital
University of Sydney
Sydney, NSW, Australia

John G. McHutchison, MD

Senior Vice President, Liver Disease Therapeutics
Gilead Sciences, Inc.
Foster City, CA, USA

Jean-Michel Pawlotsky, MD, PhD

Director, French National Reference Center for Viral Hepatitis B, C and delta
Head, Department of Virology, Bacteriology, and Hygiene
INSERM U955
Hôpital Henri Mondor
Université Paris Est
Créteil, France

WILEY-BLACKWELL

A John Wiley & Sons, Ltd., Publication

This edition first published 2012 © 2012 by Blackwell Publishing Ltd

Blackwell Publishing was acquired by John Wiley & Sons in February 2007. Blackwell's publishing program has been merged with Wiley's global Scientific, Technical and Medical business to form Wiley-Blackwell.

Registered office: John Wiley & Sons, Ltd, The Atrium, Southern Gate, Chichester, West Sussex, PO19 8SQ, UK

Editorial offices: 9600 Garsington Road, Oxford, OX4 2DQ, UK
The Atrium, Southern Gate, Chichester, West Sussex, PO19 8SQ, UK
111 River Street, Hoboken, NJ 07030-5774, USA

For details of our global editorial offices, for customer services and for information about how to apply for permission to reuse the copyright material in this book please see our website at www.wiley.com/wiley-blackwell.

The right of the author to be identified as the author of this work has been asserted in accordance with the UK Copyright, Designs and Patents Act 1988.

Library of Congress Cataloging-in-Publication Data
Advanced therapy for hepatitis C / edited by Geoffrey W. McCaughan, John G. McHutchison, Jean-Michel Pawlotsky.
  p. ; cm.
Includes bibliographical references and index.
ISBN-13: 978-1-4051-8745-9 (hardcover : alk. paper)
ISBN-10: 1-4051-8745-X (hardcover : alk. paper)
ISBN-13: 978-1-4443-4631-2 (ePDF)
ISBN-13: 978-1-4443-4634-3 (Wiley Online Library)
[etc.]
  1. Hepatitis C–Treatment.   2. Antiviral agents.   I. McCaughan, Geoffrey W.   II. McHutchison, J. G.   III. Pawlotsky, Jean-Michel.
[DNLM: 1. Hepatitis C–therapy.   2. Antiviral Agents–therapeutic use.
WC 536]
RC848.H425A38 2012
616.3′62306–dc23
                                                                                2011016561

A catalogue record for this book is available from the British Library.

This book is published in the following electronic formats: ePDF 9781444346312; Wiley Online Library 9781444346343; ePub 9781444346329; Mobi 9781444346336

Set in 9.25/11.5pt Minion by Aptara® Inc., New Delhi, India
Printed and bound in Malaysia by Vivar Printing Sdn Bhd

1 2012

Contents

Contributors

Nezam H. Afdhal MD
Beth Israel Deaconess Medical Center
Boston, MA, USA

Angelo Andriulli MD
Gastroenterology Department
IRRCS Casa Sollievo della Sofferenza
San Giovanni Rotondo, Italy

Martin Baril PhD
Research Associate
Institut de Recherche en Immunologie
et Cancérologie (IRIC)
Montréal, Québec, Canada

Michael R. Beard PhD
Head, Hepatitis C Virus Research Laboratory
School of Molecular and Biomedical Science
The University of Adelaide & Center for Cancer Biology,
SA Pathology
Adelaide, SA, Australia

Thomas Berg MD
Professor
Department of Gastroenterology and Rheumatology
Division of Hepatology
University of Leipzig
Leipzig, Germany

David G. Bowen MBBS, PhD
Sydney Medical School, University of Sydney
Royal Prince Alfred Hospital
Sydney, NSW, Australia

Patrice Cacoub MD, PhD
Professor
Department of Internal Medicine
Groupe Hospitalier Pitié-Salpêtrière
Université Pierre et Marie Curie
Paris, France

Laurent Chatel-Chaix PhD
Post-doctoral Fellow
Institut de Recherche en Immunologie
et Cancérologie (IRIC)
Montréal, Québec, Canada

Grace M. Chee PharmD
Hepatology Department
Cedars-Sinai Medical Center
Los Angeles, CA, USA

Stéphane Chevaliez PharmD, PhD
National Reference Center for Viral Hepatitis B, C
and delta
Department of Virology & INSERM U955
Hôpital Henri Mondor
Université Paris-Est
Créteil, France

Lotte Coelmont PhD
Laboratory of Virology and Chemotherapy
Rega Institute for Medical Research
University of Leuven
Leuven, Belgium

Antonio Craxì, MD
Full Professor of Gastroenterology
Sezione di Gastroenterologia, Di.Bi.M.I.S. Policlinico
Paolo Giaccone
University of Palermo
Palermo, Italy

Leen Delang PhD
Laboratory of Virology and Chemotherapy
Rega Institute for Medical Research
University of Leuven
Leuven, Belgium

Gregory J. Dore BSc, MBBS, MPH, PhD, FRACP
Professor and Head, Viral Hepatitis Clinical
Research Program
National Centre in HIV Epidemiology and
Clinical Research
The University of New South Wales;
Infectious Diseases Physician
St Vincent's Hospital
Sydney, NSW, Australia

**Mark W. Douglas BSc (Med)(Hons), MBBS (Hons),
PhD, FRACP**
Senior Lecturer, Hepatology and Virology
Storr Liver Unit, Westmead Millennium Institute
Sydney Emerging Infections and Biosecurity Institute
University of Sydney
Sydney, NSW, Australia

Xavier Forns MD, PhD
Liver Senior Specialist
Liver Unit, Hospital Clinic
IDIBAPS and Ciberehd (Centro de Investigación en Red
de Enfermedades Hepáticas y Digestivas)
Barcelona, Spain

Mathy Froeyen PhD
Assistant Professor of Pharmacy
Laboratory of Medicinal Chemistry
Rega Institute for Medical Research
University of Leuven
Leuven, Belgium

Ed Gane MB ChB, MD, FRACP
Associate Professor and Hepatologist
New Zealand Liver Transplant Unit
Auckland City Hospital
Auckland, New Zealand

Jacob George MBBS (Hons), FRACP, PhD
Director of Gastroenterology and Hepatic Services
Storr Liver Unit, Westmead Millenium Institute
University of Sydney
Sydney, NSW, Australia

Rebekah G. Gross MD
Assistant Professor of Medicine
Division of Gastroenterology and Hepatology
Weill Cornell Medical College
New York, NY, USA

Piet Herdewijn PhD
Professor of Pharmacy
Laboratory of Medicinal Chemistry
Rega Institute for Medical Research
University of Leuven
Leuven, Belgium

Ira M. Jacobson MD
Vincent Astor Professor of Medicine
Chief, Division of Gastroenterology and Hepatology
Division of Gastroenterology and Hepatology
Weill Cornell Medical College
New York, NY, USA

Sanaa M. Kamal MD, PhD
Department of Gastroenterology and Liver Disease
Ain Shams Faculty of Medicine
Cairo, Egypt;
Department of Gastroenterology
Tufts School of Medicine
Boston, MA, USA

Daniel Lamarre PhD
Full Professor, Department of Medicine
Faculty of Medicine
Institute for Research in Immunology and Cancer (IRIC)
Université de Montréal
Montréal, Québec, Canada

Alessandra Mangia MD
Liver Unit
IRRCS Casa Sollievo della Sofferenza
San Giovanni Rotondo, Italy

Diarmuid S. Manning MB, BCh
Beth Israel Deaconess Medical Center
Harvard Medical School
Boston, MA, USA

Stella Martínez MD
Liver Unit, Hospital Clinic
IDIBAPS and Ciberehd (Centro de Investigación en Red
de Enfermedades Hepáticas y Digestivas)
Barcelona, Spain

Gail V. Matthews MBChB, MRCP (UK), FRACP, PhD
Clinical Academic
National Centre in HIV Epidemiology and Clinical
Research
University of New South Wales
Sydney, NSW, Australia

Geoffrey W. McCaughan MBBS, PhD, FRACP
Head of Liver Immunobiology Program
Centenary Research Institute
A.W. Morrow Professor of Medicine
Director A.W. Morrow GE/Liver Center
Director Australian Liver Transplant Unit
Royal Prince Alfred Hospital
University of Sydney
Sydney, NSW, Australia

John G. McHutchison, MD
Senior Vice President, Liver Disease Therapeutics
Gilead Sciences, Inc.
Foster City, CA, USA

Leonardo Mottola PhD
Liver Unit
IRRCS Casa Sollievo della Sofferenza
San Giovanni Rotondo, Italy

Andrew J. Muir MD MHS
Director, Gastroenterology/Hepatology Research
Duke Clinical Research Institute
Duke University Medical Center
Durham, NC, USA

Johan Neyts PhD
Professor of Virology
Laboratory of Virology and Chemotherapy
Rega Institute for Medical Research
University of Leuven
Leuven, Belgium

Venessa Pattullo MBBS, FRACP
Storr Liver Unit, Westmead Millennium Institute
University of Sydney, Sydney, NSW, Australia;
Division of Gastroenterology
Toronto Western Hospital
University Health Network, University of Toronto
Toronto, Ontario, Canada

Jean-Michel Pawlotsky MD, PhD
Director, French National Reference Center for Viral
Hepatitis B, C and delta
Head, Department of Virology, Bacteriology, and
Hygiene
INSERM U955
Hôpital Henri Mondor
Université Paris Est
Créteil, France

Salvatore Petta MD, PhD
Sezione di Gastroenterologia, Di.Bi.M.I.S. Policlinico
Paolo Giaccone
University of Palermo
Palermo, Italy

Fred Poordad MD
Associate Professor of Medicine
David Geffen School of Medicine at UCLA;
Chief, Hepatology and Liver Transplantation
Cedars-Sinai Medical Center
Los Angeles, CA, USA

Scott A. Read MSc
Storr Liver Unit, Westmead Millennium Institute
University of Sydney
Sydney, NSW, Australia

Jose María Sánchez-Tapias MD, PhD
Senior Consultant
Liver Unit, Hospital Clinic
IDIBAPS and Ciberehd (Centro de Investigación en Red
de Enfermedades Hepáticas y Digestivas)
Barcelona, Spain

Kathleen B. Schwarz MD
Director, Pediatric Liver Center
Division of Pediatric Gastroenterology and Nutrition
Professor of Pediatrics
Johns Hopkins University School of Medicine
Baltimore, MD, USA

Mitchell L. Shiffman MD
Director
Liver Institute of Virginia
Bon Secours Virginia Health System
Richmond and Newport News, VA, USA

Benjamin Terrier MD
Department of Internal Medicine
Groupe Hospitalier Pitié-Salpêtrière
Université Paris 6 Pierre et Marie Curie
Paris, France

Alexander J. Thompson MD, PhD
St. Vincent's Hospital Melbourne, University of
Melbourne, Melbourne, VIC, Australia;
Victorian Infectious Diseases Reference Laboratory
(VIDRL), North Melbourne, VIC, Australia;
Department of Gastroenterology and Duke Clinical
Research Institute
Duke University
Durham, NC, USA

Edmund Tse MBBS, FRACP
School of Molecular and Biomedical Science
The University of Adelaide and the Center for Cancer
Biology
SA Pathology
Adelaide, SA, Australia

Heiner Wedemeyer MD
Professor
Department of Gastroenterology, Hepatology and
Endocrinology
Medizinische Hochschule Hannover
Hannover, Germany

Johannes Wiegand MD
Private Lecturer
Department of Gastroenterology and Rheumatology
Division of Hepatology
University of Leipzig
Leipzig, Germany

Kenneth Yan MBBS, Mmed (Clin Epi), FRACP
Conjoint Associate Lecturer
St George Clinical School
Faculty of Medicine
University of New South Wales
Sydney, NSW, Australia

Amany Zekry MBBS, PhD, FRACP
Department of Gastroenterology and Hepatology
Clinical School of Medicine
St George Hospital
Sydney, NSW, Australia

Preface

Hepatitis C virus results in chronic liver disease in over 170 million people worldwide. This book arrives at a watershed in the history of antiviral treatment of the hepatitis C virus. It is the beginning of the end of non-specific antiviral approaches via interferon-based therapies. From now on the field will be dominated by the arrival of HCV-specific direct antiviral agents. Initially these agents will still require interferon and ribavirin but already clinical trials are under way that do not include either of these agents.

This publication outlines the current standard of care up until this time and includes therapeutic approaches to wide patient groups. We believe that the structure of the book will remain relevant for future editions as the new therapies are gradually rolled out across these patient groups, as well as across an increasing number of countries.

G.W.M.
J.G.M.
J-M.P.

Foundations for Understanding Antiviral Therapies in HCV

1 HCV Replication

Michael R. Beard

School of Molecular and Biomedical Science, University of Adelaide, and Centre for Cancer Biology, SA Pathology, Adelaide, SA, Australia

Introduction

Hepatitis C virus (HCV) is classified in the *Hepacivirus* genus within the family *Flaviviridae* and is the leading cause of chronic hepatitis and liver disease related morbidity worldwide. With an estimated 170 million people infected worldwide and the ability of the virus to establish a chronic infection in approximately 70% of cases, it is not surprising that HCV represents a major cause of global suffering and morbidity and a burden to many public health systems. Chronic HCV infection is often associated with development of serious liver disease, including cirrhosis, liver failure, and hepatocellular carcinoma. Accordingly, a thorough understanding of the life cycle and molecular biology of HCV and its interaction with the host are essential in the development of treatment and vaccine strategies. Although these studies have been hampered by the lack of a small-animal model and, until recently, a lack of a tissue culture system that accurately reflects the life cycle of HCV, significant progress has been made in the understanding of HCV molecular biology and pathogenesis. In this chapter we discuss recent advances in models to study HCV replication and the HCV life cycle.

The HCV Genome

HCV possesses a 9.6 kb single-stranded, positive-sense RNA genome composed of a 5′ UTR (untranslated region), a long open-reading frame (ORF) encoding a polyprotein of approximately 3000 amino acids, and a 3′ UTR (Figure 1.1). The polyprotein can be divided into three segments based on the functional aspects of the proteins: the NH2 terminal region comprises the structural proteins (core, E1, and E2); a central region consists of two proteins (p7 and NS2) that are not involved in HCV replication or are structural components of the virus, but probably play a role in virion morphogenesis; and the COOH-terminal proteins (NS3, NS4A, NS4B, NS5A, and NS5B) that are required for HCV replication (Figure 1.1). A detailed description and function of the HCV proteins can be found in an excellent review from Moradpour and colleagues [1]. After release of the HCV genome into the cytoplasm the genome is exposed to the host cellular machinery for translation of the viral polyprotein. The 5′ and 3′ UTRs are highly conserved and critical to viral genome replication and translation of the viral polyprotein. The 5′ UTR is approximately 341 nucleotides long and contains a highly structured RNA element known as the internal ribosome entry site (IRES) that is recognized by the cellular 40S ribosomal subunit to initiate translation of the RNA genome in a cap-independent manner. The importance of the secondary and tertiary structure of the IRES domain for initiation of translation has been demonstrated by mutational analysis. However, the primary sequence, particularly in stem-loop IIId and IIIe, is also critical for efficient HCV IRES activity [2,3]. Recently, the structural nature of HCV IRES interactions with the 40S ribosomal subunit and the eIF3 complex has been revealed by cryo-electron microscopy [4,5]. Preceding the IRES at the extreme 5′ end are elements required for viral replication that overlap partially with the IRES region (domain II), leading to speculation that this region is involved in regulation of a viral translation to replication switch [6]. Consistent with this speculation is the recent observation that a short highly conserved RNA segment at the 5′ end of the HCV genome binds a liver-specific

Advanced Therapy for Hepatitis C, First Edition. Edited by Geoffrey W. McCaughan, John G. McHutchison and Jean-Michel Pawlotsky.
© 2012 Blackwell Publishing Ltd. Published 2012 by Blackwell Publishing Ltd.

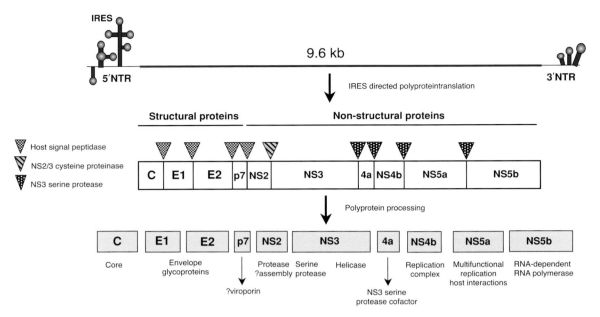

Figure 1.1 Genomic organization and polyprotein processing of the HCV genome. The HCV genome consists of a positive-stranded RNA genome that is flanked by 5′ and 3′ UTRs of highly ordered secondary structure. The polyprotein is cleaved by either host- or viral-encoded proteases (depicted by triangles) to liberate the mature structural and non-structural proteins.

microRNA, miR-122, that is required for efficient HCV replication in cultured hepatoma cells [7]. However, in the HCV-infected liver no correlation was noted between miR-122 abundance and levels of HCV RNA in the liver or serum, which suggests that the impact of miR-122 may be less prominent *in vivo* than *in vitro* [8]. miR-122 may impact HCV replication indirectly through stimulation of translation of the viral polyprotein by enhancing association of ribosomes with the IRES [9]. Although more work is required to determine its role in the HCV life cycle and pathogenesis, modulation of miR-122 expression and activity presents as an attractive target for future therapy.

Like the 5′ UTR, the 3′ UTR of the HCV genome contains a high degree of secondary structure. This region is 200–300 nucleotides in length and is comprised of three major elements involved in replication: (i) a variable region (30–50 nucleotides), which directly follows the NS5B stop codon; (ii) a polyuridine (U/C) tract (20–200 nucleotides); and (iii) a highly conserved region (98 nucleotides), known as the 3′ X region, which forms a three stem-loop structure [10–12]. Mutational analysis has revealed that the poly-U/C tract and the 3′ X region play a more important role than the variable region in the synthesis of negative-strand RNA [13].

Models to Study HCV Replication

HCV Replicons

The development of the subgenomic HCV replicon system, first reported in 1999, significantly enabled the study of HCV replication in cultured cells for the first time [14]. Replicons represent autonomously replicating HCV RNAs, and typically contain an in-frame insertion of a selectable antibiotic marker (e.g., neomycin phosphotransferase: G418) within the amino terminal HCV core sequence, followed downstream by a heterologous IRES from encephalomyocarditis virus (EMCV), a picornavirus, to drive internal translation of the downstream HCV open reading frame (NS2 to NS5B) (Figure 1.2). The minimal requirements for a viable HCV replicon are HCV-derived 5′ and 3′ ter-mini and the non-structural proteins (NS3 to NS5B) that form the replication complex, however, replication-competent HCV replicons encoding the complete HCV polyprotein are viable [15,16]. Transfection of Huh-7 (hepatoma-derived) cells with synthetically derived transcripts followed by selection with G418 results in the establishment of cell lines that harbor autonomous

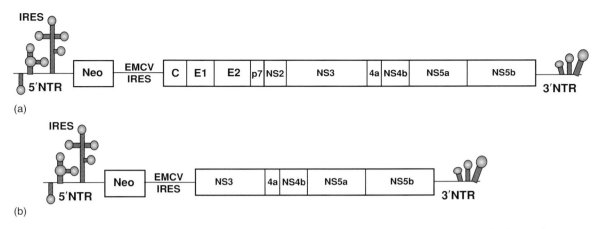

Figure 1.2 Schematic diagram of the organization of the (a) genomic and (b) subgenomic HCV replicons. In both cases the HCV IRES drives expression of the neomycin phosphotransferase gene while the EMCV IRES drives expression of the HCV proteins.

replication of the virus. HCV RNA isolated from cell lines under antibiotic selection often contains cell-culture adapted mutations that greatly enhance replication, although the molecular basis for this increased replication is unclear [15,17,18]. These adaptive mutations often map to the NS5A protein and may potentially influence phosphorylation, resulting in a hypophosphorylated state and increased replication. Adaptive mutations have also been mapped to NS3, NS4A, NS4B, and NS5B. Interestingly, these replication-adaptive cell-culture mutations have been shown to reduce *in vivo* infectivity in chimpanzees, highlighting the adaptive nature of these viruses derived from cell culture [19]. HCV replicons are not restricted to Huh-7 cells, and other cell lines such as HeLa and cells of murine origin have also yielded selected clones of replicating HCV, highlighting that HCV replication is not restricted to liver-derived cells of human origin [20,21].

The antibiotic selection process not only selects for HCV genomes with high replication capacity but also clones of Huh-7 cells that are highly permissive for HCV infection. One such cell line, Huh-7.5, has been "cured" of HCV by treatment with low doses of interferon-α, is hyperpermissive for HCV replication [22], and is clearly enriched for factors that promote replication and/or defects in innate viral sensing pathways. For example, Huh-7.5 cells have a spontaneous knockout of the dsRNA cellular sensing protein RIG-1 and do not mount a robust antiviral response to viral infection that allows for HCV replication. This highlights the importance of innate immune sensing in HCV infection and is con-

sistent with the ability of the HCV NS3/4A protein to cleave IPS-1, which is integral to the innate immune RIG-I pathway [23].

HCV replicons have been valuable tools for studying numerous aspects of the HCV life cycle and interaction with the host cell. However, their major limitation has been inability to produce infectious virus particles even when the complete complement of HCV proteins is expressed, for reasons that are not entirely clear [15,16,22]. The original replicon concept has undergone evolution and replicons are now available that contain various markers (e.g., GFP, luciferase) that allow quantitative assessment of HCV replication and have been useful in high-throughput screening of antiviral compounds.

Productive Viral Infection in Cell Culture

The recent identification in 2005 of a cloned HCV genome (genotype 2a), known as JFH-1, that is capable of initiating high-level replication in cell culture *and* production of infectious virus particles represents a major breakthrough in the pursuit of a cell-culture model for HCV [24,25]. In contrast to HCV replicon systems, transfection of Huh-7 cells with RNA synthesized *in vitro* from the cloned JFH-1 cDNA genome and a related genotype 2a chimera, FL-J6/JFH replicate efficiently in Huh-7 cells without the need for cell-culture adaptive mutations. Moreover, virus particles produced by these cells are infectious in chimpanzees and can be serially passaged *in vivo* [25] while the FL-J6/JFH virus can infect mice containing human liver grafts [24]. Interestingly, virus produced *in vivo* has a lower buoyant density than virus produced in cell culture, suggesting association with low-density lipids [26]. This system represents a major advance in the study of virus-host interactions and the virus life cycle, all in the context of replicating virus. Similarly, the highly adapted genotype 1a HCV isolate known as H77-S (derived from the H77 isolate) [27] is also capable of instigating HCV RNA replication and production of infectious virus particles [28]. This represents another breakthrough in the generation of tools to study the HCV life cycle, particularly because this genotype is more prevalent worldwide and is associated with more significant liver disease. Intragenotypic and intergenotypic chimeras of HCV that contain the non-structural protein-encoding regions of JFH-1 and the structural protein-encoding regions of other HCV genomes may help define regions of structural proteins that influence the efficiency of virus particle synthesis and secretion [29]. This relatively new cell-culture model system will be invaluable in the study of many aspects of virus-host interaction, including viral entry, and assembly and release, which were previously inaccessible to manipulation.

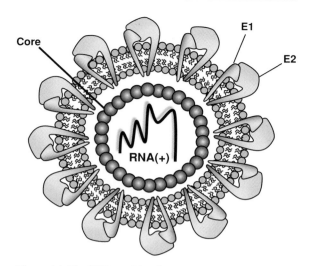

Figure 1.3 The HCV particle. The RNA genome is encapsidated by the icosahedral nucleocapsid consisting of the core protein. The nucleocapsid is enveloped by a host-derived spherical lipid bilayer that is enriched with heterodimers of the envelope glycoproteins E1 and E2.

The HCV Virion and Entry

The relatively low levels of HCV in plasma samples have hampered visualization of viral particles; however, virus-like particles have been identified by electron microscopy, which has indicated that infectious HCV virions are roughly spherical particles of diameter 55–65 nm with fine projections of approximately 6 nm ([25] and references therein). The major protein constituents of the host-derived lipid bilayer envelope are the highly glycosylated HCV envelope glycoproteins E1 and E2 that surround the viral nucleocapsid, composed of many copies of the HCV core protein and the genomic HCV RNA (Figure 1.3). HCV from serum and plasma fractionates with a wide range of buoyant densities that can be attributed to association of the virus with lipoproteins, in particular apolipoprotein-B (Apo-B) and apolipoprotein-E (Apo-E), which are components of host low density lipoprotein (LDL, Apo-B) and very low density lipoprotein (VLDL, Apo-B, Apo-E) and suggest a close association with circulating LDL/VLDL [26]. The physiological association of HCV with LDL/VLDL remains unexplained mechanistically; however, it could be involved in viral uptake (see below), or alternatively the association of Apo-B with HCV virions may indicate a role for the hepatic LDL/VLDL secretory pathway in release of the virus.

Hepatocytes are the main target for infection with HCV; however, identification of the cellular receptors responsible for HCV entry has proven difficult due to the lack of appropriate model systems. However, using a combination of HCV pseudotyped particles (HCVpp) [30,31] and cell-culture-derived HCV (HCVcc) [25], the complement of HCV receptors now seems complete.

The 25 kDa tetraspanin molecule CD81 and the human scavenger receptor class B type I (SR-BI) both bind HCV E2 and are necessary but not sufficient for HCV entry [32]. For example, CD81 ectopic expression in hepatocyte-derived cell lines that are negative for CD81 confers susceptibility to HCVpp and HCVcc; however, expression of both factors in non-hepatocyte-derived cell lines does not concur infectivity [24,30]. Clearly additional hepatocyte factors are required for HCV entry. Using an interactive cloning and expression approach, the tight junction protein claudin-1 (CLDN1) was recently identified as an HCV co-receptor [33]. CLDN1 was found to be essential for entry into hepatic cells and rendered non-hepatic cells susceptible to infection. However, despite the identification of CD81, SR-B1, and CLDN1 as essential HCV entry co-factors, a number of human cell lines and those of non-primate origin remained resistant to HCV infection, suggesting an additional entry factor. Using a cyclic lentivirus-based screen of a cDNA library derived from a highly HCV-permissive hepatocarcinoma cell line (Huh-7.5) for genes that render the non-permissive CD81+, SR-BI+ 293T cell line infectable with HCVpp, the remaining crucial factor was recently identified as occludin (OCLN), also a tight junction protein [34]. Although expression of all four entry factors (CD81, SR-B1, CLDN1, OCLN) renders mouse cell lines susceptible to HCVpp infection, these cells could not support HCVcc infection. This is not surprising given past reports of inefficient replication of HCV RNA in mouse cell lines, and suggests that specific hepatocyte factors are crucial for efficient HCV replication. The identification of CD81 and OCLN as the minimal human-specific entry factors (HCV can bind to murine SR-B1 and CLDN1) not only significantly advances our understanding of the molecular mechanisms of HCV entry but also provides important steps for the development of a mouse model of HCV infection and provides an attractive target for the development of novel antiviral strategies.

Other molecules have been suggested to be involved in HCV entry. The association of HCV virions in serum with LDL and VLDL suggests that the LDL receptor (LDLR) may be an attractive candidate receptor. However, its precise role remains to be determined [26,35]. LDLR is not sufficient itself for entry and it does not bind directly to HCV E2 [30]. Together with the glycosaminoglycans, the LDLR in concert with other cell-surface proteins may serve to collect HCV at the cell surface and facilitate binding with receptors crucial for HCV entry. Consistent with this, a role has been proposed for L-SIGN and DC-SIGN in HCV attachment although they do not seem to mediate cell entry of HCV and their role is unclear [36].

The precise molecular events underlying HCV binding and entry are not well understood. However, HCV binding to the cell surface is thought to occur in a stepwise process by binding to several receptors followed by transfer to the tight junction proteins CLDN1 and OCLN that may facilitate cellular uptake (Figure 1.4). Similar to other flaviviruses, HCV entry is thought to be mediated by clathrin-mediated endocytosis with delivery of the nucleocapsid from the endosome in a pH-dependent manner [37–39]. Furthermore, the E1 and E2 proteins are class II fusion proteins that result from the production of a fusion pore in the endosome membrane that facilitates genome release to the cytoplasm [40].

HCV Replication

The HCV replication process is summarized in Figure 1.5. After translation of the HCV proteins from the positive-sense RNA genome by direct interaction of the host 40S ribosomal subunit with the IRES within the 5′ UTR of the genome, HCV replication begins. This IRES-directed translation is cap-independent and enables virus translation/replication to continue even after host cell cap-dependent translation has been shut down in response to viral infection.

Similar to other positive-stranded viruses, HCV is believed to replicate in association with intracellular membranes in a complex called the membranous web, although the exact details of this association are not well understood. It is thought that the association predominantly with endoplasmic reticulum (ER) membranes may provide support for the organization of the replication complex, compartmentalization of the viral products, concentration of lipid constituents important for replication, and protection of the viral RNA from host-mediated innate immune defenses. This membranous web was first noticed in cultured cells harboring HCV replicons and contains detectable concentrations of the non-structural proteins NS3, NS4A, NS4B, NS5A, and NS5B, and is very similar to sponge-like inclusions noted in liver tissue from HCV-infected chimpanzees [41–44]. Expression of NS4B alone induces the formation of the membranous web, and recent work has shown that membrane association is facilitated by amino acids 40 to 69 of the N-terminal region of NS4B [45].

The phosphorylation status of NS5A appears to be a determinant of HCV RNA replication with mutations that reduce hyperphosphorylation of NS5A dramatically enhancing HCV RNA replication [46,47]. In this manner, hyperphosphorylation of NS5A may induce a switch from genome replication to viral protein translation. NS5A also interacts with several host proteins that may be important in HCV replication through formation of the replication complex or facilitating assembly. NS5A interacts with the SNARE-like vesicle-associated membrane host proteins, VAP-A and VAP-B [48]. NS5A also interacts with geranylgeranylated F-box protein, FBL2, which is essential for replication and seems to be part of the replication complex [49]. How this interaction contributes to replication is unclear but it may help anchor the replicase complex to membranes. Its involvement in the replication process highlights the close interaction between HCV replication and the host cholesterol biosynthetic pathway [50]. Another host factor, cyclophilin B, has also been implicated in HCV replication through interaction with NS5B and stabilization of RNA binding, and was originally discovered through the ability of the powerful immuno-suppressive drug cyclosporin A (CsA) to inhibit HCV replication [51]. However, more recent work suggests that

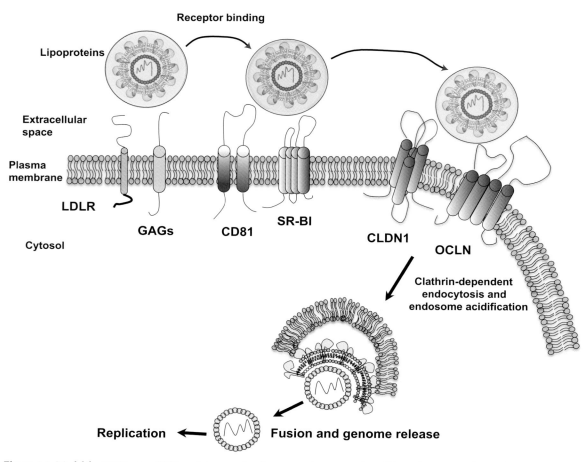

Figure 1.4 Model for HCV entry. HCV particles associated with LDL and VLDL are thought to be tethered to the hepatocyte surface by the LDL-R and GAGs and subsequent stepwise interactions with CD81 and SR-B1. HCV is transferred to the tight junction proteins OCLN and CLDN-1 from where virus enters the cell by endocytosis. Release of the HCV core containing the RNA is mediated by fusion of the E1 and E2 proteins with the endosome. The relative roles and the spatial distributions of each of the HCV receptors remain to be determined.

cyclophilin A plays a critical role in cleavage of NS5A/5B and assembly of the replication complex [52,53]. CsA analogs are currently being developed as antivirals against HCV [54].

The precise details of the HCV RNA replication process are still unclear but comparison with other flaviviruses suggests that the positive-stranded genome serves as a template for the synthesis of negative-strand RNA. Components of the membrane-bound replication complex associate with the 3′ end of the positive strand of the genome, with NS5B at the catalytic core, and initiate *de novo* synthesis of negative-strand RNA. These two strands remain base-paired, which results in the formation of a double-stranded RNA molecule that is copied multiple times by semiconservative replication by the RNA-dependent RNA polymerase (RdRp) NS5B to generate multiple progeny, positive-strand viral RNA genomes. Importantly, the NS5B RdRp has no proofreading capacity and as such is error prone. This lack of proofreading ability results in the generation of many different but closely related genomes, often referred to as quasispecies. This genetic diversity is ideally suited to escape of immune control and is a significant factor in the generation of antiviral resistance to select antiviral agents. While a proportion of new positive-strand genomes serve as templates for viral protein translation, others associate with

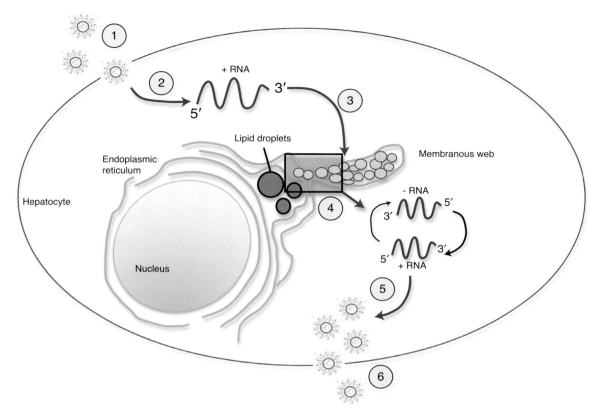

Figure 1.5 Lifecycle of HCV. 1, Virus binding and internalization; 2, release of HCV RNA and translation of viral proteins; 3, association of HCV proteins in ER and formation of the replication complex in association with lipid droplets, replication of HCV RNA; 5, virion maturation and packaging of RNA; 6, release of virions.

the core protein and form dimers within core-protein-enriched nucleocapsids. The association of the core protein with cytoplasmic lipid droplets has emerged as a critical determinant of nucleocapsid and infectious viral particle assembly. It is thought that the core uses this platform to recruit replication complexes and associated new genomes from closely associated ER-derived "lipid-droplet-associated membranes" in the assembly process [55,56]. Core particles may then become enveloped via budding through the ER where viral glycoproteins (E1/E2 heterodimers) become embedded. Little is known about the process of viral particle egress except that particles change in their biophysical properties (increased density) upon exit. Recent studies have indicated that the processes of HCV particle assembly, maturation, and secretion are dependent upon the machinery involved in the assembly and secretion of VLDL by hepatocytes [57].

The development and use of *in vitro* cell-culture model systems described above has been and continues to be fundamental in dissecting the stages of HCV replication and identification of viral-host interactions at the molecular level (Figure 1.5). While these studies are important for our understanding of HCV biology, they also provide specific targets for the development of novel therapeutics designed to completely eradicate HCV infection across all genotypes. Current therapies for HCV focus on modulation of the host immune response. However, with a greater understanding of HCV replication and host interactions, we are currently in a phase of developing therapeutics that directly target various stages of the HCV life cycle. Drugs targeting HCV entry and fusion, viral helicase, and polymerase or protease function are all under clinical investigation, with some showing exceptional promise. These targeted therapies when used in combination with the current therapeutic regime of Peg-IFN alfa-2 and rib-avirin will provide the foundation for systemic eradication of HCV in infected persons. Furthermore, defining novel host factors essential for HCV replication and a greater understanding of the immunological correlates of immunity to HCV will provide the cornerstone for further development of novel therapeutics to combat HCV infection.

References

1. Moradpour D, Penin F, Rice CM. Replication of hepatitis C virus. *Nat Rev Microbiol* 2007;5(6):453–63.

2. Kieft JS, Zhou K, Jubin R, *et al.* The hepatitis C virus internal ribosome entry site adopts an ion-dependent tertiary fold. *J Mol Biol* 1999;292(3):513–29.

3. Psaridi L, Georgopoulou U, Varaklioti A, Mavromara P. Mutational analysis of a conserved tetraloop in the 5′ untranslated region of hepatitis C virus identifies a novel RNA element essential for the internal ribosome entry site function. *FEBS Lett* 1999;453(1–2):49–53.

4. Siridechadilok B, Fraser CS, Hall RJ, *et al.* Structural roles for human translation factor eIF3 in initiation of protein synthesis. *Science* 2005;310(5753):1513–15.

5. Spahn CM, Kieft JS, Grassucci RA, *et al.* Hepatitis C virus IRES RNA-induced changes in the conformation of the 40s ribosomal subunit. *Science* 2001;291(5510):1959–62.

6. Appel N, Schaller T, Penin F, Bartenschlager R. From structure to function: new insights into hepatitis C virus RNA replication. *J Biol Chem* 2006;281(15):9833–6.

7. Jopling CL, Yi M, Lancaster AM, *et al.* Modulation of hepatitis C virus RNA abundance by a liver-specific MicroRNA. *Science* 2005;309(5740):1577–81.

8. Sarasin-Filipowicz M, Krol J, Markiewicz I, *et al.* Decreased levels of microRNA miR-122 in individuals with hepatitis C responding poorly to interferon therapy. *Nat Med* 2009;15(1):31–3.

9. Henke JI, Goergen D, Zheng J, *et al.* MicroRNA-122 stimulates translation of hepatitis C virus RNA. *EMBO J* 2008;27(24):3300–10.

10. Blight KJ, Rice CM. Secondary structure determination of the conserved 98-base sequence at the 3′ terminus of hepatitis C virus genome RNA. *J Virol* 1997;71(10): 7345–52.

11. Kolykhalov AA, Feinstone SM, Rice CM. Identification of a highly conserved sequence element at the 3′ terminus of hepatitis C virus genome RNA. *J Virol* 1996;70(6):3363–71.

12. Tanaka T, Kato N, Cho MJ, *et al.* Structure of the 3′ terminus of the hepatitis C virus genome. *J Virol* 1996;70(5): 3307–12.

13. Yi M, Lemon SM. 3′ nontranslated RNA signals required for replication of hepatitis C virus RNA. *J Virol* 2003;77(6): 3557–68.

14. Lohmann V, Korner F, Koch J, *et al.* Replication of subgenomic hepatitis C virus RNAs in a hepatoma cell line. *Science* 1999;285(5424):110–13.

15. Ikeda M, Yi M, Li K, Lemon SM. Selectable subgenomic and genome-length dicistronic RNAs derived from an infectious molecular clone of the HCV-N strain of hepatitis C virus replicate efficiently in cultured Huh7 cells. *J Virol* 2002;76(6):2997–3006.

16. Pietschmann T, Lohmann V, Kaul A, *et al.* Persistent and transient replication of full-length hepatitis C virus genomes in cell culture. *J Virol* 2002;76(8):4008–21.

17. Blight KJ, Kolykhalov AA, Rice CM. Efficient initiation of HCV RNA replication in cell culture. *Science* 2000;290(5498):1972–4.

18. Lohmann V, Korner F, Dobierzewska A, Bartenschlager R. Mutations in hepatitis C virus RNAs conferring cell culture adaptation. *J Virol* 2001;75(3):1437–49.

19. Bukh J, Pietschmann T, Lohmann V, *et al.* Mutations that permit efficient replication of hepatitis C virus RNA in Huh-7 cells prevent productive replication in chimpanzees. *Proc Natl Acad Sci U S A* 2002;99(22):14416–21.

20. Kato T, Date T, Miyamoto M, *et al.* Nonhepatic cell lines HeLa and 293 support efficient replication of the hepatitis C virus genotype 2a subgenomic replicon. *J Virol* 2005;79(1):592–6.

21. Zhu Q, Guo JT, Seeger C. Replication of hepatitis C virus subgenomes in nonhepatic epithelial and mouse hepatoma cells. *J Virol* 2003;77(17):9204–10.

22. Blight KJ, McKeating JA, Rice CM. Highly permissive cell lines for subgenomic and genomic hepatitis C virus RNA replication. *J Virol* 2002;76(24):13001–14.

23. Foy E, Li K, Wang C, *et al.* Regulation of interferon regulatory factor-3 by the hepatitis C virus serine protease. *Science* 2003;300(5622):1145–8.

24. Lindenbach BD, Evans MJ, Syder AJ, *et al.* Complete replication of hepatitis C virus in cell culture. *Science* 2005;309(5734):623–6.

25. Wakita T, Pietschmann T, Kato T, *et al.* Production of infectious hepatitis C virus in tissue culture from a cloned viral genome. *Nat Med* 2005;11(7):791–6.

26. Nielsen SU, Bassendine MF, Burt AD, *et al.* Association between hepatitis C virus and very-low-density lipoprotein (VLDL)/LDL analyzed in iodixanol density gradients. *J Virol* 2006;80(5):2418–28.

27. Kolykhalov AA, Agapov EV, Blight KJ, *et al.* Transmission of hepatitis C by intrahepatic inoculation with transcribed RNA. *Science* 1997;277(5325):570–74.

28. Yi M, Villanueva RA, Thomas DL, *et al.* Production of infectious genotype 1a hepatitis C virus (Hutchinson strain) in cultured human hepatoma cells. *Proc Natl Acad Sci U S A* 2006;103(7):2310–15.

29. Pietschmann T, Kaul A, Koutsoudakis G, *et al.* Construction and characterization of infectious intragenotypic and intergenotypic hepatitis C virus chimeras. *Proc Natl Acad Sci U S A* 2006;103(19):7408–13.

30. Bartosch B, Dubuisson J, Cosset FL. Infectious hepatitis C virus pseudo-particles containing functional E1-E2 envelope protein complexes. *J Exp Med* 2003;197(5):633–42.

31. Drummer HE, Maerz A, Poumbourios P. Cell surface expression of functional hepatitis C virus E1 and E2 glycoproteins. *FEBS Lett* 2003;546(2–3):385–90.

32. Pileri P, Uematsu Y, Campagnoli S, *et al.* Binding of hepatitis C virus to CD81. *Science* 1998;282(5390):938–41.

33. Evans MJ, von Hahn T, Tscherne DM, *et al.* Claudin-1 is a hepatitis C virus co-receptor required for a late step in entry. *Nature* 2007;446(7137):801–5.

34. Ploss A, Evans MJ, Gaysinskaya VA, *et al.* Human occludin is a hepatitis C virus entry factor required for infection of mouse cells. *Nature* 2009;457(7231):882–6.

35. Agnello V, Abel G, Elfahal M, *et al.* Hepatitis C virus and other flaviviridae viruses enter cells via low density lipoprotein receptor. *Proc Natl Acad Sci U S A* 1999;96(22):12766–71.

36. Lozach PY, Amara A, Bartosch B, *et al.* C-type lectins L-SIGN and DC-SIGN capture and transmit infectious hepatitis C virus pseudotype particles. *J Biol Chem* 2004;279(31):32035–45.

37. Blanchard E, Belouzard S, Goueslain L, *et al.* Hepatitis C virus entry depends on clathrin-mediated endocytosis. *J Virol* 2006;80(14):6964–72.

38. Koutsoudakis G, Kaul A, Steinmann E, *et al.* Characterization of the early steps of hepatitis C virus infection by using luciferase reporter viruses. *J Virol* 2006;80(11):5308–20.

39. Tscherne DM, Jones CT, Evans MJ, *et al.* Time- and temperature-dependent activation of hepatitis C virus for low-pH-triggered entry. *J Virol* 2006;80(4):1734–41.

40. Drummer HE, Poumbourios P. Hepatitis C virus glycoprotein E2 contains a membrane-proximal heptad repeat sequence that is essential for E1E2 glycoprotein heterodimerization and viral entry. *J Biol Chem* 2004;279(29):30066–72.

41. Egger D, Wolk B, Gosert R, *et al.* Expression of hepatitis C virus proteins induces distinct membrane alterations including a candidate viral replication complex. *J Virol* 2002;76(12):5974–84.

42. Gosert R, Egger D, Lohmann V, *et al.* Identification of the hepatitis C virus RNA replication complex in Huh-7 cells harboring subgenomic replicons. *J Virol* 2003;77(9):5487–92.

43. Moradpour D, Brass V, Bieck E, *et al.* Membrane association of the RNA-dependent RNA polymerase is essential for hepatitis C virus RNA replication. *J Virol* 2004;78(23):13278–84.

44. Moradpour D, Gosert R, Egger D, *et al.* Membrane association of hepatitis C virus nonstructural proteins and identification of the membrane alteration that harbors the viral replication complex. *Antivir Res* 2003;60(2):103–9.

45. Gouttenoire J, Montserret R, Kennel A, *et al.* An amphipathic {alpha}-helix at the C terminus of hepatitis C virus nonstructural protein 4B mediates membrane association. *J Virol* 2009;83(21):11378–84.

46. Appel N, Pietschmann T, Bartenschlager R. Mutational analysis of hepatitis C virus nonstructural protein 5A: potential role of differential phosphorylation in RNA replication and identification of a genetically flexible domain. *J Virol* 2005;79(5):3187–94.

47. Evans MJ, Rice CM, Goff SP. Phosphorylation of hepatitis C virus nonstructural protein 5A modulates its protein interactions and viral RNA replication. *Proc Natl Acad Sci U S A* 2004;101(35):13038–43.

48. Hamamoto I, Nishimura Y, Okamoto T, *et al.* Human VAP-B is involved in hepatitis C virus replication through interaction with NS5A and NS5B. *J Virol* 2005;79(21):13473–82.

49. Wang C, Gale M, Jr., Keller BC, *et al.* Identification of FBL2 as a geranylgeranylated cellular protein required for hepatitis C virus RNA replication. *Mol Cell* 2005;18(4):425–34.

50. Ye J, Wang C, Sumpter R, Jr., Brown MS, *et al.* Disruption of hepatitis C virus RNA replication through inhibition of host protein geranylgeranylation. *Proc Natl Acad Sci U S A* 2003;100(26):15865–70.

51. Watashi K, Ishii N, Hijikata M, *et al.* Cyclophilin B is a functional regulator of hepatitis C virus RNA polymerase. *Mol Cell* 2005;19(1):111–22.

52. Kaul A, Stauffer S, Berger C, *et al.* Essential role of cyclophilin A for hepatitis C virus replication and virus production and possible link to polyprotein cleavage kinetics. *PLoS Pathog* 2009;5(8):e1000546.

53. Liu Z, Yang F, Robotham JM, Tang H. Critical role of cyclophilin A and its prolyl-peptidyl isomerase activity in the structure and function of the hepatitis C virus replication complex. *J Virol* 2009;83(13):6554–65.

54. Flisiak R, Feinman SV, Jablkowski M, *et al.* The cyclophilin inhibitor Debio 025 combined with PEG IFNalpha2a significantly reduces viral load in treatment-naive hepatitis C patients. *Hepatology* 2009;49(5):1460–68.

55. Miyanari Y, Atsuzawa K, Usuda N, *et al.* The lipid droplet is an important organelle for hepatitis C virus production. *Nat Cell Biol* 2007;9(9):1089–97.

56. Shavinskaya A, Boulant S, Penin F, *et al.* The lipid droplet binding domain of hepatitis C virus core protein is a major determinant for efficient virus assembly. *J Biol Chem* 2007;282(51):37158–69.

57. Gastaminza P, Cheng G, Wieland S, *et al.* Cellular determinants of hepatitis C virus assembly, maturation, degradation, and secretion. *J Virol* 2008;82(5):2120–29.

2 Hepatitis C Virus Genotypes

Scott A. Read and Mark W. Douglas
Storr Liver Unit, Westmead Millennium Institute, University of Sydney at Westmead Hospital, NSW, Australia

Introduction

The hepatitis C virus (HCV) was cloned by Choo *et al.* in 1989 [1]. Like most RNA viruses, the genome exhibits a high degree of genetic variability. Thus, it soon became evident that a unified classification scheme was required and a consensus paper was published in 1994 [2]. This scheme identified 6 HCV genotypes and 11 subtypes, based on phylogenetic analysis of the NS5B region, and is still used today (Figure 2.1). More than 75 confirmed and provisional subtypes of HCV have now been identified, which are still grouped into 6 major genotypes (Table 2.1).

HCV genetic variability is seen at all levels of classification: between genotypes, within genotypes (subtypes), and within the infected individual (quasispecies). HCV genotypes differ from each other at the nucleotide level by over 30%; subtypes by 20–25%; and quasispecies by up to 10% [4,5]. This degree of polymorphism results from the error-prone viral RNA polymerase and many years of divergent evolution within different human populations. The resulting HCV genotypes have unique distributions, but all share similar gene arrangement, viral replication, and the ability to establish persistent infection. This chapter will focus on genetic differences among HCV genotypes and genotype-specific differences in disease pathogenesis and treatment response.

HCV Genotypes and Subtypes

Although HCV genotypes differ by up to one third overall, sequence divergence is not uniform across the genome. The most conserved region is the 5′ untranslated region (UTR), where RNA secondary structure forms the internal ribosomal entry site (IRES) that initiates replication [6]. In contrast, the most diverse genes are for the envelope glycoproteins E1 and E2, which under immune pressure have evolved nine times faster than the 5′ UTR [7].

Each HCV genotype contains distinct subtypes, the geographic distributions of which reflect local social and medical practices, as well as host genetics. Contaminated blood products and needle sharing have allowed widespread dissemination of genotypes 1a, 1b, and 3a, which together account for over 80% of HCV infections worldwide [3]. Focal outbreaks have led to high local prevalence of certain subtypes, such as subtype 4a, which accounts for over 50% of HCV cases in Egypt. This followed mass parenteral antischistosomal therapy (PAT) administration in the latter half of the twentieth century [8]. In contrast, geographic isolation and/or inefficient sexual transmission routes in parts of South-East Asia have kept genotype 6 subtypes geographically restricted.

Intergenotypic Recombinants

With 3% of the world's population infected with an ever-increasing number of HCV genotypes and subtypes [9], the emergence of intergenotypic recombinants was virtually inevitable. During co-infection with multiple genotypes, subtypes, or strains of HCV, template switching can occur during replication, resulting in a recombinant virus containing two (or more) parental portions in its genome. This process is not site-specific and has been reported for the *E1*, *E2*, *NS2*, *NS3*, and *NS5A* genes [10–13]. Recently Sentandreu *et al.* estimated that intrasubtype recombination occurs in over 10% of HCV infected patients [11], but the rate of recombination between genotypes is probably much less, due to their divergent sequences.

Advanced Therapy for Hepatitis C, First Edition. Edited by Geoffrey W. McCaughan, John G. McHutchison and Jean-Michel Pawlotsky.
© 2012 Blackwell Publishing Ltd. Published 2012 by Blackwell Publishing Ltd.

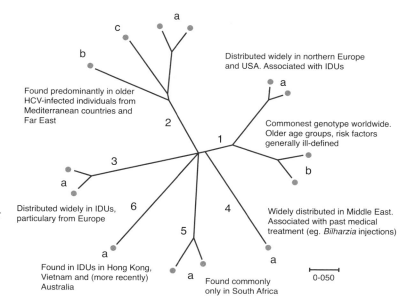

Figure 2.1 Evolutionary tree of the major subtypes of HCV. Subtypes can be differentiated by their distribution, risk groups and epidemiology. IDU, injecting drug user. Reproduced from [3], with permission from the Society for General Microbiology.

Quasispecies

The HCV RNA polymerase lacks proofreading ability, resulting in a high frequency of point mutations. The production of 10^{10} to 10^{12} new viral genomes per day [14], with a mutation rate of 1.5–2.0×10^{-3} sites per genome per year [15], results in a "swarm" of different HCV quasispecies in chronically infected individuals. Host immunity exerts the main selection pressure *in vivo*, resulting in

Table 2.1 Defined HCV genotypes and their representative subtypes.

Genotype	Assigned subtypes[a]
1	**a**, **b**, **c**, d, e, f, g, h, **i**, j, **k**, l, m
2	**a**, **b**, **c**, d, e, f, g, h, **i**, j, **k**, l, m, n, o, p, q, r
3	**a**, **b**, c, d, e, f, g, h, i, **k**, l
4	**a**, b, c, d, e, f, g, h, k, l, m, n, o, p, q, r, s, t
5	**a**
6	**a**, **b**, c, **d**, e, **f**, **g**, **h**, i, j, **k**, l, m, n, o, p, q, r, s, t, u
7	a

[a] Bold indicates confirmed subtype designation demonstrated by the coding sequences of two or more variants that are epidemiologically independent.
Source: http://hcv.lanl.gov/content/sequence/HCV/classification/genotable.html

mutants that replicate efficiently and evade the adaptive and innate immune responses. Genetic diversity is also thought to play a role in antiviral resistance as patients with higher pre-treatment quasispecies diversity are less likely to respond to interferon and ribavarin [16].

Genotype-Specific Effects of HCV Proteins on Response to Antiviral Therapy

The effectiveness of interferon-based therapy depends on HCV genotype [17]; less than 50% of patients with genotype 1 infection obtain a sustained virologic response (SVR) on current treatment regimens, compared to 75% or 80% with genotypes 2 and 3 [18,19]. Interactions have been observed between HCV E2, core, NS3/4A, and NS5A proteins and the innate immune system, so diversity among these proteins may influence treatment response.

The HCV E2 protein contains a 12 amino acid sequence that closely mimics the double-stranded RNA protein kinase (PKR) autophosphorylation site and translation initiation factor 2 (eIF2) phosphorylation site, termed the PKR-eIF2a phosphorylation homology domain (PePHD) [20]. It has been suggested that the degree of E2-PKR homology may correlate with resistance to treatment [20], but other studies have produced conflicting results [21,22]. Larger studies are thus required.

Core protein has been shown *in vitro* to up-regulate suppressor of cytokine signaling 3 (SOCS3), a key negative regulator of the interferon-stimulated JAK-STAT signaling pathway [23]. Hepatic expression of SOCS3 is higher in patients who do not respond to interferon-based therapy [24] and SOCS3 levels are higher in genotype 1 infection than genotype 2, consistent with genotype-specific variations in treatment response [24].

The NS3/4A complex forms a viral protease that cleaves non-structural proteins from the HCV polyprotein [25]. NS3/4A also cleaves the signaling molecules TRIF and Cardif, ablating pattern recognition receptor (PRR) signaling from Toll-like receptor-3 (TLR3) and RIG-I, respectively [26,27]. Franco *et al.* compared NS3 protease activity between 12 HCV isolates and showed up to a six-fold variation, with the highest activity in genotype 1 isolates [28].

NS5A is the most promiscuous HCV protein, interacting with key components of metabolic, growth, and immune signaling cascades [29]. NS5A interacts with PKR to prevent autophosphorylation and subsequent eIF2 phosphorylation, in part via a 40 amino acid segment in the C-terminal domain called the interferon sensitivity-determining region (ISDR) [30]. Enomoto *et al.* showed that genotype 1b strains with mutations in this region responded better to treatment [31]. Reports vary [32,33], but a meta-analysis found a positive correlation between the number of ISDR mutations and response to therapy [34]. NS5A is a highly immunogenic protein, so Simmonds has proposed a balance between optimal function and immune evasion [3]. NS5A from genotype 2 and 3 isolates may be more immunogenic than genotypes 1 and 4, so under increased selection pressure it becomes less efficient at suppressing innate immunity, resulting in better treatment outcomes.

Elevated hepatic basal interferon-stimulated genes (ISG) expression is seen in patients who do not respond to interferon therapy, blunting their interferon response [17,35]. Interestingly, pre-treatment ISG levels are higher in genotype 1 and 4 infections than genotype 2 and 3, perhaps contributing to genotype-specific response rates [17].

Insulin Resistance

HCV genotype 1 and 4 infections are associated with insulin resistance [36,37], which reduces the response to interferon-based therapy [38], as discussed in Chapter 23 and reviewed recently [39]. Differential effects of geno-

types 1 and 3 core on insulin signaling have been observed [40], and may partially explain genotype-specific differences in treatment response.

Steatosis

HCV affects lipid metabolism in a genotype-specific manner, with a strong association between genotype 3 and steatosis [41,42]. Genotype 3-associated steatosis appears to be a direct viral effect, as it occurs in the absence of other metabolic risk factors [43,44], correlates with increased viral load [41,45], and improves following successful antiviral therapy [46–48]. In contrast, patients infected with non-3 genotypes develop steatosis in association with HCV-induced insulin resistance and other metabolic abnormalities [45,49].

Conclusion

The HCV genome, although highly diverse overall, remains constrained by its host in many key areas. The error-prone RNA polymerase has allowed HCV to diversify among populations, resulting in various genotypes and subtypes, and to adapt quickly to an individual host through quasispecies diversity. Hypervariable regions in immunogenic proteins allow the virus to escape the host immune system, while regions essential for viral structure and replication remain conserved.

The complex interactions between HCV and its human host vary among genotypes, providing significant challenges for interferon-based therapies. A number of specific HCV polymerase and protease inhibitors are in phase III clinical trials, but they are rarely effective against all genotypes, and resistance emerges rapidly [50]. It is therefore likely that a multifaceted treatment approach is required to eradicate this virus, which has demonstrated the ability to securely embed itself within the liver interactome.

References

1. Choo QL, Kuo G, Weiner AJ, *et al.* Isolation of a cDNA clone derived from a blood-borne non-A, non-B viral hepatitis genome. *Science* 1989;244(4902):359–62.
2. Simmonds P, Alberti A, Alter HJ, *et al.* A proposed system for the nomenclature of hepatitis C viral genotypes. *Hepatology* 1994;19(5):1321–4.
3. Simmonds P. Genetic diversity and evolution of hepatitis C virus – 15 years on. *J Gen Virol* 2004;85(Pt 11):3173–88.

4. Simmonds P, Holmes EC, Cha TA, *et al.* Classification of hepatitis C virus into six major genotypes and a series of subtypes by phylogenetic analysis of the NS-5 region. *J Gen Virol* 1993;74(Pt 11):2391–9.

5. Maggi F, Fornai C, Vatteroni ML, *et al.* Differences in hepatitis C virus quasispecies composition between liver, peripheral blood mononuclear cells and plasma. *J Gen Virol* 1997;78(Pt 7):1521–5.

6. Spahn CM, Kieft JS, Grassucci RA, *et al.* Hepatitis C virus IRES RNA-induced changes in the conformation of the 40s ribosomal subunit. *Science* 2001;291(5510):1959–62.

7. Salemi M, Vandamme AM. Hepatitis C virus evolutionary patterns studied through analysis of full-genome sequences. *J Mol Evol* 2002;54(1):62–70.

8. Frank C, Mohamed MK, Strickland GT, *et al.* The role of parenteral antischistosomal therapy in the spread of hepatitis C virus in Egypt. *Lancet* 2000;355(9207):887–91.

9. Shepard CW, Finelli L, Alter MJ. Global epidemiology of hepatitis C virus infection. *Lancet Infect Dis* 2005;5(9): 558–67.

10. Kageyama S, Agdamag DM, Alesna ET, *et al.* A natural intergenotypic (2b/1b) recombinant of hepatitis C virus in the Philippines. *J Med Virol* 2006;78(11):1423–8.

11. Sentandreu V, Jimenez-Hernandez N, Torres-Puente M, *et al.* Evidence of recombination in intrapatient populations of hepatitis C virus. *PLoS ONE* 2008;3(9):e3239.

12. Kalinina O, Norder H, Mukomolov S, Magnius LO. A natural intergenotypic recombinant of hepatitis C virus identified in St. Petersburg. *J Virol* 2002;76(8):4034–43.

13. Legrand-Abravanel F, Claudinon J, Nicot F, *et al.* New natural intergenotypic (2/5) recombinant of hepatitis C virus. *J Virol* 2007;81(8):4357–62.

14. Neumann AU, Lam NP, Dahari H, *et al.* Hepatitis C viral dynamics in vivo and the antiviral efficacy of interferon-alpha therapy. *Science* 1998;282(5386):103–7.

15. Bukh J, Miller RH, Purcell RH. Genetic heterogeneity of hepatitis C virus: quasispecies and genotypes. *Semin Liver Dis* 1995;15(1):41–63.

16. Morishima C, Polyak SJ, Ray R, *et al.* Hepatitis C virus-specific immune responses and quasi-species variability at baseline are associated with nonresponse to antiviral therapy during advanced hepatitis C. *J Infect Dis* 2006;193(7): 931–40.

17. Sarasin-Filipowicz M, Oakeley EJ, Duong FH, *et al.* Interferon signaling and treatment outcome in chronic hepatitis C. *Proc Natl Acad Sci U S A* 2008;105(19):7034–9.

18. Fried MW, Shiffman ML, Reddy KR, *et al.* Peginterferon alfa-2a plus ribavirin for chronic hepatitis C virus infection. *N Engl J Med* 2002;347(13):975–82.

19. Hadziyannis SJ, Sette H, Jr., Morgan TR, *et al.* Peginterferon-alpha2a and ribavirin combination therapy in chronic hepatitis C: a randomized study of treatment duration and ribavirin dose. *Ann Intern Med* 2004;140(5): 346–55.

20. Taylor DR, Shi ST, Romano PR, *et al.* Inhibition of the interferon-inducible protein kinase PKR by HCV E2 protein. *Science* 1999;285(5424):107–10.

21. Munoz de Rueda P, Casado J, Paton R, *et al.* Mutations in E2-PePHD, NS5A-PKRBD, NS5A-ISDR, and NS5A-V3 of hepatitis C virus genotype 1 and their relationships to pegylated interferon-ribavirin treatment responses. *J Virol* 2008;82(13):6644–53.

22. Ukai K, Ishigami M, Yoshioka K, *et al.* Mutations in carboxy-terminal part of E2 including PKR/eIF2alpha phosphorylation homology domain and interferon sensitivity determining region of nonstructural 5A of hepatitis C virus 1b: their correlation with response to interferon monotherapy and viral load. *World J Gastroenterol* 2006;12(23):3722–8.

23. Bode JG, Ludwig S, Ehrhardt C, *et al.* IFN-alpha antagonistic activity of HCV core protein involves induction of suppressor of cytokine signaling-3. *FASEB J* 2003;17(3):488–90.

24. Persico M, Capasso M, Persico E, *et al.* Suppressor of cytokine signaling 3 (SOCS3) expression and hepatitis C virus-related chronic hepatitis: insulin resistance and response to antiviral therapy. *Hepatology* 2007;46(4):1009–15.

25. Failla C, Tomei L, De Francesco R. Both NS3 and NS4A are required for proteolytic processing of hepatitis C virus nonstructural proteins. *J Virol* 1994;68(6):3753–60.

26. Li K, Foy E, Ferreon JC, *et al.* Immune evasion by hepatitis C virus NS3/4A protease-mediated cleavage of the Toll-like receptor 3 adaptor protein TRIF. *Proc Natl Acad Sci U S A* 2005;102(8):2992–7.

27. Breiman A, Grandvaux N, Lin R, *et al.* Inhibition of RIG-I-dependent signaling to the interferon pathway during hepatitis C virus expression and restoration of signaling by IKKepsilon. *J Virol* 2005;79(7):3969–78.

28. Franco S, Clotet B, Martinez MA. A wide range of NS3/4A protease catalytic efficiencies in HCV-infected individuals. *Virus Res* 2008;131(2):260–70.

29. Macdonald A, Harris M. Hepatitis C virus NS5A: tales of a promiscuous protein. *J Gen Virol* 2004;85(Pt 9):2485–502.

30. Gale M, Jr., Blakely CM, Kwieciszewski B, *et al.* Control of PKR protein kinase by hepatitis C virus nonstructural 5A protein: molecular mechanisms of kinase regulation. *Mol Cell Biol* 1998;18(9):5208–18.

31. Enomoto N, Sakuma I, Asahina Y, *et al.* Comparison of full-length sequences of interferon-sensitive and resistant hepatitis C virus 1b. Sensitivity to interferon is conferred by amino acid substitutions in the NS5A region. *J Clin Invest* 1995;96(1):224–30.

32. Rispeter K, Lu M, Zibert A, *et al.* The "interferon sensitivity determining region" of hepatitis C virus is a stable sequence element. *J Hepatol* 1998;29(3):352–61.

33. Stratidaki I, Skoulika E, Kelefiotis D, *et al.* NS5A mutations predict biochemical but not virological response to interferon-alpha treatment of sporadic hepatitis C virus infection in European patients. *J Viral Hepatitis* 2001;8(4):243–8.

34. Pascu M, Martus P, Hohne M, *et al*. Sustained virological response in hepatitis C virus type 1b infected patients is predicted by the number of mutations within the NS5A-ISDR: a meta-analysis focused on geographical differences. *Gut* 2004;53(9):1345–51.

35. Chen L, Borozan I, Feld J, *et al*. Hepatic gene expression discriminates responders and nonresponders in treatment of chronic hepatitis C viral infection. *Gastroenterology* 2005;128(5):1437–44.

36. Hui JM, Sud A, Farrell GC, *et al*. Insulin resistance is associated with chronic hepatitis C virus infection and fibrosis progression. *Gastroenterology* 2003;125(6):1695–704.

37. Moucari R, Asselah T, Cazals-Hatem D, *et al*. Insulin resistance in chronic hepatitis C: association with genotypes 1 and 4, serum HCV RNA level, and liver fibrosis. *Gastroenterology* 2008;134(2):416–23.

38. Conjeevaram HS, Kleiner DE, Everhart JE, *et al*. Race, insulin resistance and hepatic steatosis in chronic hepatitis C. *Hepatology* 2007;45(1):80–87.

39. Douglas MW, George J. Molecular mechanisms of insulin resistance in chronic hepatitis C. *World J Gastroenterol* 2009;15(35):4356–64.

40. Pazienza V, Clement S, Pugnale P, *et al*. The hepatitis C virus core protein of genotypes 3a and 1b downregulates insulin receptor substrate 1 through genotype-specific mechanisms. *Hepatology* 2007;45(5):1164–71.

41. Rubbia-Brandt L, Quadri R, Abid K, *et al*. Hepatocyte steatosis is a cytopathic effect of hepatitis C virus genotype 3. *J Hepatol* 2000;33(1):106–15.

42. Mihm S, Fayyazi A, Hartmann H, Ramadori G. Analysis of histopathological manifestations of chronic hepatitis C virus infection with respect to virus genotype. *Hepatology* 1997;25(3):735–9.

43. Hui JM, Kench J, Farrell GC, *et al*. Genotype-specific mechanisms for hepatic steatosis in chronic hepatitis C infection. *J Gastroenterol Hepatol* 2002;17(8):873–81.

44. Cua IH, Hui JM, Kench JG, George J. Genotype-specific interactions of insulin resistance, steatosis, and fibrosis in chronic hepatitis C. *Hepatology* 2008;48(3):723–31.

45. Adinolfi LE, Gambardella M, Andreana A, *et al*. Steatosis accelerates the progression of liver damage of chronic hepatitis C patients and correlates with specific HCV genotype and visceral obesity. *Hepatology* 2001;33(6):1358–64.

46. Kumar D, Farrell GC, Fung C, George J. Hepatitis C virus genotype 3 is cytopathic to hepatocytes: reversal of hepatic steatosis after sustained therapeutic response. *Hepatology* 2002;36(5):1266–72.

47. Patton HM, Patel K, Behling C, *et al*. The impact of steatosis on disease progression and early and sustained treatment response in chronic hepatitis C patients. *J Hepatol* 2004;40(3):484–90.

48. Poynard T, Ratziu V, McHutchison J, *et al*. Effect of treatment with peginterferon or interferon alfa-2b and ribavirin on steatosis in patients infected with hepatitis C. *Hepatology* 2003;38(1):75–85.

49. Hezode C, Roudot-Thoraval F, Zafrani ES, *et al*. Different mechanisms of steatosis in hepatitis C virus genotypes 1 and 3 infections. *J Viral Hepatitis* 2004;11(5):455–8.

50. Kieffer TL, Sarrazin C, Miller JS, *et al*. Telaprevir and pegylated interferon-alpha-2a inhibit wild-type and resistant genotype 1 hepatitis C virus replication in patients. *Hepatology* 2007; 46(3):631–9.

3

Immune Responses to HCV: Implications for Therapy

David G. Bowen

Sydney Medical School, University of Sydney, and Royal Prince Alfred Hospital, Sydney, NSW, Australia

Introduction

Successful clearance of the hepatitis C virus (HCV) in the minority of infected individuals who resolve infection has been shown to require broad, sustained virus-specific immune responses. However, even in those individuals developing chronic infection, persisting virus-specific immunity often remains detectable. Although the mechanisms by which HCV establishes and maintains persistent infection remain incompletely understood, the virus appears to subvert both innate (non-antigen-specific) and adaptive (antigen-specific) components of the immune response. In this chapter, interactions between the immune response and HCV will be discussed, as will key implications of these interactions for anti-HCV therapy.

Humoral Immune Responses to HCV

Although antibodies to HCV are usually detectable within 10–12 weeks of infection, the role of the humoral immune response in the control of viral replication remains to be determined, with investigations hampered until recently by a lack of small-animal models and *in vitro* infection systems. Early experiments in the chimpanzee model provided examples of *in vitro* antibody-mediated neutralization of HCV prior to inoculation [1]. However, further studies have indicated that sterilizing immunity does not necessarily occur following resolution of infection, and that reinfection is possible following the development of anti-HCV antibodies, even with homologous virus [1]. In addition, although studies have indicated that antibody-mediated immune selection pressure can occur early in infection [2,3], spontaneous resolution of infection without the development of detectable antibodies has been documented in chimpanzees [1], and has been observed in individuals with hypogammaglobulinemia [4]. Furthermore, while some investigators have described the development of neutralizing antibodies in association with the spontaneous resolution of HCV infection [3,5], others have found neutralizing antibodies in persistently infected individuals, rather than in those with spontaneously resolving infection [1]. A study performed in a single individual with well-characterized infection suggests that although neutralizing antibodies can develop during chronic infection, the virus may continually escape these humoral responses [6]. From available data, it is thus apparent that the virus-specific antibody response exerts immune pressure on HCV; however, the role of this response in control of infection remains to be determined.

Adaptive Cellular Immune Responses to HCV

T Cell Immunity in Acute HCV

Effective, sustained HCV-specific cellular immune responses are critical for resolution of infection. Failure to develop a CD4+ (helper) T cell response is associated with HCV persistence, while recrudescence of viral replication has been described following loss of previously strong HCV-specific CD4+ T cell responses [1]. Conversely, viral clearance during acute infection is associated with a broad, vigorous, and sustained CD4+ T cell response; memory responses remain readily detectable for many years post-resolution [1,7]. Experiments in which persistent infection developed on homologous HCV rechallenge of CD4+ T cell-depleted chimpanzees following previously

Advanced Therapy for Hepatitis C, First Edition. Edited by Geoffrey W. McCaughan, John G. McHutchison and Jean-Michel Pawlotsky.
© 2012 Blackwell Publishing Ltd. Published 2012 by Blackwell Publishing Ltd.

resolved infection have reinforced the importance of this cellular subset to infection resolution [8].

In addition to a strong CD4+ T cell response, an early, vigorous, and multi-specific CD8+ T cell or cytotoxic T lymphocyte (CTL) response is required for viral clearance [1,7]. However, while individuals lacking a strong acute CTL response appear to progress to chronic infection, strong multi-specific CD8+ T cell responses have also been recorded in early infection in individuals who subsequently develop chronic infection [1,9]. As observed with the CD4+ T cell response, in those individuals who clear infection, antiviral CTL responses can still be detected many years later [1]. CD8+ T cell depletion studies in chimpanzees have also indicated a central role for CTLs in viral clearance [10].

In a number of published studies, initial serum transaminase increases, onset of CTL responses, and viral control all occurred simultaneously [1,7], suggesting that not only do CD8+ T cells contribute to the control of viral replication, but that acute hepatitis C is an immunopathological process. However, HCV infection can resolve spontaneously without a significant transaminase increase [11], and it has been suggested that the lack of liver damage observed in these instances could reflect non-cytopathic control of viral replication, perhaps through a mediator such as interferon gamma (IFN-γ), as occurs in hepatitis B infection. Studies in cell culture of both subgenomic and genomic replicons and in human hepatocyte chimeric mice indicate that IFN-γ may inhibit HCV replication [1,12]. However, it should be noted that the number of cells replicating HCV in the acutely infected liver is not known, but may vary widely between individuals, and could range from 5% to 50% of hepatocytes [7]. Thus, especially as transaminase increases are a relatively crude tool in the assessment of hepatocellular injury, the alternative possibility exists that spontaneous resolution of acute hepatitis C without biochemical evidence of liver injury rather reflects cytolytic control of replication in a relatively small number of infected hepatocytes [1]. Alternatively, it has been suggested that in individuals where virus is controlled with negligible rises in transaminases, viral clearance is associated with apoptosis of infected cells, with minimal occurrence of necrosis [13].

T Cell Immunity in Chronic Hepatitis C

The fate of T lymphocytes in persisting HCV infection has been difficult to delineate, with studies complicated somewhat by the localization of most surviving HCV-specific populations to the liver. A number of studies have detected weak or narrowly focused peripheral blood HCV-specific CTL responses in chronic infection, although others have found multi-specific responses to be present, although often at low frequencies [1,7]. In contrast, studies of intrahepatic T cells have demonstrated HCV-specific CTLs within the liver in long-term chronic infection, with multiple epitopes targeted in at least some individuals [1,7].

In contrast to persisting CD8+ T cell responses that may be observed in HCV persistence, chronic HCV infection is associated with the loss of detectable virus-specific CD4+ T cell responses within the peripheral blood [1,7]. Function methods of CD4+ T cell identification demonstrate weak or absent responses [1,7]; however, it remains unclear whether virus-specific CD4+ T cells are present but functionally impaired, or are truly absent. Studies employing a limited range of major histocompatibility complex (MHC) class II tetramers for identification of antigen-specific cells independent of function have demonstrated HCV-specific CD4+ T cells in the blood of subjects with resolved HCV infection; however, these populations were poorly detectable in those with persistent viremia [1,14,15]. The relative difficulty in direct detection of CD4+ T cells suggests that they are lost earlier in infection or are somewhat more impaired in frequency and function that CD8+ T cells. It should be noted, however, that HCV-specific CD4+ T cells have been identified in the livers of chronically HCV infected individuals [16,17], indicating that, as with CD8+ T cells, HCV-specific CD4+ T cells may be sequestered to this compartment in chronic infection. Loss of virus-specific CD4+ T cells may also depend on which viral protein is targeted, with cells specific for the core antigen being more readily detected that those directed against the non-structural proteins [1]. It is also possible that HCV-specific CD4+ T cells persisting in chronic infection possess altered patterns of cytokine production [1].

It is thus apparent that HCV can persistently replicate despite long-lived and, at least in some individuals, broadly directed CD8+ T cell responses that are unable to clear the infection, perhaps at least in part because of a paucity of CD4+ T cell help. A number of mechanisms may explain immune evasion by this virus.

HCV and Immune Evasion: Mechanisms of Viral Persistence

A wide variety of mechanisms have been postulated to underlie the establishment of persistent infection by HCV, including inhibition of the innate immune response, with

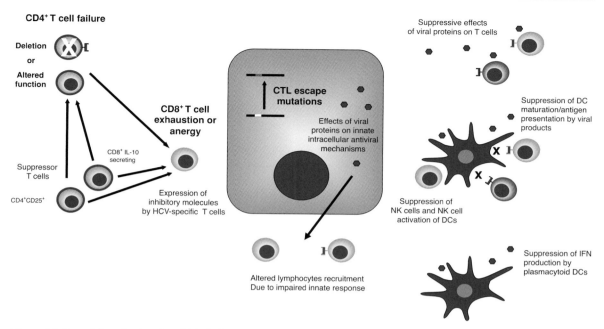

Figure 3.1 Potential mechanisms by which the hepatitis C virus subverts the immune response to establish chronic infection. It is likely that failure of the virus-specific CD4+ T cell response is central to HCV persistence, while dysfunction of the CTL response and viral evasion of intracellular innate immune pathways are also likely key factors. How the various elements of immune evasion interplay remains to be determined. Modified from [1].

likely resultant defective priming of adaptive immune responses; impairment of function of HCV-specific T cells; the development of regulatory T cell responses modulating antiviral immunity; and viral escape from T cell responses. It is likely that a combination of these factors, which are outlined in Figure 3.1 and are discussed below, contribute to the persistence of HCV infection.

Effects of HCV on the Innate Immune Response

Unusually, cellular immune responses to HCV appear delayed for several weeks, even in the setting of demonstrable viremia. Production of cytokines such as type I IFNs, including the IFN-αs and IFN-β, by virally infected cells and cells of the innate immune system may not only have direct antiviral effects, but function as an important component in triggering the antigen-specific immune response. As discussed below and summarized in Table 3.1, a number of mechanisms have been described by which HCV may interefere not only with cytokine signaling by infected cells, but also with other important components of the innate immune response.

Table 3.1 Effects of HCV on the innate immune response.

Inhibition of type I IFN signaling
NS3/4A inhibition of TLR-3 and RIG-I signaling
HCV core protein inhibition of JAK-STAT pathway
NS5A induction of IL-8, an inhibitor of IFN activity

Effects on dendritic cells
Plasmacytoid DCs
Reduced numbers in chronic infection
Impairment of function by viral proteins and cell-culture-derived virus

Conventional DCs
Possible infection of DCs
Potential effects on antigen presentation and cytokine function

Effects on DCs in chronic infection controversial

NK cells
Potential down-regulation of NK cell function by viral E2 protein

Down-regulation of NK cell activation of DCs

HCV and IFN Signaling

Available data, largely from *in vitro* analyses, indicate that HCV may interfere with IFN signaling via a number of pathways (reviewed in [18,19]). HCV core protein may inhibit IFN signaling via the JAK-STAT pathway [20], while expression of the HCV protein NS5A has been show to induce IL-8 [18], which inhibits IFN activity *in vitro*. Of much recent interest has been the ability of the HCV NS3/4A protease to inhibit production of type I IFN by infected cells via cleavage of adaptor proteins in the signaling pathways of pathogen-associated molecular pattern (PAMP) receptors. Replicating HCV RNA can be recognized by the intracellular PAMP receptor retinoic-acid-inducible gene I (RIG-I) and Toll-like receptor-3 (TLR), a major receptor for double stranded RNA [18]. The HCV protease NS3/4A inhibits the activation of interferon regulatory factor-3 (IRF-3) [21], a critical transcription factor in type I IFN production, by cleavage of adaptor proteins in the RIG-I [22] and TLR-3 pathways [23]. However, it should be noted that other hepatotropic viruses that do not exhibit propensity to chronic infection have also recently been demonstrated to possess similar capacity [24,25]. In addition, microarray analysis of mRNA expression in chimpanzees has revealed that acute infection is associated with increased expression of IFN-stimulated genes [18]. Thus the extent to which type I IFN production is inhibited in HCV infection and the significance of this phenomenon remain to be determined.

HCV and Dendritic Cells

In addition to possible effects on innate immune responses by infected cells, some studies have indicated that HCV might affect the function of dendritic cells (DCs), the major professional antigen-presenting cell for lymphocytes. Reduced numbers of plasmacytoid DCs, a major source of type I IFNs, have been reported in chronic HCV infection, and *in vitro* data suggests that HCV proteins or cell-culture-derived virus can inhibit the ability of this cell type to secrete these cytokines [26,27]. Studies have indicated that HCV might infect DCs [28], although this finding remains controversial [29,30], and there is also *in vitro* evidence that HCV-derived proteins may affect the ability of DCs to efficiently present antigen in HCV-infected individuals, or may result in the production of cytokines by DCs that may inhibit the antiviral immune response [1,19]. However, data as to whether DC function is impaired in chronically HCV infected individuals have been inconsistent [1]. Importantly, in the absence of advanced liver disease, the immune defect associated with HCV is virus specific. Thus, although transient early defects in DC function cannot be excluded as a mechanism of persistence, the induction of ongoing generalized defects in DC function lasting into chronic infection is not consistent with the observed clinical phenotype.

HCV and the NK Cell Response

Genetic studies have demonstrated an association between the clearance of HCV infection and expression of NK cell receptor and ligand combinations that are associated with lower levels of NK cell inhibition [31], thus implying a significant role for this cellular subset in anti-HCV immunity. Various studies have suggested a range of mechanisms by which HCV might inhibit NK cells [1], although *in vitro* studies indicating inhibition of NK cell function by viral E2 protein have not been borne out by experiments using infectious viral particles [32]. Whether NK cells are dysfunctional in HCV infection thus remains controversial [19].

Anergy or Exhaustion of the HCV-Specific CTL Response

Data from studies in which HCV-specific CD8+ T cells have been directly identified in the blood via the use of MHC class I tetramers have indicated that these cells may be present but functionally deficient in chronic disease, with phenotype characteristic of early stages of differentiation [1,7]. More recently, HCV-specific CD8+ T cells have been demonstrated to express a range of co-inhibitory molecules in chronic infection, including programmed death 1 (PD-1) [33,34], cytotoxic T lymphocyte antigen-4 (CTLA-4) [35], and T cell immunoglobulin and mucin domain-containing molecule 3 (Tim-3) [36]; these observations are consistent with T cell "exhaustion," or loss of function. Furthermore, the demonstration that the inhibition of interaction between PD-1 and one of its ligands, PD-ligand 1 (PD-L1), leads to improved CD8+ T cell function and reduced viral titers in a mouse model of chronic infection [37] and that PD-1 blockade improves survival in SIV infection in macaques [38], has led to much interest in the role of these inhibitory receptors in chronic HCV infection. While a number of studies have demonstrated improved function of HCV-specific CD8+ T cells following blockade of these receptors, either alone or in combination [33–35], the *in vivo* effects of such strategies remain to be determined in HCV infection.

Regulatory T Cells

Another mechanism by which immunity to HCV may be subverted is by control of antiviral responses by regulatory T cell subsets (Tregs). A number of investigators have reported that the frequency of CD4+CD25+ Tregs present in the peripheral circulation of patients with chronic HCV infection is significantly increased over that observed in recovered or uninfected individuals, although this finding has not been universal [1]. In *in vitro* studies, the presence of CD4+CD25+ Tregs from chronically HCV-infected individuals suppressed HCV-specific immune responses; however, the significance of this observation remains uncertain, as such suppression was also shown to affect CD8+ T cell populations specific for cytomegalovirus, Epstein-Barr virus, and influenza virus [1]. Furthermore, similar findings have been made in chimpanzees that resolve infection [39], and Treg function in acute infection does not appear to differ between individuals who resolve infection and those who develop chronic infection [40]. Whether specificity might be conferred by increased frequencies of such Treg populations within the secondary lymphoid organs or liver in chronic HCV infection, where antigen-specific interactions are more likely to occur, is yet to be determined.

In addition to CD4+ Tregs, CD8+ T cells may also secrete regulatory cytokines that may affect the antiviral immune response. CD8+ T cells have been cloned from the livers of chronically HCV-infected individuals who elaborated the cytokine interleukin-10 (IL-10) [1], which has suppressive effects on the cell-mediated immune response. Virus-specific IL-10 producing cells have also been directly identified within the liver parenchyma [41]. Following HCV-specific stimulation, this subpopulation can suppress the *in vitro* proliferative responses of liver-derived lymphocytes in an IL-10 dependent manner [1]. This finding has led to the hypothesis that the generation of such antigen-specific intrahepatic regulatory CD8+ T cell populations may impair the function of virus-specific CTLs, thus contributing to viral persistence.

Immunomodulatory Activity by HCV Proteins

A range of studies have suggested that HCV proteins may possess immunomodulatory activity, and have direct effects on T cells. In particular, HCV core protein has been shown to bind to the Clq complement receptor, gC1qR, with subsequent inhibition of T cell proliferative responses [42], and is known to inhibit virus-specific T cell responses *in vitro* [43]. Cross-linking of the HCV E2 protein has been shown *in vitro* to lead to co-stimulation of T cells [44], potentially altering responses, and may inhibit migration and chemokine secretion [45]. However, while such predominantly *in vitro* data indicates that HCV proteins may affect HCV-specific T cells, it should be noted

that as these proteins are likely to be ubiquitously present, such interactions have the potential to influence all T cell responses, a possibility that is difficult to reconcile with the observed lack of generalized immunosuppression in this infection [1].

Cytotoxic T Lymphocyte Escape Mutation

"Escape mutations," where Darwinian selection pressures exerted by the adaptive immune response confer replicative advantages on viral subpopulations in which the genome encodes mutations that impair presentation or recognition of epitopes, have long been known to occur in infections with highly mutable RNA viruses such as HIV. As an RNA virus with an error-prone RNA polymerase, HCV also exhibits a marked propensity for mutation. This, in combination with high viral production rates, leads to significant generation of minor viral variants or "quasispecies." Evidence that immune pressure may play a role in the selection of such variants in HCV infection and lead to the development of escape mutations was first obtained in the chimpanzee, the only animal model of infection, where CTL escape mutations were found to occur early in infection and remain fixed in circulating quasispecies for many years [46]. More recent human studies in which viral sequence was available either from the inoculum or early in infection have confirmed the development of escape mutations in individuals who evolve to chronic infection (reviewed in [46]). However, it remains unclear whether the development of CTL escape mutations is a cause or an epiphenomenon of chronic HCV infection. Determining the role of CTL escape mutation in HCV persistence will require future studies closely relating their development to the virus-specific T cell response.

Although examples of mutations in CD4+ T cell epitopes leading to altered function have been described in HCV [1], recent evidence indicates that escape mutations in MHC class II restricted epitopes occur rarely in comparison to those in MHC class I restricted epitopes targeted by CTLs [47]. It is thus apparent that escape mutation does not play a major role in the failure of virus-specific CD4+ T cell responses in chronic HCV.

Other Potential Mechanisms

In addition to the above-discussed mechanisms, it has been hypothesized that the hepatotropic hepatitis C virus may take advantage of the unusual tolerogenic properties of the liver to facilitate chronic infection [48].

However, although this possibility is suggested by data derived from small-animal studies, there is as yet no direct evidence for the involvement of such mechanisms in HCV persistence.

Immune Responses to HCV: Implications for HCV Therapy

The effects of existing therapy on HCV-specific immune responses and their role in clearance under treatment remain unclear, with conflicting data available [49]. Although it is appealing to hypothesize that successful antiviral therapy with interferon-based approaches would be associated with the induction or enhancement of HCV T cell specific responses, this has not been a consistent finding in studies. Indeed, in some reports, sustained virologic response (SVR) was associated with a loss of anti-HCV specific T cell responses. Nevertheless, a number of aspects of the nature of immune responses to HCV and the putative mechanisms by which HCV evades these responses to persist in the infected host hold significant implications for HCV therapy. Importantly, the ability of this virus to subvert innate immune responses, and hence both their direct antiviral effects and their role in triggering of virus-specific immune responses, presents a factor potentially alterable by antiviral therapy. In particular, in the light of data indicating the ability of the NS3A/4 protease to interrupt IFN signaling, the development of protease inhibitors has aroused much interest as to whether successful blockade of this viral protein will not only directly inhibit viral replication, but also enhance this pathway, thus potentially enhancing both the innate immune response and potentiating adaptive immune responses [19].

The demonstrated persistence of HCV-specific CTL responses even years into chronic infection also holds potential implications for HCV therapies. CTL populations may persist targeting not only epitopes that have developed escape mutations, but also non-mutated epitopes. Although exhibiting exhausted phenotype and likely impaired function directly *ex vivo*, these populations have long been shown to be expandable at least *in vitro*, demonstrating cytolytic function and the ability to secrete potentially antiviral cytokines *in vitro* following such expansion [1,7]. More recent demonstrations of functional improvement of HCV-specific CTLs following *in vitro* blockade of inhibitory T cell receptors has further enhanced interest as to whether strategies to enhance HCV-specific immune responses may be tenable *in vivo*.

Indeed, phase 1 studies of blockade of PD-1 in HCV are being undertaken, while monoclonal antibodies directed against other co-inhibitory molecules are under development or in clinical trials [50]. In addition, the presence of persisting, albeit dysfunctional, HCV-specific T cells in chronic infection raises the possibility that such responses may be rescued via other strategies *in vivo*. Should ongoing inhibition of HCV-specific T cells by virally encoded factors prove to play a role in mediating their dysfunction, this could potentially include antivirals directly suppressing HCV replication.

Concluding Remarks

The adaptive immune response appears to be the critical mediator via which natural resolution of HCV infection occurs. However, our understanding of the mechanisms of immune control and clearance of HCV remains incomplete, as does our knowledge of how such responses are frequently subverted by this virus. Ongoing research, particularly in the areas of interactions between HCV and the innate immune response and mechanisms of failure of the virus-specific CD4+ T cell response, will likely yield new data important for both our understanding of existing and candidate HCV therapies, as well as facilitate design of possible future therapies.

References

1. Bowen DG, Walker CM. Adaptive immune responses in acute and chronic hepatitis C virus infection. *Nature* 2005; 436(7053):946–52.
2. Farci P, Shimoda A, Coiana A, *et al.* The outcome of acute hepatitis C predicted by the evolution of the viral quasispecies. *Science* 2000;288(5464):339–44.
3. Dowd KA, Netski DM, Wang XH, *et al.* Selection pressure from neutralizing antibodies drives sequence evolution during acute infection with hepatitis C virus. *Gastroenterology* 2009;136(7):2377–86.
4. Semmo N, Lucas M, Krashias G, *et al.* Maintenance of HCV-specific T-cell responses in antibody-deficient patients a decade after early therapy. *Blood* 2006;107(11):4570–1.
5. Pestka JM, Zeisel MB, Blaser E, *et al.* Rapid induction of virus-neutralizing antibodies and viral clearance in a single-source outbreak of hepatitis C. *Proc Natl Acad Sci U S A* 2007;104(14):6025–30.
6. von Hahn T, Yoon JC, Alter H, *et al.* Hepatitis C virus continuously escapes from neutralizing antibody and T-cell responses during chronic infection in vivo. *Gastroenterology* 2007;132(2):667–78.

7. Shoukry NH, Cawthon AG, Walker CM. Cell-mediated immunity and the outcome of hepatitis C virus infection. *Annu Rev Microbiol* 2004;58:391–424.

8. Grakoui A, Shoukry NH, Woollard DJ, *et al.* HCV persistence and immune evasion in the absence of memory T cell help. *Science* 2003;302(5645):659–62.

9. Kaplan DE, Sugimoto K, Newton K, *et al.* Discordant role of CD4 T-cell response relative to neutralizing antibody and CD8 T-cell responses in acute hepatitis C. *Gastroenterology* 2007;132(2):654–66.

10. Shoukry NH, Grakoui A, Houghton M, *et al.* Memory CD8+ T cells are required for protection from persistent hepatitis C virus infection. *J Exp Med* 2003;197(12):1645–55.

11. Thimme R, Bukh J, Spangenberg HC, *et al.* Viral and immunological determinants of hepatitis C virus clearance, persistence, and disease. *Proc Natl Acad Sci U S A* 2002; 99(24):15661–8.

12. Ohira M, Ishiyama K, Tanaka Y, *et al.* Adoptive immunotherapy with liver allograft-derived lymphocytes induces anti-HCV activity after liver transplantation in humans and humanized mice. *J Clin Invest* 2009;119(11):3226–35.

13. Spengler U, Nattermann J. Immunopathogenesis in hepatitis C virus cirrhosis. *Clin Sci (Lond)* 2007;112(3):141–55.

14. Ulsenheimer A, Lucas M, Seth NP, *et al.* Transient immunological control during acute hepatitis C virus infection: ex vivo analysis of helper T-cell responses. *J Viral Hepatitis* 2006;13(10):708–14.

15. Lucas M, Ulsenheimer A, Pfafferot K, *et al.* Tracking virus-specific CD4+ T cells during and after acute hepatitis C virus infection. *PLoS ONE.* 2007;2: e649.

16. Schirren CA, Jung MC, Gerlach JT, *et al.* Liver-derived hepatitis C virus (HCV)-specific CD4(+) T cells recognize multiple HCV epitopes and produce interferon gamma. *Hepatology* 2000;32(3):597–603.

17. Rico MA, Quiroga JA, Subira D, *et al.* Features of the CD4 +T-cell response in liver and peripheral blood of hepatitis C virus-infected patients with persistently normal and abnormal alanine aminotransferase levels. *J Hepatol* 2002;36(3):408–16.

18. Gale M, Jr., Foy EM. Evasion of intracellular host defence by hepatitis C virus. *Nature* 200518;436(7053):939–45.

19. Rehermann B. Hepatitis C virus versus innate and adaptive immune responses: a tale of coevolution and coexistence. *J Clin Invest* 2009;119(7):1745–54.

20. Lin W, Kim SS, Yeung E, *et al.* Hepatitis C virus core protein blocks interferon signaling by interaction with the STAT1 SH2 domain. *J Virol* 2006;80(18):9226–35.

21. Foy E, Li K, Wang C, *et al.* Regulation of interferon regulatory factor-3 by the hepatitis C virus serine protease. *Science* 2003;300(5622):1145–8.

22. Meylan E, Curran J, Hofmann K, *et al.* Cardif is an adaptor protein in the RIG-I antiviral pathway and is targeted by hepatitis C virus. *Nature* 2005;437(7062):1167–72.

23. Li K, Foy E, Ferreon JC, *et al.* Immune evasion by hepatitis C virus NS3/4A protease-mediated cleavage of the Toll-like receptor 3 adaptor protein TRIF. *Proc Natl Acad Sci U S A* 2005;102(8):2992–7.

24. Chen Z, Benureau Y, Rijnbrand R, *et al.* GB virus B disrupts RIG-I signaling by NS3/4A-mediated cleavage of the adaptor protein MAVS. *J Virol* 2007;81(2):964–76.

25. Yang Y, Liang Y, Qu L, *et al.* Disruption of innate immunity due to mitochondrial targeting of a picornaviral protease precursor. *Proc Natl Acad Sci U S A* 2007;104(17): 7253–8.

26. Dolganiuc A, Chang S, Kodys K, *et al.* Hepatitis C virus (HCV) core protein-induced, monocyte-mediated mechanisms of reduced IFN-alpha and plasmacytoid dendritic cell loss in chronic HCV infection. *J Immunol* 2006;177(10): 6758–68.

27. Shiina M, Rehermann B. Cell culture-produced hepatitis C virus impairs plasmacytoid dendritic cell function. *Hepatology* 2008;47(2):385–95.

28. Goutagny N, Fatmi A, De Ledinghen V, *et al.* Evidence of viral replication in circulating dendritic cells during hepatitis C virus infection. *J Infect Dis* 2003;187(12):1951–8.

29. Mellor J, Haydon G, Blair C, *et al.* Low level or absent in vivo replication of hepatitis C virus and hepatitis G virus/GB virus C in peripheral blood mononuclear cells. *J Gen Virol* 1998;79(Pt 4):705–14.

30. Rollier C, Drexhage JA, Verstrepen BE, *et al.* Chronic hepatitis C virus infection established and maintained in chimpanzees independent of dendritic cell impairment. *Hepatology* 2003;38(4):851–8.

31. Khakoo SI, Thio CL, Martin MP, *et al.* HLA and NK cell inhibitory receptor genes in resolving hepatitis C virus infection. *Science* 2004;305(5685):872–4.

32. Yoon JC, Shiina M, Ahlenstiel G, Rehermann B. Natural killer cell function is intact after direct exposure to infectious hepatitis C virions. *Hepatology* 2009;49(1):12–21.

33. Urbani S, Amadei B, Tola D, *et al.* PD-1 expression in acute hepatitis C virus (HCV) infection is associated with HCV-specific CD8 exhaustion. *J Virol* 2006;80(22):11398–403.

34. Radziewicz H, Ibegbu CC, Fernandez ML, *et al.* Liver-infiltrating lymphocytes in chronic human hepatitis C virus infection display an exhausted phenotype with high levels of PD-1 and low levels of CD127 expression. *J Virol* 2007; 81(6):2545–53.

35. Nakamoto N, Cho H, Shaked A, *et al.* Synergistic reversal of intrahepatic HCV-specific CD8 T cell exhaustion by combined PD-1/CTLA-4 blockade. *PLoS Pathog* 2009;5(2): e1000313.

36. McMahon RH, Golden-Mason L, Nishimura MI, *et al.* Tim-3 expression on PD-1+ HCV-specific human CTLs is associated with viral persistence, and its blockade restores hepatocyte-directed in vitro cytotoxicity. *J Clin Invest* 2010; 120(12):4546–57.

37. Barber DL, Wherry EJ, Masopust D, *et al.* Restoring function in exhausted CD8 T cells during chronic viral infection. *Nature* 2006;439(7077):682–7.

38. Velu V, Titanji K, Zhu B, *et al.* Enhancing SIV-specific immunity in vivo by PD-1 blockade. *Nature* 2009;458(7235): 206–10.

39. Manigold T, Shin EC, Mizukoshi E, *et al.* Foxp3+CD4+ CD25+ T cells control virus-specific memory T cells in chimpanzees that recovered from hepatitis C. *Blood* 2006; 107(11):4424–32.

40. Smyk-Pearson S, Golden-Mason L, Klarquist J, *et al.* Functional suppression by FoxP3+CD4+CD25(high) regulatory T cells during acute hepatitis C virus infection. *J Infect Dis* 2008;197(1):46–57.

41. Abel M, Sene D, Pol S, *et al.* Intrahepatic virus-specific IL-10-producing CD8 T cells prevent liver damage during chronic hepatitis C virus infection. *Hepatology* 2006;44(6):1607–16.

42. Yao ZQ, Ray S, Eisen-Vandervelde A, *et al.* Hepatitis C virus: immunosuppression by complement regulatory pathway. *Viral Immunol* 2001;14(4):277–95.

43. Accapezzato D, Francavilla V, Rawson P, *et al.* Subversion of effector CD8+ T cell differentiation in acute hepatitis C virus infection: the role of the virus. *Eur J Immunol* 2004; 34(2):438–46.

44. Soldaini E, Wack A, D'Oro U, *et al.* T cell costimulation by the hepatitis C virus envelope protein E2 binding to CD81 is mediated by Lck. *Eur J Immunol* 2003;33(2):455–64.

45. Volkov Y, Long A, Freeley M, *et al.* The hepatitis C envelope 2 protein inhibits LFA-1-transduced protein kinase C signaling for T-lymphocyte migration. *Gastroenterology* 2006; 130(2):482–92.

46. Bowen DG, Walker CM. Mutational escape from CD8+ T cell immunity: HCV evolution, from chimpanzees to man. *J Exp Med* 2005;201(11):1709–14.

47. Fuller MJ, Shoukry NH, Gushima T, *et al.* Selection-driven immune escape is not a significant factor in the failure of CD4 T cell responses in persistent hepatitis C virus infection. *Hepatology* 2010;51(2):378–87.

48. Bowen DG, McCaughan GW, Bertolino P. Intrahepatic immunity: a tale of two sites? *Trends Immunol* 2005;26(10): 512–7.

49. Feld JJ, Hoofnagle JH. Mechanism of action of interferon and ribavirin in treatment of hepatitis C. *Nature* 2005; 436(7053):967–72.

50. Crawford A, Wherry EJ. Editorial: Therapeutic potential of targeting BTLA. *J Leukoc Biol* 2009;86(1):5–8.

4

Mechanisms of Action of Antiviral Drugs: The Interferons

Edmund Tse and Michael R. Beard

School of Molecular and Biomedical Science, University of Adelaide, and Centre for Cancer Biology, SA Pathology, Adelaide, SA, Australia

Introduction

The type 1 interferons (IFN; IFN-α and -β) are key innate immune cytokines produced by most cells to combat viral infection and are rapidly induced following viral infection through a series of intricate sensory mechanisms. This increase in IFN production in turn results in induction of a large number of genes collectively known as interferon-stimulated genes (ISGs), and it is through the action of these genes that IFN exerts its antiviral effect. It is this antiviral property of IFN in part that is exploited in the current therapy for chronic hepatitis C. While IFN has multiple immunomodulatory functions, the induction of ISGs is thought to be fundamental to controlling HCV infection. The ISGs responsible for the anti-HCV effect are not well understood, although the roles of a number of ISGs are emerging as well as anti-HCV effectors. In this chapter the events leading to the induction of type 1 IFN following HCV infection and IFN action are outlined. Furthermore, the current state of known ISGs to control HCV replication, as well as their ability as a predictor of IFN therapeutic outcome, will also be discussed.

Hepatocyte Response to HCV Infection

Viral infections including HCV initiate a series of intracellular events that culminate in the generation of an antiviral state directly within the infected cell and indirectly within the surrounding tissue [1] (Figure 4.1). The host response is triggered when a pathogen-associated molecular pattern (PAMP) presented by the infecting virus is recognized and engaged by specific PAMP receptors expressed by the host cell. This in turn activates a number of signaling cascades that culminate in the expression of antiviral effector genes collectively termed ISGs, including type I IFNs as well as proinflammatory cytokines [2–4]. For RNA viruses, the products of viral infection and replication, such as viral proteins and/or either single-stranded (ss) or double-stranded (ds) RNA, have been identified as viral PAMPs. These are engaged by specific toll-like receptors (TLR) or nucleic acid binding proteins that serve as PAMP receptors [5,6]. Two such PAMP receptors that play a role in sensing infection of hepatocytes with HCV are the retanoic-acid-inducible gene I (RIG-I) and TLR-3, which recognizes dsRNA. There is increasing evidence, however, that RIG-I is the major PAMP associated with innate immune activation in HCV infection of hepatocytes. Engagement of these PAMPs by dsRNA sets in motion a complex signaling cascade that results in the phosphorylation of the latent transcription factor IRF3 and NFκB and their translocation from the cytoplasm to the nucleus, whereby they bind to the IFN-β promoter, leading to a transcriptional response that produces secreted IFN-β from the infected cell (Figure 4.1). IFN-β can act in an autocrine or paracrine manner through binding of the type I IFN receptor present on most cell types. This results in the activation of the JAK-STAT pathway, in which the receptor-associated JAK1 and Tyk2 protein kinases catalyze the phosphorylation of STAT 1 and 2 proteins on critical serine and tyrosine residues and facilitate dimerization and association with IRF9 (Figure 4.1). This transcription factor complex, now termed ISGF3, translocates to the nucleus and binds to the IFN-stimulated response element within the promoter/enhancer region

Advanced Therapy for Hepatitis C, First Edition. Edited by Geoffrey W. McCaughan, John G. McHutchison and Jean-Michel Pawlotsky.
© 2012 Blackwell Publishing Ltd. Published 2012 by Blackwell Publishing Ltd.

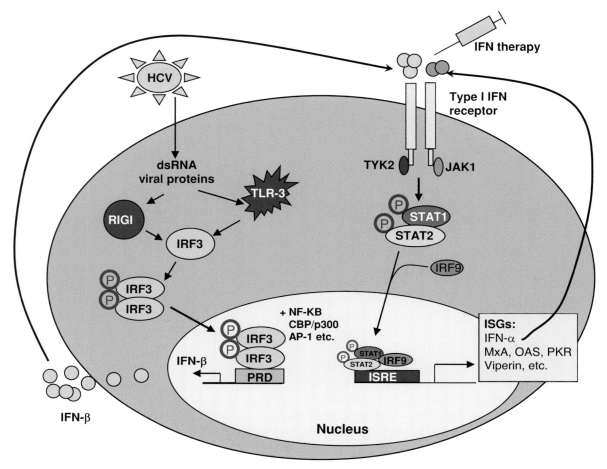

Figure 4.1 HCV induction of IFN-α/β.

of ISGs including IFN-α and induces expression of hundreds of ISGs. For the purposes of this chapter, the discussion of the signaling pathways at play in recognition of viral PAMPs is brief and a more detailed account can be found in the following excellent review articles [7,8]. It is the expression of these ISGs that imparts the antiviral activity of IFN on a wide range of viruses, including HCV. However, expression of the type I IFNs has much greater effects than just ISG expression, as it is known to modulate several aspects of the adaptive immunity, including establishment of cytotoxic T cell responses, generation of natural killer cells, and B-cell differentiation. As such, activation of the early innate response to viral infection provides a strong primer for the induction of the adaptive immune response and, while often discussed separately,

the innate and adaptive immune responses are intimately linked. Furthermore, the importance of this early IFN response to viral infection is highlighted by the fact that most viruses, including HCV, have evolved strategies to combat either IFN production or IFN action [9].

Recognition of HCV by RIG-I and TLR-3

The importance of the RIG-I and TLR-3 pathways of PAMP recognition in HCV infection is highlighted by the fact that HCV can specifically block these pathways, resulting in control of type I IFN expression and action. However, the relative roles that RIG-I and TLR-3 play in recognition of HCV PAMPs is not firmly established, although there is evidence to suggest that RIG-I plays a major role. To date no HCV PAMP has been shown to activate the TLR-3 pathway *in vitro*, and while hepatocytes do express TLR-3, they do so at extremely low levels. Furthermore, TLR-3 is a transmembrane protein associated with endosomes and as such detection of HCV by TLR-3 would likely require phagocytosis of virus or virus-infected cells to initiate activation. In this sense the TLRs present in other resident cells of the liver may act as secondary sensors of HCV through sensing viral products in phagocytosed cells. So how does RIG-I specifically detect HCV PAMPs given the abundance of cellular RNA (ds and ss) within the cell? RIG-I specifically recognizes cytoplasmic ssRNA containing 5' triphosphate (ppp), short dsRNA, and uridine- or adenosine-rich viral RNA motifs [10]. Not surprisingly the HCV genome contains several of these motifs that facilitate recognition by RIG-I. As with cellular mRNA, the HCV RNA genome is not capped and hence the HCV RNA contains a 5' ppp to facilitate engagement with RIG-I. The 3' non-coding region of HCV contains the primary HCV PAMP that activates RIG-I signaling. The HCV 3' NCR contains a variable region containing ds stem-loop structures, a poly U-rich region that is single stranded, and a conserved "X" region that also contains significant secondary structure. It was predicted that the ds regions of the 3' NCR would facilitate RIG-I activation, however, this was not the case, with the polyU/UC region found to be a potent activator of RIG-I [10]. These unique features of the HCV PAMP discriminate it from cellular RNAs and demonstrate the ability of RIG-I to distinguish "self" (cellular RNA) from "non-self" (viral RNA).

Activation and Antagonism of HCV Recognition Pathways

So how do the HCV PAMPs activate RIG-I? This is a complex process and not fully understood and a full description is beyond the scope of this chapter. Briefly, RIG-I exists in an inactive conformation facilitated by intramolecular interaction between the N-terminal CARD domain and the C-terminal RD, which suppresses ATP-ase activity of RIG-I [11,12]. Following engagement of the HCV PAMP with RIG-I, there is a conformational change that results in oligomerization and exposure of the CARD domain for interaction with the CARD domain of the adaptor protein IFN promoter-stimulating factor-1 (IPS-1, also known as cardif, VISA, and MAVS). This inter-

action occurs on the outer mitochondrial membrane and results in activation of downstream signaling molecules, resulting in IRF3 activation and expression of a specific set of genes, including IFN-β (Figure 4.2). Secreted IFN-β then acts locally and systemically via the JAK-STAT pathway for the induction of hundreds of ISGs, one of which is IFN-α, which in turn amplifies the innate antiviral response. The importance of this pathway in HCV pathogenesis is exemplified in the fact that HCV has evolved a mechanism to disrupt RIG-I signaling, with the net result to prevent type I IFN expression (Figure 4.2). This is achieved though the action of the HCV NS3/4A protein, whose normal function as a protease is to cleave the HCV polyprotein and release mature non-structural viral proteins. However, NS3/4A also cleaves IPS-1, releasing it from the mitochondrial membrane and rendering it inactive, resulting in abolished IRF3 activation and attenuated gene expression [4,13–15]. In addition to IPS-1, NS3/4A has also shown to cleave TRIFF (Toll/interleukin-1 receptor/assistance domain containing adaptor protein), the signaling adaptor molecule for TLR3-mediated antiviral signaling [4]. However the importance and the role of the TLR-3 pathway in innate immunity is not well defined. Interestingly, IPS-1 is cleaved in the liver biopsies of HCV-infected individuals and in those patients with high levels of cleaved IPS-1 there was a reduction in the activation of the JAK-STAT pathway and the expression of a panel of ISGs [16]. Clearly, IPS-1 cleavage noted *in vitro* also occurs in the HCV-infected liver and may suggest in part how HCV evades the innate immune system, leading to persistence. However, another hepatitis virus, hepatitis A virus, which almost always results in an acute self-limiting infection, also cleaves IPS-1, indicating that chronicity of HCV is a complex, multifaceted process [17–19].

Antagonism of RIG-I is not the only mechanism whereby HCV disrupts innate immune activation (Figure 4.2). The JAK-STAT signal transduction pathway is another target, although its importance in the context of the HCV-infected liver requires validation. Expression of the core protein alone can bind STAT1, preventing phosphorylation and subsequent activation of downstream anti-HCV ISGs [20]. Furthermore, it has also been shown that core can induce the expression of the suppressor of cytokine signaling-3 (SOCS-3), a negative regulator of the JAK-STAT pathway, resulting in decreased STAT1 activation. The HCV proteins NS5A and E2 directly interfere with the antiviral actions of ISGs, including PKR, while NS5A also blocks the action of the well-described antiviral protein 2-5 OAS via a direct interaction. Furthermore NS5A induces the expression and secretion of IL-8, which

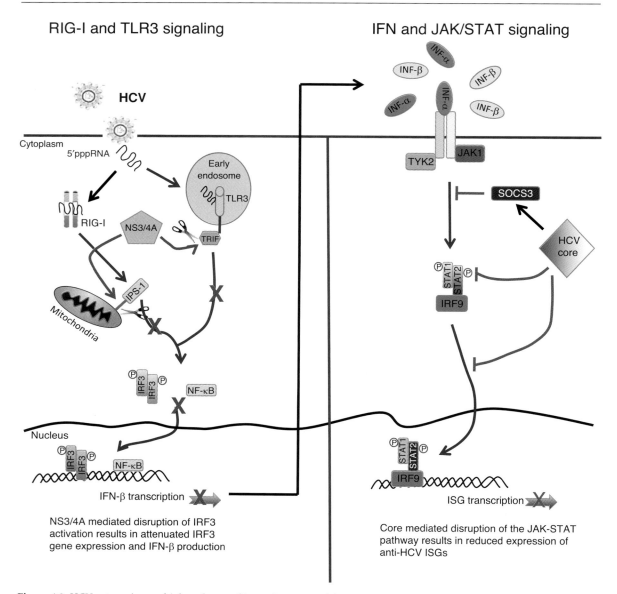

RIG-I and TLR3 signaling

IFN and JAK/STAT signaling

NS3/4A mediated disruption of IRF3
activation results in attenuated IRF3
gene expression and IFN-β production

Core mediated disruption of the JAK-STAT
pathway results in reduced expression of
anti-HCV ISGs

Figure 4.2 HCV antagonizes multiple pathways of innate immune activity.

serves to reduce the expression of ISGs [21]. IL-8 levels are increased in HCV-infected individuals who do not respond to IFN therapy, suggesting that NS5A may directly modulate ISG expression. Clearly HCV, as do most viruses, has evolved multiple mechanisms to evade the innate response to viral infection although the relative contributions of each of these mechanisms in the infected individual remains to be elucidated.

Interferon-stimulated Genes and HCV Control

ISGs are a spectrum of genes that are up-regulated as a result of IFN stimulation. It is these genes that carry out the antiviral action of IFN proteins. Although activation of the JAK-STAT pathway by IFN has been well defined, many of the actions of these hundreds of genes known to be up-regulated by IFN remain relatively unknown. Some of the better defined ISGs and their role in controlling HCV are discussed below.

ISG15

ISG15 is a 17 kDa ubiquitin-like protein which is markedly induced by IFN stimulation, TLR activation, and viral infections [22,23]. ISG15 works in conjunction with a number of other type I inducible proteins, namely E1 (ISG15 activating enzyme), E2 (1SG15 conjugating enzyme), and E3 (ISG15 ligase), to conjugate ISG15 to many cellular and viral proteins in a process termed ISGylation. While not completely understood, ISGylation most likely works by conjugation of ISG15 to cellular proteins preventing proteosomal degradation [24] or targeting protein activity [25].

While ISG15 has been associated with an antiviral effect against a number of viruses such as influenza, herpes, and HIV, its role in controlling HCV is controversial. One report suggests that ISG15 promotes HCV replication through exploiting ISGylation as a host immune evasion strategy to decrease the anti-HCV activity of IFN [26]. Conversely, Kim and colleagues showed that ISGylation of the HCV NS5A protein inhibits HCV replication [27]. NS5A is a key protein involved in HCV replication and viral assembly, and ISGylation may disrupt its normal function in the virus life cycle. What are the reasons for this discordance? This may be reflected in different model systems of HCV replication used and different HCV genotypes investigated. Nevertheless, it seems that ISG15 has a role in the HCV lifecycle and further experiments are required to determine its role in HCV pathogenesis. Interestingly, ISG15 expression is increased in patients who do not respond to treatment with PegIFN and ribavirin [28–31], suggesting it may play a role in the HCV-infected liver to control IFN responses.

USP18

USP18 is also induced by IFN stimulation and is biochemically linked to USP15 (see above). USP18 is an ubiquitin-specific protease that cleaves ISG15 from its cellular targets. USP18 has been shown to play a critical role in the antiviral activity of IFN-α against HCV in an *in vitro* model system. Knock down of USP18 potentiated the ability of IFN-α to inhibit HCV replication and infectious particle production [32], as well as a concurrent increase in cellular protein ISGylation in response to IFN-α. Furthermore, USP18 is up-regulated in HCV-infected liver samples, correlating with non-response to antiviral therapy [28].

ISG20

ISG20 is an IFN inducible 3′-5′ exonuclease that inhibits several human and animal RNA viruses. It is strongly induced in many viral infections, including hepatitis C in humans [33] and experimental infection of chimpanzees, as well as following administration of IFN [34,35]. Recent work has suggested that ISG20 exerts its antiviral effect against HCV via its 3′-5′ exonuclease activity, although this does not seem to involve the degradation of HCV RNA. Thus the exact mechanism of ISG20 action remains unresolved [36]. ISG20 also demonstrated antiviral activity against yellow fever virus, hepatitis A virus, and hepatitis B virus, indicating its broad range of specificity.

PKR

The IFN-inducible protein kinase RNA activated or protein kinase R (PKR) is a double-stranded RNA-dependent protein kinase that targets the eukaryotic translation ignition factor 2 (eIF-2alpha) for phosphorylation at Ser51, leading to reduction of cellular and viral protein translation [37,38]. PKR appears to have antiviral properties toward HCV infection, as PKR-deficient cell lines confer HCV replicon growth advantage [36]. However, this antiviral property is seen only in infection naïve cells, suggesting protection from cell to cell spread rather than replication [36].

Despite its antiviral properties, HCV has also adopted tactics to overcome this defense mechanism. HCV-NS5A seems to enhance HCV replication by binding and inhibiting PKR activity through the PKR binding domain and subsequently blocking the phosphorylation of eIF2 [39–43]. Furthermore, the unglycosylated form of the HCV envelope protein E2 was also able to stop translation inhibition of HCV protein by binding to PKR [44–46].

ISG56

ISG56 (p56) is a target gene of IRF3 and is activated by HCV replication and IFN [3,38,47–50]. ISG56 suppresses HCV replication through disruption of HCV polyprotein production, via an interaction with the translational machinery that binds the HCV internal ribosome entry site (IRES). ISG56 binds to the 'e' subunit of human eIF3, reducing the recruitment of ribosome complex to the HCV IRES, resulting in protein translation inhibition of viral and cellular RNA.

It has been shown that HCV, through adaptive mechanisms and immune selective pressure, can improve replication through suppression of ISG56. Marked suppression of ISG56 has been shown in the Huh-7 cell line harboring an evolved strain of a replication-efficient HCV type 1b subgenomic RNA replicon [47], either through viral-induced reduction of promoter activity or stability of ISG56 mRNA. This is seen to be independent of an IFN mediating effect. This is likely secondary to attenuation by one or more viral products and not through deregulation of the IFN-stimulated pathway. Furthermore, in this replication-efficient replicon model, there was also reduction of interaction between ISG56 and eIF3, leading to increased ribosomal recruitment and increased viral RNA translation [47].

Viperin

Viperin is an IFN-stimulated protein which in addition to its anti-HCV properties [33,36] also inhibits HCMV, influenza, dengue, and HIV [51–53]. It can be significantly up-regulated by direct dsRNA stimulation, leading to activation of IRF3 independently of IFN [33,50]. Viperin inhibits influenza replication through disruption of cell membrane and lipid raft integrity, leading to reduced virion budding [52]. In regards to HCV, viperin seems to be acting through a different mechanism. Viperin has been shown to associate with lipid droplets, which are integral to HCV replication [54]. HCV core and NS5A proteins localize to lipid droplets in a process that is thought to facilitate assembly [55]. It is possible that at the surface of lipid droplets, viperin may disrupt HCV RNA NS5A/core interactions. In individuals with chronic HCV infection (CHC), global gene expression studies have shown there is a marked up-regulation of viperin mRNA from pretreatment liver biopsy samples [33]. This suggests that HCV itself and the associated type I IFN response strongly induce viperin expression *in vivo*.

Table 4.1 summarizes the role of these ISGs in controlling HCV.

Ribavirin and its Relation to ISG Expression

Ribavirin is an integral component to the treatment of CHC infection along with pegylated IFN-α. Ribavirin is a guanosine analog, with antiviral activities to both DNA and RNA viruses [56]. It has been shown that ribavirin enhances the antiviral activity of IFN, but the exact mechanism of action remains unclear. Thomas and colleagues have shown that ribavirin may enhance IFN activity through ISG up-regulation [57]. Gene array analysis from liver biopsy samples revealed that those HCV-infected individuals taking combination therapy of ribavirin and pegylated IFN had higher up-regulation of

Table 4.1 Known ISGs that control HCV replication.

Interferon-stimulated gene	Mechanism of action	References
ISG15	Conjugation to numerous cellular proteins preventing target protein degradation or blocking activity	[23–27]
	Activation of cytotoxic T cells; dentritic cell maturation and neutrophil recruitment	
	May also have a negative regulator of IFN pathway	
USP18 (*UBP43*)	Displace ISG15 from cellular target proteins	[28,32]
	Independent negative regulator of IFN pathway	
ISG20	3′-5′ exonuclease leading to viral RNA degradation	[33–36]
	Possible indirect activities on viral replication or transcription	
	Facilitating adaptive T cell response	
PKR	Phosphorylates translation ignition factor eIF2α leading to reduction of viral protein translation	[36–43]
ISG56	Disruption of HCV IRES translation	[38,47–50]
	Binding to eIF3 leading to protein translation inhibition	
Viperin	?N terminal amphipathic α helix that binds to lipid droplets disrupting HCV replication assembly	[33,36,51–53]

the ISGs IRF7 and IRF9 at the messenger RNA level. *In vitro*, ribavirin has been shown to up-regulate a narrow spectrum of ISGs in Huh-7.5.1 cells, including IRF7, IRF9, and ISG15, compared to IFN. Furthermore, actions of ribavirin and IFN-α appear to be synergistic, with marked increased ISG expression compared with either agent alone. This up-regulation of ISG may be secondary to ribavirin's inhibition of a transcriptional repressor. This implies that transcriptional repressors may be important factors in ISG regulation [58].

ISGs and Prediction of Treatment Outcome in CHC Infection

Pegylated IFN-α and ribavirin is currently the treatment of choice for CHC infection. Multiple host and viral factors have been shown to affect treatment outcome, including genotype, viral load, race, and liver fibrosis score. The mechanism of how these viral and clinical factors affect treatment outcome remains unclear. Treatment with pegylated IFN-α and ribavirin is associated with numerous side effects and treatment outcome is not straightforward to predict prior to commencement of therapy. However, studies using core liver biopsy from HCV-infected individuals have shown a pattern of ISG expression that may predict treatment outcome prior to therapy.

Chen and colleagues were one of the first groups to suggest that ISG profiling of liver biopsy could be used to predict treatment outcomes prior to IFN therapy [28]. They demonstrated a set of 18 genes, which differed consistently between 31 patients who were responders or nonresponders to pegylated IFN and ribavirin therapy. They noted that gene expression in responders was closer to that of normal livers, whereas in non-responders, a general up-regulation of gene expression was observed. Genes that differed between responders and non-responders include IFN-sensitive genes as well as two genes, *ISG15* and *IFI15*, thought to be important in IFN regulatory pathway [28]. Using a subset of eight of these genes, the authors were able to predict treatment outcomes in 30 out of 31 patients, independent of classical treatment prognosticators such as genotype, fibrosis score, and viral load. Similar results were found for ISG expression in treatment studies. Although absolute ISG expression was similar between rapid responders and slow responders, baseline ISG levels in rapid responders were lower and with greater fold changes compared to slow responders [29].

Peripheral blood mononuclear cells (PBMC) is an attractive way of studying HCV pathogenesis and clinical response to IFN therapy. This is due to the ease of acquiring PBMC samples for ISG profiling prior to treatment, as well as periodically throughout IFN therapy, which is not the case for liver biopsies.

Gene expression studies have been performed on PBMC in CHC infection. One particular study investigated ISG profiling with racial origin (Caucasians versus African American), which is a known clinical factor predictive of treatment response [59]. Those with a positive response (>3.5 log drop in viral load) had greater numbers of gene up- and down-regulated compared with those who had minimal viral response (<1.4 log drop in viral load). Furthermore, most of these changes occurred very early, within the 24-hour mark from starting treatment. Most of these genes were ISGs, including genes such as *IRF7* and viperin, but none of which were specifically associated with treatment outcome or racial differences alone. Gene expression between racial groups was not significantly different in this study. It is believed that those with poor response to exogenous IFN stimulation must have a physiological defect leading to a blunted or defective pathway [59]. These results were substantiated by another group, who showed sustained virological response (SVR) after combination therapy was associated with increased transcriptional response to *ex vivo* stimulation of pre-treatment PBMC with IFN [60]. In particular, there was a positive correlation between ISG up-regulation and STAT1 activation, a key signaling molecule in the JAK-STAT pathway. Furthermore, STAT1 activation and levels of ISG induction were higher among Caucasians than among African Americans. This finding differed from data previously obtained from Taylor and colleagues; however, it may provide an insight into understanding why certain ethnic groups respond better to treatment compared with others [60].

However, the use of PBMCs is questionable as there is evidence to suggest that the pattern of ISG expression in PBMCs is different from that of the liver, and may not predict HCV treatment outcome as previous thought. In a study from Sarasin-Filipowicz *et al.*, mRNA from liver biopsy tissue showed at least a 2-fold change in 252 genes in rapid responders, compared to only 36 genes in non-rapid responders [31]. Most of the gene alterations were observed in ISGs. The absolute expression levels of these genes were similar in the rapid and non-rapid responders. In terms of PBMCs, unlike what is seen in liver tissue, there was no appreciable pre-activation of ISG compared to post-therapy with IFN between rapid and non-rapid responders. Furthermore, gene expression occurred in rapid and non-rapid responders universally when IFN therapy was given. This study confirmed that treatment failure of HCV infection with IFN-based therapy is highly associated with pre-activation of ISGs in liver tissue [31]. Furthermore, it would appear that treatment-resistant patients are refractory to further exogenous IFN as the IFN signaling cascade is already saturated.

Thus, while ISG expression in the liver may provide a means to predict treatment response, the difficulty in obtaining liver biopsy samples may limit its usefulness as a clinical diagnostic predictor of treatment outcome.

IL28B and its Prediction to CHC Treatment Response and Spontaneous Clearance

Recent data have shown that host genetic makeup may affect treatment response to CHC infection. It has been hypothesized that the basis of IFN-based treatment success is largely based on the host's immune response to the virus. Furthermore, a higher number of non-responders in African Americans compared with Americans of European descent, also suggests genetic makeup of individuals may play a role in achieving SVR [60]. However, the exact genetic mechanism leading to viral clearance remains elusive.

It is clear that ISG expression can be used to predict treatment response [28,29,31]. ISG expression is a phenotypic response to an infection state. Recently it has been shown that genetic makeup can also be used to predict not only treatment response, but also the spontaneous clearance of HCV infection. Genome-wide studies have shown that single nucleotide polymorphisms, found upstream of the *IL28B* gene, are critical in determining spontaneous clearance as well as predicting treatment response to CHC infection. *IL28B* encodes the type III IFN-λ3 protein, which activates the well-described JAK-STAT pathway, leading to transcription of ISGs; however, *IL28B* and its associated activation of cellular pathways and ISG expression is much less developed than for type I IFNs. Ge and colleagues have shown it to have a strong association of more than 2-fold positive response to antiviral treatment against CHC infection [61]. Two other researchers have confirmed this observation of genetic variation with treatment response in patients with genotype 1 CHC infection [62,63]. Furthermore, single nucleotide polymorphism (SNP) of the IL28B allele has been shown to be

a better predictor of null virologic response (OR 37.68), compared to more conventional treatment prediction factors, including fibrosis grade and viral load [63]. Furthermore, those with the favorable SNP allele, are much more likely to undergo spontaneous clearance in the setting of acute HCV infection, compared to those with homologous unfavorable haplotype (OR 0.29) or heterozygote haplotype (OR 0.35) [64].

It is then possible that such genetic expression can be used to predict treatment outcomes and hopefully avoid the burden of IFN-induced side effects. Furthermore, based on the gene product of IL28B, IFN-λ3 could be used as an alternate treatment agent in anti-HCV therapy, potentially achieving a higher rate of SVR with fewer side effects.

Despite the above overwhelming evidence for the predictive value of IL28 genotype, recent data has suggested that ISG may have better prediction in treatment response to CHC infection compared to IL28B. In the cohort of patients of Dill and colleagues, ISG expression was significant higher in non-responders and patients who relapsed, compared to those with SVR. On the contrary, expression of IL28A, IL28B, IL29, IL28RA, and IL10RB did not differ between SVR and non-SVR groups [65]. Furthermore, patients with the same *IL28B* genotype had variable expression of ISG, suggesting a poor correlation between genotype and this phenotype. Furthermore, those with SVR has comparable ISG profiles but with varying *IL28B* genotype. This suggests that ISG and *IL28B*, although both are treatment prediction parameters, are likely to be independent of each other [65].

Concluding Remarks

The innate immune response to HCV infections is a critical part of the host response to controlling HCV infections. This is reinforced by the fact that HCV has evolved multiple mechanisms to subvert this response culminating in an abrogated early host response to infections. The importance of this is further exemplified in that the type and breadth of this response to viral infection shapes the magnitude of the adaptive immune response, which is critical for viral clearance. Ongoing research into the ISGs that control HCV replication, from both endogenous and exogenous administered IFN, is rapidly expanding. It is hoped that an understanding of the mechanisms responsible for anti-HCV action of ISGs will facilitate the design of novel therapeutic strategies to combat hepatitis C.

References

1. Stark GR, Kerr IM, Williams BR, *et al.* How cells respond to interferons. *Annu Rev Biochem* 1998;67:227–64.
2. Yoneyama M, Kikuchi M, Natsukawa T, *et al.* The RNA helicase RIG-I has an essential function in double-stranded RNA-induced innate antiviral responses. *Nat Immunol* 2004;5(7):730–37.
3. Sumpter R, Jr., Loo YM, Foy E, *et al.* Regulating intracellular antiviral defense and permissiveness to hepatitis C virus RNA replication through a cellular RNA helicase, RIG-I. *J Virol* 2005;79(5):2689–99.
4. Li K, Foy E, Ferreon JC, *et al.* Immune evasion by hepatitis C virus NS3/4A protease-mediated cleavage of the Toll-like receptor 3 adaptor protein TRIF. *Proc Natl Acad Sci U S A* 2005;102(8):2992–7.
5. Iwasaki A, Medzhitov R. Toll-like receptor control of the adaptive immune responses. *Nat Immunol* 2004;5(10):987–95.
6. Cook DN, Pisetsky DS, Schwartz DA. Toll-like receptors in the pathogenesis of human disease. *Nat Immunol* 2004; 5(10):975–9.
7. Gale M, Jr., Foy EM. Evasion of intracellular host defence by hepatitis C virus. *Nature* 2005;436(7053):939–45.
8. Horner SM, Gale M, Jr. Intracellular innate immune cascades and interferon defenses that control hepatitis C virus. *J Interferon Cytokine Res* 2009;29(9):489–98.
9. Katze MG, He, Y, Gale M, Jr. Viruses and interferon: a fight for supremacy. *Nat Rev Immunol* 2002;2(9):675–87.
10. Saito T, Owen DM, Jiang F, *et al.* Innate immunity induced by composition-dependent RIG-I recognition of hepatitis C virus RNA. *Nature* 2008;454(7203):523–7.
11. Saito T, Hirai R, Loo YM, *et al.* Regulation of innate antiviral defenses through a shared repressor domain in RIG-I and LGP2. *Proc Natl Acad Sci U S A* 2007;104(2):582–7.
12. Gee P, Chua PK, Gevorkyan J, *et al.* Essential role of the N-terminal domain in the regulation of RIG-I ATPase activity. *J Biol Chem* 2008;283(14):9488–96.
13. Foy E, Li K, Sumpter R, Jr., *et al.* Control of antiviral defenses through hepatitis C virus disruption of retinoic acid-inducible gene-I signaling. *Proc Natl Acad Sci U S A,* 2005;102(8):2986–91.
14. Loo YM, Owen DM, Li K, *et al.* Viral and therapeutic control of IFN-beta promoter stimulator 1 during hepatitis C virus infection. *Proc Natl Acad Sci U S A* 2006;103(15):6001–6.
15. Meylan E, Curran J, Hofmann K, *et al.* Cardif is an adaptor protein in the RIG-I antiviral pathway and is targeted by hepatitis C virus. *Nature* 2005;437(7062):1167–72.
16. Bellecave P, Sarasin-Filipowicz M, Donzé O, *et al.* Cleavage of mitochondrial antiviral signaling protein in the liver of patients with chronic hepatitis C correlates with a reduced activation of the endogenous interferon system. *Hepatology* 2010;51(4):1127–36.
17. Lemon SM. Induction and evasion of innate antiviral responses by hepatitis C virus. *J Biol Chem* 285(30): 22741–7.
18. Qu L, Lemon SM. Hepatitis A and hepatitis C viruses: divergent infection outcomes marked by similarities in induction and evasion of interferon responses. *Semin Liver Dis* 2010;30(4):319–32.
19. Yang Y, Liang Y, Qu L, *et al.* Disruption of innate immunity due to mitochondrial targeting of a picornaviral protease precursor. *Proc Natl Acad Sci U S A* 2007;104(17):7253–8.
20. Suthar MS, Gale M, Jr., Owen DM. Evasion and disruption of innate immune signalling by hepatitis C and West Nile viruses. *Cell Microbiol* 2009;11(6):880–88.
21. Polyak SJ, Khabar KS, Paschal DM, *et al.* Hepatitis C virus nonstructural 5A protein induces interleukin-8, leading to partial inhibition of the interferon-induced antiviral response. *J Virol* 2001;75(13):6095–106.
22. Der SD, Zhou A, Williams BR, Silverman RH. Identification of genes differentially regulated by interferon alpha, beta, or gamma using oligonucleotide arrays. *Proc Natl Acad Sci U S A* 1998;95(26):15623–8.
23. Potter JL, Narasimhan J, Mende-Mueller L, Haas AL. Precursor processing of pro-ISG15/UCRP, an interferon-beta-induced ubiquitin-like protein. *J Biol Chem* 1999; 274(35):25061–8.
24. Liu M, Li XL, Hassel BA. Proteasomes modulate conjugation to the ubiquitin-like protein, ISG15. *J Biol Chem* 2003;278(3):1594–602.
25. Lenschow DJ. Antiviral properties of ISG15. *Viruses* 2010;2:2154–68.
26. Chen L, Sun J, Meng L, *et al.* ISG15, a ubiquitin-like interferon-stimulated gene, promotes hepatitis C virus production in vitro: implications for chronic infection and response to treatment. *J Gen Virol* 2010;91(Pt 2):382–8.
27. Kim MJ, Hwang SY, Imaizumi T, Yoo JY. Negative feedback regulation of RIG-I-mediated antiviral signaling by interferon-induced ISG15 conjugation. *J Virol* 2008;82(3):1474–83.
28. Chen L, Borozan I, Feld J, *et al.* Hepatic gene expression discriminates responders and nonresponders in treatment of chronic hepatitis C viral infection. *Gastroenterology* 2005;128(5):1437–44.
29. Feld JJ, Nanda S, Huang Y, *et al.* Hepatic gene expression during treatment with peginterferon and ribavirin: identifying molecular pathways for treatment response. *Hepatology* 2007;46(5):1548–63.
30. Asselah T, Bièche I, Sabbagh A, *et al.* Gene expression and hepatitis C virus infection. *Gut* 2009;58(6):846–58.
31. Sarasin-Filipowicz M, Oakeley EJ, Duong FH, *et al.* Interferon signaling and treatment outcome in chronic hepatitis C. *Proc Natl Acad Sci U S A* 2008;105(19):7034–9.
32. Randall G, Chen L, Panis M, *et al.* Silencing of USP18 potentiates the antiviral activity of interferon against hepatitis C virus infection. *Gastroenterology* 2006;131(5):1584–91.

33. Helbig KJ, Lau DT, Semendric L, *et al.* Analysis of ISG expression in chronic hepatitis C identifies viperin as a potential antiviral effector. *Hepatology* 2005;42(3):702–10.

34. Bigger CB, Brasky KM, Lanford RE, DNA microarray analysis of chimpanzee liver during acute resolving hepatitis C virus infection. *J Virol* 2001;75(15):7059–66.

35. Lanford RE, Guerra B, Lee H, *et al.* Genomic response to interferon-alpha in chimpanzees: implications of rapid downregulation for hepatitis C kinetics. *Hepatology* 2006;43(5):961–72.

36. Jiang D, Guo H, Xu C, *et al.* Identification of three interferon-inducible cellular enzymes that inhibit the replication of hepatitis C virus. *J Virol* 2008;82(4):1665–78.

37. Dey M, Cao C, Dar AC, *et al.* Mechanistic link between PKR dimerization, autophosphorylation, and eIF2alpha substrate recognition. *Cell* 2005;122(6):901–13.

38. Wang C, Pflugheber J, Sumpter R, Jr., *et al.* Alpha interferon induces distinct translational control programs to suppress hepatitis C virus RNA replication. *J Virol*, 2003;77(7):3898–912.

39. Gale M, Jr., Blakely CM, Kwieciszewski B, *et al.* Control of PKR protein kinase by hepatitis C virus nonstructural 5A protein: molecular mechanisms of kinase regulation. *Mol Cell Biol* 1998;18(9):5208–18.

40. Gale MJ, Jr., Korth MJ, Katze MG. Repression of the PKR protein kinase by the hepatitis C virus NS5A protein: a potential mechanism of interferon resistance. *Clin Diagn Virol* 1998;10(2–3):157–62.

41. Gale M, Jr., Katze MG. Molecular mechanisms of interferon resistance mediated by viral-directed inhibition of PKR, the interferon-induced protein kinase. *Pharmacol Ther* 1998;78(1):29–46.

42. Gale MJ, Jr., Korth MJ, Tang NM, *et al.* Evidence that hepatitis C virus resistance to interferon is mediated through repression of the PKR protein kinase by the nonstructural 5A protein. *Virology* 1997;230(2):217–27.

43. Noguchi T, Satoh S, Noshi T, *et al.* Effects of mutation in hepatitis C virus nonstructural protein 5A on interferon resistance mediated by inhibition of PKR kinase activity in mammalian cells. *Microbiol Immunol* 2001;45(12):829–40.

44. Pavio N, Romano PR, Graczyk TM, *et al.* Protein synthesis and endoplasmic reticulum stress can be modulated by the hepatitis C virus envelope protein E2 through the eukaryotic initiation factor 2alpha kinase PERK. *J Virol* 2003;77(6):3578–85.

45. Pavio N, Taylor DR, Lai MM. Detection of a novel unglycosylated form of hepatitis C virus E2 envelope protein that is located in the cytosol and interacts with PKR. *J Virol* 2002;76(3):1265–72.

46. Taylor DR, Shi ST, Romano PR, *et al.* Inhibition of the interferon-inducible protein kinase PKR by HCV E2 protein. *Science* 1999;285(5424):107–10.

47. Sumpter R, Jr., Wang C, Foy E, *et al.* Viral evolution and interferon resistance of hepatitis C virus RNA replication in a cell culture model. *J Virol* 2004;78(21):11591–604.

48. Zhu H, Zhao H, Collins CD, *et al.* Gene expression associated with interferon alfa antiviral activity in an HCV replicon cell line. *Hepatology* 2003;37(5):1180–88.

49. Guo J, Peters KL, Sen GC. Induction of the human protein P56 by interferon, double-stranded RNA, or virus infection. *Virology* 2000;267(2):209–19.

50. Grandvaux N, Servant MJ, tenOever B, *et al.* Transcriptional profiling of interferon regulatory factor 3 target genes: direct involvement in the regulation of interferon-stimulated genes. *J Virol* 2002;76(11):5532–9.

51. Hinson ER, Joshi NS, Chen JH, *et al.* Viperin is highly induced in neutrophils and macrophages during acute and chronic lymphocytic choriomeningitis virus infection. *J Immunol* 2010;184(10):5723–31.

52. Wang X, Hinson ER, Cresswell P. The interferon-inducible protein viperin inhibits influenza virus release by perturbing lipid rafts. *Cell Host Microbe* 2007;2(2):96–105.

53. Rivieccio MA, Suh HS, Zhao Y, *et al.* TLR3 ligation activates an antiviral response in human fetal astrocytes: a role for viperin/cig5. *J Immunol* 2006;177(7):4735–41.

54. Hinson ER, Cresswell P. The antiviral protein, viperin, localizes to lipid droplets via its N-terminal amphipathic alpha-helix. *Proc Natl Acad Sci U S A* 2009;106(48):20452–7.

55. Miyanari Y, Atsuzawa K, Usuda N, *et al.* The lipid droplet is an important organelle for hepatitis C virus production. *Nat Cell Biol* 2007;9(9):1089–97.

56. Sidwell RW, Huffman JH, Khare GP, *et al.* Broad-spectrum antiviral activity of Virazole: 1-beta-D-ribofuranosyl-1,2,4-triazole-3-carboxamide. *Science* 1972;177(50):705–6.

57. Thomas E, Feld JJ, Li Q, *et al.* Ribavirin potentiates interferon action by augmenting interferon-stimulated gene induction in hepatitis C virus cell culture models. *Hepatology* 2011;53(1):32–41.

58. Hu S, Xie Z, Onishi A, *et al.* Profiling the human protein-DNA interactome reveals ERK2 as a transcriptional repressor of interferon signaling. *Cell* 2009;139(3):610–22.

59. Taylor MW, Tsukahara T, Brodsky L, *et al.* Changes in gene expression during pegylated interferon and ribavirin therapy of chronic hepatitis C virus distinguish responders from nonresponders to antiviral therapy. *J Virol* 2007;81(7):3391–401.

60. He XS, Ji X, Hale MB, *et al.* Global transcriptional response to interferon is a determinant of HCV treatment outcome and is modified by race. *Hepatology* 2006;44(2):352–9.

61. Ge D, Fellay J, Thompson AJ, *et al.* Genetic variation in IL28B predicts hepatitis C treatment-induced viral clearance. *Nature* 2009;461(7262):399–401.

62. Suppiah V, Moldovan M, Ahlenstiel G, *et al.* IL28B is associated with response to chronic hepatitis C interferon-alpha and ribavirin therapy. *Nat Genet* 2009;41(10):1100–4.

63. Tanaka Y, Nishida N, Sugiyama M, *et al.* Genome-wide association of IL28B with response to pegylated interferon-alpha and ribavirin therapy for chronic hepatitis C. *Nat Genet* 2009;41(10):1105–9.

64. Thomas DL, Thio CL, Martin MP, *et al.* Genetic variation in IL28B and spontaneous clearance of hepatitis C virus. *Nature* 2009;461(7265):798–801.

65. Dill MT, Duong FH, Vogt JE, *et al.* Interferon-induced gene expression is a stronger predictor of treatment response than IL28B genotype in patients with hepatitis C. *Gastroenterology* 2011;140(3):1021–31.

5 Pharmacology and Mechanisms of Action of Antiviral Drugs: Ribavirin Analogs

Fred Poordad and Grace M. Chee

Cedars-Sinai Medical Center, Los Angeles, CA, USA

Introduction

The current standard of care for the treatment of chronic hepatitis C (HCV) since 2001 has been pegylated interferon (Peg-IFN) and ribavirin (RBV) in combination for 24–48 weeks depending on viral genotype. This will likely remain the backbone of therapy for the next several years. The next phase of HCV treatment will involve direct-acting oral antivirals such as protease and polymerase inhibitors. To date, attempts to minimize RBV or eliminate it have been unsuccessful with both standard of care therapy and in early phase trials using direct acting antivirals. The desire to eliminate RBV centers largely around the predominant adverse event of anemia; in mild cases, this requires dose reduction, but occasionally requires blood transfusions or erythropoietic stimulating factors. As a result, analogs of RBV with a better toxicity profile have been sought. To a large extent this has yielded little to date. The following summarizes some of the compounds that have been developed with the goal of replacing RBV.

Ribavirin

The history of RBV began more than 30 years ago when it was first described in the early 1970s. RBV (1-β-D-ribofuranosyl-1H-1,2,4-triazole-3-carboxamide) is a purine ribonucleoside analog with a spectrum of activity against RNA and DNA viruses. While it did not have adequate efficacy against most viruses, it was FDA approved for the treatment of respiratory syncytial virus in aerosolized form. The use of RBV for HCV began in the 1990s, and as monotherapy had little effect on viral decline, but improved aminotransferases. It was the combination with interferon alfa (IFN-α) that led to approval for the treatment of HCV.

The Pharmacokinetics of Ribavirin

RBV is rapidly absorbed following oral administration, reaching maximum plasma concentrations within 2 hours. The distribution of the compound is vast with an estimated volume of distribution greater than 2000 liters. Steady state is achieved in roughly 4 weeks, with a terminal half-life of 298 hours (~12 days), indicating that daily administration may be feasible. The drug is eliminated via the renal pathway, and requires dose modification with impaired renal function.

The mechanisms by which RBV works in HCV remain unclear. Several modes of action have been postulated, but none has been proven (Table 5.1). Both direct and indirect antiviral activities have been proposed. It is known that RBV is phosphorylated to ribavirin 5′-triphosphate (RTP) via host cellular kinases. The monophosphorylated RMP is a competitive inhibitor of inosine monophosphate dehydrogenase (IMPDH), an enzyme required for the phosphorylation of guanosine monophosphate to guanosine triphosphate (GTP), which is needed for viral replication. Depleted stores of GTP may therefore inhibit viral replication. Other putative mechanisms of RBV include impairing translation of viral RNA by RBV substitutions in the mRNA 5′ cap structure and mismatch mutations in viral RNA [1]. Indirect mechanisms of action are

---

Advanced Therapy for Hepatitis C, First Edition. Edited by Geoffrey W. McCaughan, John G. McHutchison and Jean-Michel Pawlotsky.
© 2012 Blackwell Publishing Ltd. Published 2012 by Blackwell Publishing Ltd.

Table 5.1 Proposed mechanisms of action of ribavirin

Mechanism	Immune modulator	Inhibition of inosine 5'-monophosphate dehydrogenase (IMPDH)	Inhibition of NS5B RNA-dependent RNA polymerase	Incorporation into viral genome via the NS5B polymerase
Action	Up-regulation of intrahepatocyte T-helper 1 (Th1) response, down-regulation of Th2 response	Inhibition of guanine phosphorylation, which is required for viral replication	Direct-acting antiviral inhibiting viral genome replication	Ribavirin triphosphate base pairs with cytidine and uridine leading to mutations in the viral genome

thought to occur via modulation of T-helper cell activity, leading to a predominant pro-inflammatory milieu [2,3]. In combination with IFN-α, most investigators believe that an intrahepatic T-cell effect with natural killer cell activation and a robust Th-1 response drives the antiviral activity [4–6].

Monotherapy with RBV appears to have a minimal and transient effect on HCV [7]. It is with monotherapy that the potential NS5B mutagenic activity of RBV is most notable, and clinically this translated into short-term decreases in viral replication [8]. This effect was less appreciable in the presence of IFN-α, particularly when the patient is interferon responsive [9,10].

In the pre-RBV era of the early 1990s, viral clearance rates were very low, particularly in genotype 1 disease, where response rates below 10% were the norm. The addition of RBV to a 48-week treatment period increased this to roughly 30% [11]. An additional 10% sustained

virologic response (SVR) was achieved in genotype 1 by changing the thrice weekly IFN-α regimen to a weekly pegylated interferon formulation [12]. The addition of RBV to pegylated interferon took the SVR in genotype 1 from 21% to 46%. Hence, RBV has had much more of an impact on the treatment of HCV than pegylation of interferon [13] (Figure 5.1).

The relevance of RBV was underscored in the early phase II clinical trials with protease inhibitor compounds such as telaprevir and boceprevir. In treatment arms with low-dose or no RBV, viral breakthrough and relapse rates were higher, with lower clearance rates [14,15].

The presence of RBV is important for the entire duration of therapy, and it is perhaps the overall exposure over the treatment course that is of most relevance in optimizing treatment outcomes. Once an appropriate dose has been selected, then exposure of greater than 80% of the intended dose is critical to minimize virologic relapse.

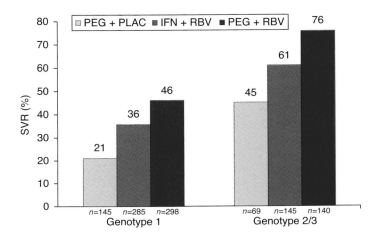

Figure 5.1 Sustained virologic response with and without ribavirin. PEG, peginterferon alfa-2a; PLAC, placebo; IFN, interferon alfa-2a; RBV, ribavirin.

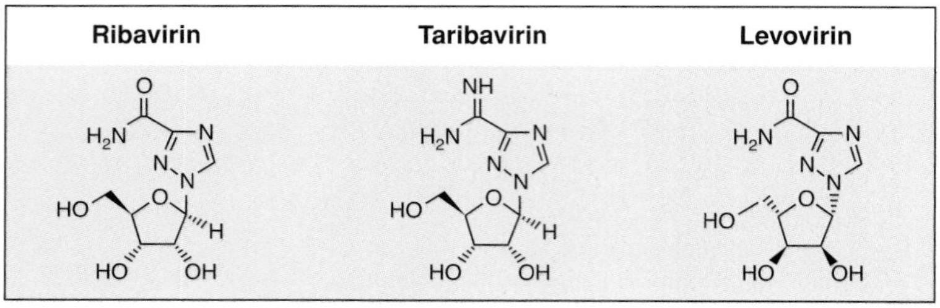

Figure 5.2 Chemical structures of ribavirin, taribavirin, and levovirin.

Indeed, an even higher exposure may be needed in certain difficult-to-cure subsets of patients, but when considered as a body, then relapse rates of 20% increase to 30–50% when cumulative exposure to RBV falls below 80% [16].

Toxicities of Ribavirin

The most problematic adverse event noted with RBV is hemolytic anemia. The mechanism of this process centers on the entry of the neutrally charged RBV into the red blood cell via the adenosine transporter. Ribavirin is preferentially phosphorylated over adenosine, leading to an energy-depleted milieu for the red cell with resultant membrane fragility and lysis. It is this adverse event that has led to the development of other molecules discussed below. The rate of anemia with the current standard of care regimens using pegylated interferon is roughly 30% [17]. Interestingly, monotherapy with RBV leads to a much lower anemia rate, indicating that the bone marrow suppressive effects of interferon dampen the compensatory reticulocytosis that follows hemolysis. The anemia rates in the emerging era of protease-interferon-ribavirin regimens are higher by an additional gram of hemoglobin, with anemia rates as high as 55% [14,15].

Ribavirin Analogs

The importance of RBV in emerging treatment regimens using direct acting antiviral agents such as protease inhibitors has been demonstrated. In the European PROVE-2 study of telaprevir, the 12-week, RBV-free arm using telaprevir/Peg achieved a 36% SVR compared to 60% in the telaprevir/Peg/RBV arm of equal duration. Additionally, the viral breakthrough rates were 24% com-

pared to less than 5%, and relapse was nearly 20% greater (48% versus 30%) [18]. Anemia will be more problematic in the new regimens and is the impetus to find analogs of RBV that are less toxic in this regard (Figure 5.2).

Levovirin

Levovirin (1-β-L-ribofuranosyl-1,2,4-triazole-3-carboxamide) is a guanosine nucleoside analog and the L-enantiomer of RBV. While RBV contains the natural D-ribose moiety, levovirin has the synthetic L-ribose. The advantage of levovirin is its lack of phosphorylation and hence lack of accumulation in the red blood cell [19]. In a small phase I study, the compound was safe and well tolerated at doses as high as 1200 mg, and no anemia was noted [20]. In a phase II trial, not yet published in manuscript form, no virologic benefit of levovirin was noted over pegylated interferon alone [21]. In a replicon assay, RBV monotherapy leads to *NS5B* mutations but levovirin does not, even at high concentrations. This may in part explain the lack of clinical efficacy of levovirin and further supports the mechanism of viral mutagen of RBV [22]. Levovirin was known to have poor oral bioavailability and this was enhanced by developing a 5'-valinate monoester prodrug called levovirin valinate hydrocholoride (R1518), which used a nutrient transporter in the intestinal epithelial cells and increased bioavailability several fold [23]. However, this could not overcome the lack of *in vitro* or *in vivo* efficacy and was not developed further.

Taribavirin

Taribavirin (1-β-D-ribofuranosyl-1,2,4-triazole-3-carboxamidine), formerly known as viramidine, is a

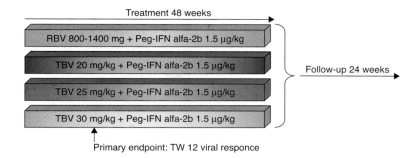

Figure 5.3 Taribavirin weight-based dosing study design. RBV, ribavirin; Peg-IFN, pegylated interferon; TBV, taribavirin; TW, treatment week.

positively charged carboxyamide prodrug of ribavirin. Taribavirin (TBV) is absorbed in the small bowel, achieving steady state in roughly 4 weeks. The deamination of TBV to RBV occurs via the adenosine deaminase enzyme, which is abundant in many tissues, but has high concentrations in the liver [24]. Early studies with monkeys revealed radiolabeled TBV accumulated at a rate that was 3-fold greater than RBV in the liver tissue after 10 days of dosing [25,26]. This initially was interpreted as a liver targeting phenomenon, but not further delineated.

The active moiety of TBV is RBV and hence the mechanism of action is thought to be the same as the postulated mechanisms of RBV. The advantage of TBV over RBV is its positive charge compared to the neutrally charged RBV, making the former less apt to enter the red blood cell via the adenosine transporter.

The Pharmacokinetics of Taribavirin

The pharmacokinetic properties of TBV have been described in greater detail elsewhere [26]. Conversion to RBV is rapid and like RBV, area under the curve concentration (AUC) is greater when taken with food. Some gender differences exist between males and females, with higher TBV AUC in females, and some ethnic differences also exist. It is not known if these differences represent adenosine deaminase activity differences, or if they are clinically relevant [27,28].

Clinical Efficacy

The safety and tolerability of TBV was demonstrated in early phase studies using single oral doses up to 1200 mg and multiple doses as high as 800 mg twice daily for 28 days [29]. Subsequently, dose ranging phase II studies using 400, 600, and 800 mg twice daily in genotypes 1, 2, and 3

revealed comparable viral efficacy to RBV 1000 or 1200 mg daily, but with less anemia (53% versus 24%, showing a >2.5 g/dl decline in hemoglobin from baseline). No clinical advantage beyond 600 mg twice daily was noted in this study and hence, that dose was chosen for the phase III trial.

Two large phase III trials were conducted using both pegylated interferon alfa-2a and -2b with TBV 600 mg b.i.d. compared to pegylated interferon and RBV 1000 or 1200 mg daily. While the primary safety endpoint of lower anemia rate was met, the non-inferiority endpoint for efficacy was not met. In a post hoc analysis of the data, patients with greater than 18 mg/kg exposure of TBV had comparable efficacy to the RBV control arms.

Based on this subset analysis of the phase III data, further investigation of weight-based dosing of TBV was initiated with another phase II trial. The final results of this trial were presented at an international congress in 2009 [30]. The primary endpoints of the study were the week-12 viral response and rate of anemia at any point during the study. Both primary endpoints were met using all three doses of TBV, compared to the control arm (Figures 5.3–5.5). The proof of concept that weight-based dosing of TBV yields comparable efficacy but less anemia compared to RBV was established in this study. The overall safety was comparable to RBV, but with more diarrhea noted with TBV. This was generally short in duration, mild, and not treatment limiting.

Inosine 5′-Monophosphate Dehydrogenase (IMPDH) Inhibitors

This class of drug inhibits the enzyme that is critical for guanine biosynthesis. One of the mechanisms

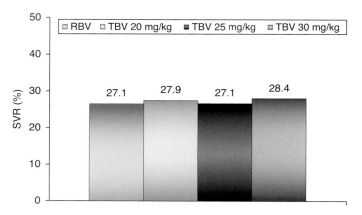

Summary

Ribavirin has been a critical partner in the dual-therapy regimens using interferons to treat chronic hepatitis C. It will remain an integral part of the coming small molecule regimens as well, since several trials seeking to either reduce the dose of RBV or remove it altogether have shown lower efficacy and higher relapse. The anemia associated with RBV has and will remain problematic and this will continue to drive drug development, particularly if the future regimens are limited by anemia. Of the RBV analogs assessed to date, only taribavirin has shown promise as a viable alternative. The issue of safety has been addressed now in two phase III trials as well as two phase II trials, all showing acceptable safety margins. The next step will be to assess TBV in the setting of direct-acting antiviral therapies to assess its efficacy and safety in the evolving new treatment paradigms.

Figure 5.4 Sustained virologic response. *No statistical difference between groups. All arms dosed with peginterferon alfa-2b 1.5 mcg/kg/week. RBV, ribavirin; TBV, taribavirin.

of RBV is thought to be through inhibition of this enzyme. The best studied compound that is a selective, non-competitive inhibitor of IMPDH is merimepodib (MMPD; (S)-N-3-[3-(3-methoxy-4-oxazol-5-yl-phenyl)-ureido]-benzyl-carbamic acid tetrahydroguran-3-yl-ester). Early studies showed it to have additive antiviral activity when combined with interferon [31]. In a phase II trial assessing efficacy, genotype 1 HCV non-responders to pegylated interferon and RBV were re-treated for up to 48 weeks if they showed viral negativity by week 24. Doses of 50 and 100 mg of MMPD were compared to placebo in addition to interferon and RBV. In this difficult to treat population, the sustained response among the three groups was 4–6%, indicating no additive efficacy over interferon and RBV alone. The adverse event profile was similar to the placebo group, but based on the apparent lack of efficacy, the compound will not be developed further [32].

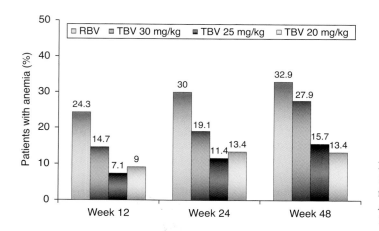

Figure 5.5 Cumulative anemia (hemoglobin < 10g/dl) at TW 12, TW 24, and TW 48. *p < 0.05 for 20 mg/kg and 25 mg/kg versus ribavirin. All arms dosed with peginterferon alfa-2b 1.5 mcg/kg/week. RBV, ribavirin; TBV, taribavirin.

References

1. Tam RC, Lau JYN, Hong J. Mechanisms of action of ribavirin in antiviral therapies. *Antiviral Chem Chemother* 2002;12: 261–72.
2. Tam RC, Pai B, Bard J, *et al.* Ribavirin polarized human T cell response towards a Type 1 cytokine profile. *J Hepatol* 1999;30: 376–82.
3. Hultgren C, Milich DR, Weiland W, Sallberg M. The antiviral compound ribavirin modulates the T helper (Th) 1/Th 2 subset balance in hepatitis B and C virus-specific immune responses. *J Gen Virol* 1998;79: 2381–91.
4. Abonyi ME, Lakatos PL. Ribavirin in the treatment of hepatitis C. *Anticancer Res* 2005;25: 1315–20.
5. Barnes E, Salio M, Cerundolo V, *et al.* Impact of alpha interferon and ribavirin on the function of maturing dendritic cells. *Antimicrob Agents Chemother* 2004;48: 3382–9.
6. Meier V, Burger, E, Mihm S, *et al.* Ribavirin inhibits DNA, RNA, and protein synthesis in PHA-stimulated human peripheral blood mononuclear cells: possible explanation for therapeutic efficacy in patients with chronic HCV infection. *J Med Virol* 2003;69: 50–58.
7. Brok J, Gluud LL, Gluud C. Ribavirin monotherapy for chronic hepatitis C infection: a Cochrane Hepato-Biliary Group systematic review and meta-analysis of randomized trials. *Am J Gastroenterol* 2006;101: 842–7.
8. Pawlotsky JM, Dahari H, Neumann AU, *et al.* Antiviral action of ribavirin in chronic hepatitis C. *Gastroenterology* 2004;126: 703–14.
9. Asahina Y, Izumi N, Enomoto N, *et al.* Mutagenic effects of ribavirin and response to interferon/ribavirin combination therapy in chronic hepatitis C. *J Hepatol* 2005;43: 623–9.
10. Hofmann WP, Polta A, Herrmann E, *et al.* Mutagenic effect of ribavirin on hepatitis C nonstructural 5B quasispecies in vitro and during antiviral therapy. *Gastroenterology* 2007;132: 921–30.
11. McHutchison JG, Gordon SC, Schiff ER, *et al.* Interferon alfa-2b alone or in combination with ribavirin as initial treatment for chronic hepatitis C. *Hepatitis Interventional Therapy Group. N Engl J Med* 1998;339(21): 1485–92.
12. Manns MP, McHutchison JG, Gordon SC, *et al.* Peginterferon alfa-2b plus ribavirin compared with interferon alfa-2b plus ribavirin for initial treatment of chronic hepatitis C: a randomised trial. *Lancet* 2001;358: 958–65.
13. Fried MW, Shiffman ML, Reddy KR, *et al.* Peginterferon alfa-2a plus ribavirin for chronic hepatitis C virus infection. *N Engl J Med* 2002;347: 975–82.
14. McHutchison JG, Everson GT, Gordon SC, *et al.* Telaprevir with peginterferon and ribavirin for chronic HCV genotype 1 infection. *N Engl J Med* 2009;360(18):1827–38.
15. Kwo P, Lawitz EJ, McCone J, *et al.* HCV SPRINT-1: Final results SVR 24 NS3 protease inhibitor boceprevir plus PegIFN alpha-2b/ribavirin HCV 1 treatment naïve patients. *J Hepatol* 2009;50(Suppl 1):S4.
16. Reddy KR, Shiffman ML, Morgan TR, *et al.* Impact of ribavirin dose reductions in hepatitis C virus genotype 1 patients completing peginterferon alfa-2a/ribavirin treatment. *Clin Gastoenterol Hepatol* 2007;5: 124–9.
17. McHutchison JG, Lawitz EJ, Shiffman ML, *et al.* Peginterferon alfa-2b or alfa-2a with ribavirin for treatment of hepatitis C infection. *N Engl J Med* 2009;361(6):580–93.
18. Hézode C, Forestier N, Dusheiko G, *et al.* Telaprevir and peginterferon with or without ribavirn for chronic HCV infection. *N Engl J Med* 2009;360(18):1839–50.
19. Lin C-C, Luu T, Lourenco D, *et al.* Absorption, pharmacokinetics and excretion of levovirin in rats, dogs and cynomolgus monkeys. *J Antimicrob Chemother* 2003;51: 93–9.
20. Rossi S, Wright T, Lin C-C, *et al.* Phase I clinical studies of levovrin – a second generation ribavirin candidate. *Hepatology* 2001;34(4 Pt 2):327A.
21. Pockros P, Pessoa M, Diago M, *et al.* Combination of levovirin and pegylated interferon alfa-2a fails to generate an induction response comparable to ribavirin and pegylated interferon alfa-2a in patients with CHC. *Antivir Ther* 2004; 9:H17 A32.
22. Hofmann WP, Polta A, Hermann E, *et al.* Mutagenic effect of ribavirin on hepatitis C nonstructural 5B quasispecies in vitro and during antiviral therapy. *Gastroenterology* 2007; 132: 921–30.
23. Huang y, Ostrowitzki S, Hill G, *et al.* Single- and multiple-dose pharmacokinetics of levorin valinate hydrochloride (R1518) in healthy volunteers. *J Clin Pharmacol* 2005;45: 578–88.
24. Wu JZ, Walker H, Lau JY, *et al.* Activation and deactivation of a broad-spectrum antiviral drug by a single enzyme: adenosine deaminase catalyzes two consecutive deamination reactions. *Antimicrob Agents Chemother* 2003;47(1):426–31.
25. Lin, C, Luu K, Lourenco D, Yeh L. Pharmacokinetics and metabolism of [14C]viramidine in rats and cynomolgus monkeys. *Antimicrobial Agents Chemother* 2003;47: 2458–63.
26. Lin C, Yeh L-T, Vitarella D, Hong Z. Taribavirin, a prodrug of ribavirin, shows better liver-targeting properties and safety profiles than ribavirin in animals. *Anitviral Chem Chemother* 2003;14: 145–52.
27. Poordad F, Chee G. Taribavirin: a potential alternative to ribavirin. *Future Virol* 2009;4(2):113–20.
28. Lin CC, Philips L, Xu C, Yeh LT. Pharmacokinetics and safety of viramidine, a prodrug of ribavirin, in healthy volunteers. *J Clin Pharmacol* 2004;44(3):265–75.
29. Aora S, Xu, C, Teng A, *et al.* Ascending multiple-dose pharmacokinetics of viramidine, a prodrug of ribavirin, in adult subjects with compensated hepatitis C infection. *J Clin Pharmacol* 2005;45: 275–85.

30. Poordad F, Lawitz E, Shiffman ML, *et al.* Virologic response rates of weight-based taribavirin versus ribavirin in treatment-naïve patients with genotype 1 chronic hepatitis C. *Hepatology* 2010;52(4):1208–15.

31. Markland W, McQuaid TJ, Jain J, *et al.* Broad-spectrum antiviral activity of the IMP dehydrogenase inhibitor VX-497: a comparison with ribavirin and demonstration of antiviral additivity with alpha interferon. *Antimicrob Agents Chemother* 2000;44(4):859–66.

32. Rustgi VK, Lee WM, Lawitz E, *et al.* Merimepodib, pegylated interferon, and ribavirin in genotype 1 chronic hepatitis C pegylated interferon and ribavirin nonresponders. *Herpatology* 2009; 50(6):1719–26.

6 Pharmacology and Mechanisms of Action of Antiviral Drugs: Polymerase Inhibitors

Lotte Coelmont,[*] Leen Delang,[*] Mathy Froeyen, Piet Herdewijn, and Johan Neyts

Rega Institute for Medical Research, K.U.Leuven, Leuven, Belgium
*These authors contributed equally to this work.

Introduction

The hepatitis C virus (HCV) NS5B RNA-dependent RNA polymerase (RdRp) catalyzes the synthesis of a complementary minus-strand RNA, using the (incoming) RNA genome as a template, and subsequently the synthesis of a new progeny genomic plus-strand RNA from the minus-strand RNA template. The structure can be compared with a right hand, where the palm domain contains the catalytic site and where the fingers and thumb are responsible for the interaction with the RNA. The fingertips are two loops that extend from the finger domain and that make contact with the thumb domain [1]. The RdRp is an excellent target for inhibition of HCV replication. Both nucleoside (NI) and non-nucleoside (NNI) polymerase inhibitors are in pre-clinical and clinical development.

Nucleoside Inhibitors

Nucleoside inhibitors need to be 5′-phosphorylated intracellular to their corresponding 5′-triphosphate, which is then recognized by the viral RdRp and incorporated in the growing RNA chain, thereby mimicking natural nucleosides. NIs with anti-HCV activity possess a 3′-hydroxyl function and may therefore not be considered as obligate chain terminators. They may act, however, as virtual chain terminators, that is, by steric hindrance exerted by, for example, the neighboring 2′-C-methyl and/or 4′-C-azido groups and/or by an increased error frequency. In general, nucleoside analogs exert comparable activity against distinct HCV genotypes, since the active site of the polymerase is well conserved. All active site inhibitors of NS5B are nucleoside analogs (Figure 6.1a).

Valopicitabine

Valopicitabine (NM283) is an oral prodrug (3′-O-valine ester) of 2′-C-methylcytidine (NM107) [2] and the first nucleoside analog inhibitor of HCV to enter clinical studies. When combined in vitro with ribavirin (RBV), a molecule believed to increase intracellular levels of CTP, an antagonistic effect was observed. The most likely explanation for this observation is competition at the level of the RdRp of the 5′-triphosphate of 2′-C-methylcytidine with the increased CTP concentration [3]. This and other 2′-C-methyl ribonucleosides were shown to be efficient chain-terminating inhibitors of HCV genome replication [4]. Replicons resistant to 2′-C-methylcytidine carry the S282T mutation in the viral polymerase and show a reduced fitness compared to wild type virus. HCV polymerase that carried the S282T mutation no longer incorporated 2′-C-methyl-CTP during the initiation step of RNA synthesis [5]. The presence of the S282T mutation results in a general reduction (5- to 20-fold) in terms of polymerase efficiency, which may translate to a decreased viral fitness [6]. In phase II clinical trials in HCV-infected patients, valopicitabine was combined for 48 weeks of treatment with pegylated interferon alfa (Peg-IFN-α). The decline in viral load was not significantly different when compared to the standard of care (SoC) group, that is,

Advanced Therapy for Hepatitis C, First Edition. Edited by Geoffrey W. McCaughan, John G. McHutchison and Jean-Michel Pawlotsky.
© 2012 Blackwell Publishing Ltd. Published 2012 by Blackwell Publishing Ltd.

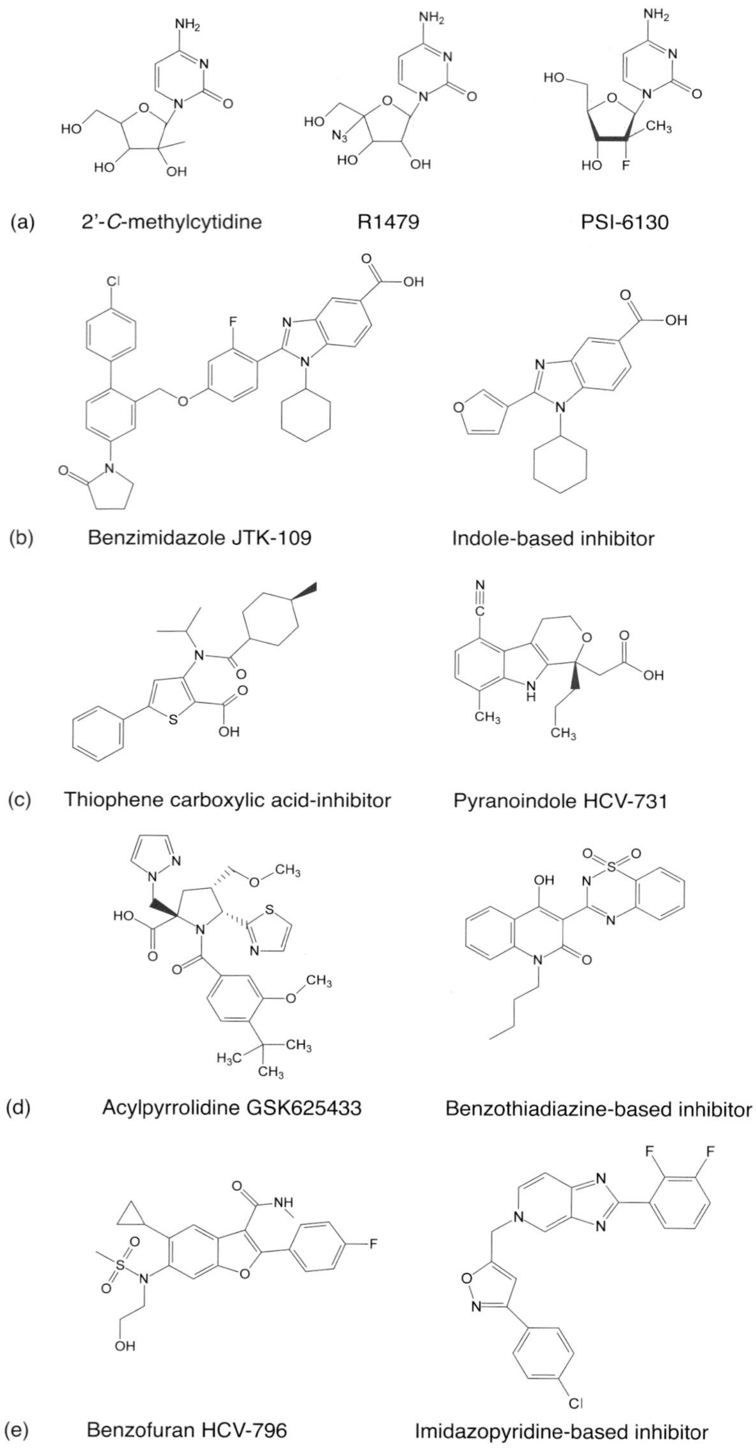

(a)   2'-*C*-methylcytidine   R1479   PSI-6130

(b)   Benzimidazole JTK-109   Indole-based inhibitor

(c)   Thiophene carboxylic acid-inhibitor   Pyranoindole HCV-731

(d)   Acylpyrrolidine GSK625433   Benzothiadiazine-based inhibitor

(e)   Benzofuran HCV-796   Imidazopyridine-based inhibitor

Figure 6.1 Structural formulae of a selection of HCV RdRp inhibitors. (a) Nucleoside inhibitors; (b) non-nucleoside inhibitors, thumb domain 1; (c) non-nucleoside inhibitors, thumb domain 2; (d) non-nucleoside inhibitors, palm domain 1; and (e) non-nucleoside inhibitors, palm domain 2.

Peg-IFN and RBV [7]. No selection of resistant viruses was observed in patients treated with this nucleoside analog [8]. Based on the overall risk-benefit profile observed in clinical trials, the development of valopicitabine was stopped.

Following 2'-C-methylcytidine, various other nucleoside analogs targeting the HCV NS5B polymerase have been reported to inhibit HCV replicon replication in vitro: these include, but are not limited to, 2'-O-methylcytidine [9], 2'-C-methyladenosine [9], 2'-C-methylguanosine [4], 7-deaza-2'-C-methyladenosine [10], 2'-deoxy-2'-fluoro-2'-C-methylcytidine (PSI-6130) [11], and 4'-azidocytidine (R1479) [12]. Except for PSI-6130, none of these nucleoside analogs is being further developed. Among the NS5B polymerase inhibitors, R7128, an ester prodrug of PSI-6130, is the most advanced.

R1626 is a prodrug (tri-isobutyl ester) of the nucleoside analog 4'-azidocytidine (R1479). The 5'-triphosphate of R1479 is incorporated into nascent RNA by the HCV polymerase and reduces further elongation with similar efficiency as the obligate chain terminator 3'-dCTP [12]. In vitro studies mapped resistance to R1479 to amino acid substitutions S96T and S96T/N142T of NS5B. Moreover, no cross-resistance could be observed between R1479 and 2'-C-methylcytidine-resistant subgenomic replicons [13]. In a phase IIa study in which patients received combined therapy of R1626 with Peg-IFN or Peg-IFN plus RBV, a high rate of HCV infection relapse on combination therapy was observed. However, during 4-week treatment in combination with SoC, no drug resistance was observed [14]. Moreover, 78% of patients treated with 3000 mg twice daily and 45% of patients treated with 1500 mg twice daily developed grade 4 neutropenia [15]. The development of R1626 was stopped at the end of 2008.

RG7128 is a di-isobutyl ester prodrug of PSI-6130, a cytidine nucleoside analog (β-D-2'-deoxy-2'-fluoro-2'-C-methylcytidine) [11]. PSI-6130 is metabolized intracellular to the 5'-triphosphate of β-D-2'-deoxy-2'-fluoro-2'-C-methylcytidine and also, following deamination, to the triphosphate of β-D-2'-deoxy-2'-fluoro-2'-C-methyluridine (PSI-6206) [16]. Both triphosphates are incorporated as non-obligate chain terminators into RNA catalyzed by purified NS5B [17]. Plasma exposure to the prodrug RG7128 is negligible; exposure to PSI-6130 and PSI-6206 increases with increasing doses of RG7128. Terminal half-life is approximately 5 h for PSI-6130 and 20 h for PSI-6206. Replicons resistant to PSI-6130 carry, as is the case for valopicitabine-resistant replicons, the S282T mutation. Interestingly, this mutation results only in a low level (3- to 4-fold) of in vitro resistance and emergence of

resistance is slower than for other classes of direct-acting antiviral agents (DAA) [18–20]. Results of a phase I study of RG7128 (500 or 1500 mg twice daily) in combination with Peg-IFN and RBV for 28 days resulted in a decrease in viral load ranging from −3.8 to −5.1 $\log_{10}$ IU/ml, respectively (−2.9 $\log_{10}$ for SoC) [21]. When HCV genotype 2 and 3 prior non-responders were treated with RG7128 (1500 mg twice a day) in combination with Peg-IFN and RBV for 28 days, a mean viral load reduction of −5.0 $\log_{10}$ was observed. In monotherapy for 2 weeks, mean viral load decreased with −2.7 $\log_{10}$ IU/ml. The drug was generally well tolerated and is currently in phase II clinical development [22]. During the INFORM-1 study, chronically infected HCV genotype 1 patients received RG7128 combined with another DAA inhibitor, RG7227 (danoprevir, a protease inhibitor). The combination of the highest doses of both compounds (1000 mg RG7128 and 900 mg danoprevir twice daily) resulted in a median decrease in viral load of −5.1 $\log_{10}$ IU/ml after 14 days of treatment. Overall this combination was generally safe and well tolerated [23]. These are promising results with the eye on a future IFN-free treatment regimen for chronic HCV.

Liver-targeted prodrugs of nucleotide polymerase inhibitors of HCV replication are designed to enhance formation of the active triphosphate in the liver while minimizing systemic exposure of the nucleotide drug and its nucleoside metabolite. Such prodrugs of nucleotide analogs (i.e., nucleoside 5'-monophosphates) are preferentially cleaved by hepatic enzymes, thereby efficiently releasing their nucleoside monophosphate in liver cells. The rate-limiting step for metabolic activation of nucleoside analogs, the initial phosphorylation to a nucleoside monophosphate, is bypassed, resulting in higher levels of nucleoside triphosphates in the cell. IDX184, a prodrug of 2'-methylguanosine monophosphate, demonstrated a modest reduction in HCV RNA in treatment-naïve genotype 1 infected patients (−0.74 $\log_{10}$, 100 mg once daily for three days) [24]. IDX184 is rapidly absorbed (median T_{max}: 0.25−0.5 h) and eliminated (mean half-life: 0.6−1 h). Plasma exposure is low and dose-related [25]. Recently, the development of IDX-184 was put on hold. PSI-7851 is a phosphoramidate prodrug of the nucleotide analog PSI-6206-MP (beta-D-2'-deoxy-2'-fluoro-2'-C-methyluridine monophosphate) [26]. In HCV subgenomic replicon, PSI-7851 demonstrated approximately 15- to 20-fold improved in vitro potency ($EC_{90} = 0.31$ μm) compared to PSI-6130 [27]. The half-life of the triphosphate in primary human hepatocytes is approximately 38 hours, which suggests the possibility for once daily dosing. In treatment-naïve patients

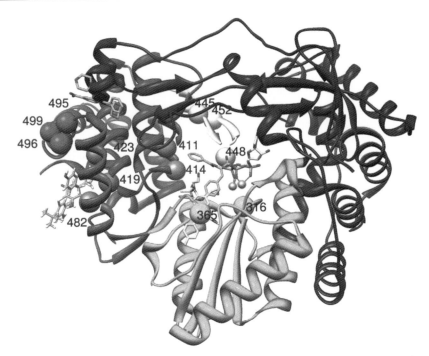

Figure 6.2 Binding sites for HCV polymerase inhibitors. This figure is created using Chimera based on superposition of different pdb structures using the Dali server [30,31]. The superimposed structures are 1GX6 (active site with UTP), 2BRK (with benzimidazole in thumb domain site 1), 1OS5 (with dihydropyranone in thumb domain 2 site), 1YVF (with benzothiadiazine in palm domain site 1), 3FQL (with benzofuran in the palm domain site 2). The palm, fingers and thumb domains are colored white, dark grey and light grey respectively. Mutations in different regions have following colors: grey for residues P495, P496, V499 in thumb domain 1 and for L419, M423, I482 in thumb domain 2, light grey for N411, M414 in palm domain 1, white for C316, S365 in palm domain 2 and for C445, Y448 and Y452 in the beta-hairpin loop.

multiple oral doses (50 mg, 100 mg, or 200 mg once daily for 3 days) resulted in a dose-dependent reduction in viral load [maximal mean reduction -1.01 $\log_{10}$ IU/ml (200 mg daily) after 3 days] [28]. A phase IIa clinical trial with PSI-7977, a chirally pure isomer of PSI-7851, in combination with the SoC, demonstrated antiviral activity following 28 days of treatment (mean -5.1 to -5.3 $\log_{10}$ IU/ml decrease in HCV RNA versus -2.8 $\log_{10}$ IU/ml for SoC) [29]. A phase IIb study of PSI-7977 in combination with RBV administered with and without Peg-IFN alfa-2a was recently initiated.

Non-Nucleoside Inhibitors

HCV NNIs act as allosteric inhibitors by binding to less conserved sites outside the active domain of the viral polymerase. Consequently, these inhibitors act in a non-competitive way with nucleotide incorporation. Since the mechanism of action of NNIs differs from that of NIs, cross-resistance between these two classes is unlikely to occur. At least four different sites are targeted by NNIs; two sites are located in the thumb domain and two others in the palm domain (Figure 6.2). In contrast to NIs, a restricted spectrum of activity of NNIs against different genotypes has been noted.

Thumb Domain 1

The first NNI that entered clinical trials was the benzimidazole JTK-003. The compound is believed to interact with an allosteric site on the surface of the thumb domain [32]. The formation of intramolecular contacts between the thumb and the finger domains may force the enzyme into an "open," inactive conformation, thereby inhibiting the viral polymerase. Drug-resistant variants carry mutations at position P495. Clinical development was halted for unknown reasons.

Another class of NNIs that interact with thumb domain 1 are indole-based inhibitors such as MK-3281 (see Figure 6.1b) [33]. *In vitro* MK-3281 resulted in equipotent antiviral activity against the RdRp of HCV genotypes 1a, 1b, and 3a, but weak activity against the RdRp of genotypes 2a and 2b [34]. Following oral administration, MK-3281 increases in plasma with median T_{max} values of 2.5–3.5 hours. Thereafter, concentrations decline in a biphasic manner with mean terminal half-time $\approx$14.3–18.6 h. MK-3281 given to genotype 1b patients as monotherapy (800 mg b.i.d. for 7 days) was well tolerated and resulted in a strong reduction of viral load ($-3.8 \pm 0.19 \log_{10}$ IU/ml). Activity against genotypes 1a and 3 was, however, limited (-1.3 ± 0.15 and $-1.2 \pm 0.16 \log_{10}$ IU/ml, respectively) [35].

Another potent thumb domain 1-targeting NNI of the HCV RdRp is BI 207127. During a phase Ib study escalating doses (100, 200, 400, or 800 mg) of BI 207127 were given orally as a monotherapy for 5 days to HCV genotype 1 infected patients. Plasma drug levels exhibited supra-proportional pharmacokinetics at steady state with 400 mg and 800 mg doses. A dose-dependent decline in viral load was noted with 5/9 patients showing a ≥ 4 $\log_{10}$ maximal drop in viral load in the group receiving 800 mg. No viral breakthrough was observed during treatment. BI 207127 was overall safe and well tolerated with the only drug-related adverse effect being a mild erythema that resolved after treatment cessation [36]. NS5B drug-resistant variants were selected in 6 out of 46 patients; the predominant mutation encoded changes at Pro^{495} [37]. During a comparative study 57 HCV genotype 1 treatment-naïve and treatment-experienced patients received escalating doses of BI 207127 (400, 600, or 800 mg, t.i.d.) in combination with the SoC. Treatment resulted in rapid and strong antiviral responses which were more pronounced in the treatment-naïve patient group (at least a drop of $\geq 3 \log_{10}$ from baseline with no evidence of virologic rebound). Five treatment-experienced patients in the highest dosage groups discontinued treatment due to mainly rash-related adverse effects [38]. During a phase Ib study, SOUND-C1, 32 treatment-naïve genotype 1 HCV patients received a combination of BI 207127 (400 mg or 600 mg doses, t.i.d.) with the protease inhibitor BI 201335 (120 mg, once daily) together with RBV for 28 days. All patients had a rapid and sharp decline in HCV viral load during the first two days, followed by a slower second phase decline. In the lower and higher dose groups, 73% and 100% of patients achieved a rapid virologic response. These initial data suggest that there is a potential to combine oral DAA inhibitors to reduce the viral load in a more tolerable, IFN-sparing regimen [39].

Thumb Domain 2

Thiophene carboxylic acid derivatives target thumb domain 2, a hydrophobic cavity located at the base of the thumb domain of NS5B (see Figure 6.1c) [40]. Thiophene carboxylic acid derivatives are non-competitive with nucleotide incorporation and inhibit the initiation step of RNA synthesis by interfering with conformational changes [41]. Thiophene-based inhibitors were found to select for Met^{423} and Leu^{419} resistant mutants in replicon cell culture experiments [42]. VX-222 had low micromolar antiviral activity ($IC_{90} = 0.03$–0.06 μm) against HCV 1a and 1b in replicon assays. Following three days of monotherapy, VX-222 achieved a mean reduction in HCV RNA ranging from -3.1 to $-3.4 \log_{10}$ with similar activity in genotype 1a and 1b infected patients [43]. No serious adverse effects were reported. The half-life of VX-222 is 4–6 hours and T_{max} was reached at 2–6 hours post-dose. VX-222 is currently studied in combination with the protease inhibitor VX-950 (Telaprevir). VX-759 was well tolerated and resulted in a significant reduction in viral load in treatment-naïve genotype 1 infected patients during a proof-of-concept study ($> 1 \log_{10}$ reduction with a mean maximal decrease of -1.9, -2.3, and $-2.5 \log_{10}$ after dosing for 10 days at, respectively, 400 mg t.i.d., 800 mg b.i.d., and 800 mg t.i.d.) [44]. On-treatment rebound of viremia suggested the emergence of resistant strains. Genotypic analysis revealed mutations at positions 419, 423, and 482. Recently phase Ib development was completed.

Two other classes of molecules have been identified to target thumb domain 2. Pyranoindole derivatives (i.e., HCV-371 and a follow-up compound HCV-086) entered clinical development but failed to demonstrate significant efficacy and development was therefore discontinued (see Figure 6.1c) [45,46]. PF-868554/Filibuvir, a dihydropyranone derivative ((R)-6-cyclopentyl-6-(2-(2,6-diethylpyridin-4-yl)ethyl)-3-((5,7-dimethyl-[1,2,4]triazolo[1,5-α]pyrimidin-2-yl)methyl)-4 hydroxy-5,6-dihydropyran-2-one), is a potent and selective HCV inhibitor *in vitro* [47]. It exerts strong *in vitro* antiviral activity against the 1b Con1 replicon (EC_{50} of 0.075 μm), and reduced activity against the 1a H77 replicon (EC_{50} of 0.39 μm). The predominant *in vitro* resistance mutation is M423T [48]. Other amino acid mutations, M426T and I482T, were detected at a much lower frequency. Absorption of PF-868554 is rapid, with maximum plasma concentrations generally achieved by approximately 1 hour post-dose. Mean apparent elimination half-life ranges from 11.1 to 11.7 hours. In treatment-naïve genotype 1 patients triple therapy [PF-868554 (200, 300, or 500 mg b.i.d.) in combination with Peg-IFN and RBV] was associated with a maximal mean reduction in HCV RNA of -4.67 $\log_{10}$ IU/ml at day 28 [49]. Currently filibuvir is in phase II of clinical development.

Palm Domain 1

Palm domain 1 is located at the junction of the palm and the thumb domains of NS5B and is in relatively close proximity to the catalytic site. The first class of palm domain 1 inhibitors reported were those with a benzothiadiazine scaffold (see Figure 6.1d). Akin to other NNIs, benzothiadiazine-based compounds inhibit RNA synthesis before formation of an elongation complex [50]. Benzothiadiazines select *in vitro* for drug-resistant mutation M414T [51]. Evaluation of ABT-333 in a phase I clinical trial was recently completed. Genotype 1 treatment-naïve patients received ABT-333 for 28 days (2 days monotherapy, 26 days in combination with the SoC), resulting in significantly greater decreases in HCV RNA when compared to the SoC + placebo (maximum HCV RNA reduction -4.0 $\log_{10}$ IU/ml versus -1.4 $\log_{10}$ IU/ml for placebo) [52]. Rat absorption, distribution, metabolism, and excretion (ADME) studies with ABT-333 show that it is eliminated primarily by biliary excretion. Mean T_{max} of ABT-333 in healthy volunteers is approximately 3–4 hours and mean terminal half-life is approximately 6–11 hours. In 2010, phase II clinical trials with ABT-333 were initiated. Another benzothiadiazine inhibitor, ANA598, exhibits nanomolar potency against genotype 1 HCV replicons (EC_{50} 1b = 3 nM, EC_{50} 1a = 50 nM) [53]. The plasma elimination half-life of ANA598 ranges from 22 to 31 hours. Biliary excretion is the major route of elimination. In phase Ib studies, ANA598, dosed at 200 mg b.i.d. for 3 days as monotherapy, resulted in a median viral load decline of -2.4 $\log_{10}$ in treatment-naïve genotype 1 infected patients [54]. At day 4, three viral variants (C316Y, Y448H, G554D) were detected in 8 of 9 patients who received ANA598 monotherapy [55]. A phase II clinical trial in which treatment-naïve genotype 1 HCV infected patients were treated with a combination of SoC and ANA598 showed that ANA598 added to SoC produced a more rapid viral clearance than SoC alone [56].

Acylpyrrolidines are yet another class of palm domain 1 binding compounds (see Figure 6.1d) [57]. The activity of acylpyrrolidines is affected by the M414T mutation, therefore suggesting that these compounds bind within palm domain 1 [58]. GSK625433 was advanced into phase I clinical trials but this study was halted because of adverse effects noted in long-term mouse carcinogenicity studies [59].

Palm Domain 2

Palm domain 2 overlaps partially with palm domain 1, in proximity to the enzyme active site and the junction between the palm and thumb domain. A class of benzofurans was identified as potent inhibitors of *in vitro* HCV replication (see Figure 6.1e) [60]. HCV-796, a potent benzofuran, selects *in vitro* for mutations at positions Leu^{314}, Cys^{316}, Ile^{363}, Ser^{365}, and Met^{414} [61]. In a combination trial of HCV-796 (doses ranging from 100 to 1000 mg, b.i.d.) with Peg-IFN and RBV, mean viral load reductions at day 14 were -2.6 to -3.2 $\log_{10}$ for genotype 1 infected patients, increasing to -3.5 to -4.8 $\log_{10}$ in non-genotype 1 infected patients [62]. The development of HCV-796 was halted, because elevated liver enzyme levels were detected in some patients after eight weeks of therapy with HCV-796 (www.fiercebiotech.com/story/wyeth-viropharma-drops-hep-c-drug/2008-04-17).

A class of imidazopyridines exerts potent *in vitro* activity against HCV (see Figure 6.1e). Drug-resistant variants select for mutations in palm domain 2 (C316Y) but also in the β-hairpin loop (C445F, Y448H, Y452H), which is in close proximity to the catalytic site. This hairpin loop is believed to be involved in primer-independent initiation of RNA replication [63]. Given the fact that the imidazopyridines do not inhibit, in contrast to other NNIs, the enzymatic activity of the purified RdRp, the precise mechanism by which this class of molecules targets the enzyme may be via a unique mechanism. GS-9190/Tegobuvir is currently being evaluated in phase II studies in combination with GS-9256, a protease inhibitor, when used as: (i) a dual antiviral therapy alone; (ii) a three-drug regimen with RBV; or (iii) a four-drug regimen with RBV and Peg-IFN. The study found that the all-oral regimen of GS-9190, GS-9256, and RBV produced substantial viral suppression, with a median maximal decline from baseline in HCV RNA of -5.1 $\log_{10}$ IU/ml during 28 days of treatment. No virologic breakthroughs were observed in patients treated with a four-drug regimen [64]. Across cohorts, the median half-life of GS-9190 was 10–15 hours.

Perspectives

The viral polymerase has, for various viruses, proven to be an excellent target for selective inhibition of viral replication. Indeed, inhibition of the HIV reverse transcriptase (by NRTIs and NNRTIs), of the herpes virus DNA polymerase (NI) and HBV reverse transcriptase/DNA polymerase (NI) have shown good antiviral efficacy. The RdRp of HCV offers, in contrast to the viral NS3 serine protease, various non- (or only partially) overlapping sites that can be targeted by selective inhibitors. Clinical efficacy has been demonstrated with both nucleoside and non-nucleoside analogs. The barrier toward drug resistance appears, in general, to be higher for nucleoside analogs than for non-nucleoside analogs. Obviously combination therapy will be needed for the efficient future management of HCV infection. Adding one potent DAA to the current SoC may possibly/hopefully suffice to result in a high rate of sustained virologic response (SVR). Combinations that would solely consist of DAAs may require two or more of such inhibitors. In theory a multitude of possibilities exist in which polymerase inhibitors can be combined with, for example, protease or NS5A inhibitors. Also a combination with host-targeting molecules (such as cyclophilin-binding compounds) can be envisaged. Given the fact that the HCV RdRp has various non-overlapping sites for inhibition of viral replication, combinations of various RdRp inhibitors may be possible. In an elegant study, Le Pogam and colleagues demonstrated that NNI RdRp inhibitors that target different allosteric sites on the RdRp delay or prevent the emergence of drug-resistant variants [65]. The genotype of double resistant variants (that occur at low frequency) is the sum of the monoresistant mutations; no novel complex genotype occurs. This is also the case in triple resistant variants that are resistant against three NNIs with a different allosteric binding site or against two different NNIs and a NI or a protease inhibitor (our unpublished results). One of the most prescribed anti-HIV drugs, Atripla, contains three reverse transcriptase inhibitors (a nucleotide, a nucleoside, and a non-nucleoside inhibitor). This triple therapy is highly effective and associated with a very low risk of resistance development. Triple HCV therapy based on the combination of three RdRp inhibitors may (in theory) also be possible. In conclusion, the HCV RdRp is an excellent target for inhibition of viral replication. RdRp inhibitors may either be used in combination with the SoC, other DAAs or host-targeting molecules.

Acknowledgments

L.D. is a fellow of the Fonds voor Wetenschappelijk Onderzoek-Vlaanderen (FWO). Lotte Coelmont is supported by the Research Fund K.U.Leuven. The original work of the authors is supported by grants from FWO (G.0728.09N) and the Geconcentreerde Onderzoeksactie (K.U.Leuven, GOA 10/014).

References

1. Bressanelli S, Tomei L, Roussel A, et al. Crystal structure of the RNA-dependent RNA polymerase of hepatitis C virus. Proc Natl Acad Sci U S A 1999;96:13034–9.
2. Pierra C, Amador A, Benzaria S, et al. Synthesis and pharmacokinetics of valopicitabine (NM283), an efficient prodrug of the potent anti-HCV agent 2'-C-methylcytidine. J Med Chem 2006;49:6614–20.
3. Coelmont L, Paeshuyse J, Windisch, MP, et al. Ribavirin antagonizes the in vitro anti-hepatitis C virus activity of 2'-C-methylcytidine, the active component of valopicitabine. Antimicrob Agents Chemother 2006;50:3444–6.
4. Migliaccio G, Tomassini JE, Carroll SS, et al. Characterization of resistance to non-obligate chain-terminating ribonucleoside analogs that inhibit hepatitis C virus replication in vitro. J Biol Chem 2003;278:49164–70.
5. Dutartre H, Bussetta C, Boretto J, Canard B. General catalytic deficiency of hepatitis C virus RNA polymerase with an S282T mutation and mutually exclusive resistance towards 2'-modified nucleotide analogues. Antimicrob Agents Chemother 2006;50:4161–9.
6. Ludmerer SW, Graham DJ, Boots E, et al. Replication fitness and NS5B drug sensitivity of diverse hepatitis C virus isolates characterized by using a transient replication assay. Antimicrob Agents Chemother 2005;49:2059–69.
7. Afdhal N, O'Brien C, Godofsky E. Valopicitabine (NM283), alone or with peginterferon, compared to peg interferon/ribavirin (pegIFN/RBV) retreatment in patients with HCV-1 infection and prior non-response to pegIFN/RBV: one-year results. J Hepat 2007;46:S5.
8. Lawitz E, Nguyen T, Younes Z, et al. Valopicitabine (NM283) plus PEG-interferon in treatment-naive hepatitis C patients with HCV genotype-1 infection: HCV RNA clearance during 24 weeks of treatment. Hepatology 2006;44:223A.
9. Carroll SS, Tomassini JE, Bosserman M, et al. Inhibition of hepatitis C virus RNA replication by 2'-modified nucleoside analogs. J Biol Chem 2003;278:11979–84.
10. Olsen DB, Eldrup AB, Bartholomew L, et al. A 7-deaza-adenosine analog is a potent and selective inhibitor of hepatitis C virus replication with excellent pharmacokinetic properties. Antimicrob Agents Chemother 2004;48:3944–53.
11. Stuyver LJ, McBrayer TR, Tharnish PM, et al. Inhibition of hepatitis C replicon RNA synthesis by beta-D-2'-deoxy-2'-fluoro-2'-C-methylcytidine: a specific inhibitor of hepatitis C virus replication. Antivir Chem Chemoth 2006;17:79–87.
12. Klumpp K, Leveque V, Le Pogam S, et al. The novel nucleoside analog R1479 (4'-azidocytidine) is a potent inhibitor

of NS5B-dependent RNA synthesis and hepatitis C virus replication in cell culture. *J Biol Chem* 2006;281:3793–9.

13. Le Pogam S, Jiang WR, Leveque V, *et al.* In vitro selected Con1 subgenomic replicons resistant to 2′-C-methyl-cytidine or to R1479 show lack of cross resistance. *Virology* 2006;351:349–59.

14. Roberts SK, Cooksley G, Dore GJ, *et al.* Robust antiviral activity of R1626, a novel nucleoside analog: a randomized, placebo-controlled study in patients with chronic hepatitis C. *Hepatology* 2008;48:398–406.

15. Pockros PJ, Nelson D, Godofsky E, *et al.* R1626 plus peginterferon Alfa-2a provides potent suppression of hepatitis C virus RNA and significant antiviral synergy in combination with ribavirin. *Hepatology* 2008;48:385–97.

16. Ma H, Jiang WR, Robledo N, *et al.* Characterization of the metabolic activation of hepatitis C virus nucleoside inhibitor beta-D-2′-deoxy-2′-fluoro-2′-C-methylcytidine (PSI-6130) and identification of a novel active 5′-triphosphate species. *J Biol Chem* 2007;282:29812–20.

17. Murakami E, Bao H, Ramesh M, *et al.* Mechanism of activation of beta-D-2′-deoxy-2′-fluoro-2′-c-methylcytidine and inhibition of hepatitis C virus NS5B RNA polymerase. *Antimicrob Agents Chemother* 2007;51:503–9.

18. Ali S, Leveque V, Le Pogam S, *et al.* Selected replicon variants with low-level in vitro resistance to the hepatitis C virus NS5B polymerase inhibitor PSI-6130 lack cross-resistance with R1479. *Antimicrob Agents Chemother* 2008; 52:4356–69.

19. Le Pogam S, Seshaadri A, Kosaka A, *et al.* Existence of hepatitis C virus NS5B variants naturally resistant to non-nucleoside, but not to nucleoside, polymerase inhibitors among untreated patients. *J Antimicrob Chemother* 2008; 61:1205–1216.

20. McCown MF, Rajyaguru S, Le Pogam S, *et al.* The hepatitis C virus replicon presents a higher barrier to resistance to nucleoside analogs than to nonnucleoside polymerase or protease inhibitors. *Antimicrob Agents Chemother* 2008;52: 1604–12.

21. Lalezari J, Gane E, Rodriguez-Torres M, *et al.* Potent antiviral activity of the HCV nucleoside polymerase inhibitor R7128 with Peg-IFN and ribavirin: interim results of R7128 500mg BID for 28 days. *J Hepatol* 2008;48:S29.

22. Le Pogam S, Seshaadri A, Ewing A, *et al.* RG7128 alone or in combination with pegylated interferon-alpha 2a and ribavirin prevents hepatitis C virus (HCV) replication and selection of resistant variants in HCV-infected patients. *J Infect Dis* 2010;202:1510–19.

23. Gane EJ, Roberts SK, Stedman CAM, *et al.* Oral combination therapy with a nucleoside polymerase inhibitor (RG7128) and danoprevir for chronic hepatitis C genotype 1 infection (INFORM-1): a randomised, double-blind, placebo-controlled, dose-escalation trial. *Lancet* 2010;376:1467–75.

24. Lalezari J, Asmuth D, Casiro A, *et al.* Antiviral activity, safety and pharmacokinetics of Idx184, a liver-targeted nucleotide

HCV polymerase inhibitor, in patients with chronic hepatitis C. *Hepatology* 2009;50:11A–12A.

25. Zhou XJ, Pietropaolo K, Chen J, *et al.* Safety and pharmacokinetics of IDX184, a liver-targeted nucleotide polymerase inhibitor of hepatitis C virus, in healthy subjects. *Antimicrob Agents Chemother* 2011;55:76–81.

26. Murakami E, Niu CR, Bao HY, *et al.* The mechanism of action of beta-D-2′-deoxy-2′-fluoro-2′-C-methylcytidme involves a second metabolic pathway leading to beta-D-2′-deoxy-2-fluoro-2′-C-methyluridine 5′-triphosphate, a potent inhibitor of the hepatitis C virus RNA-dependent RNA polymerase. *Antimicrob Agents Chemother* 2008;52: 458–64.

27. Lam AM, Murakami E, Espiritu C, *et al.* PSI-7851, a pronucleotide of beta-D-2′-deoxy-2′-fluoro-2′-C-methyluridine monophosphate, is a potent and pan-genotype inhibitor of hepatitis C virus replication. *Antimicrob Agents Chemother* 2010;54:3187–96.

28. Rodriguez-Torres M, Lawitz E, Flach S, *et al.* Antiviral activity, pharmacokinetics, safety, and tolerability of PSI-7851, a novel nucleotide polymerase inhibitor for HCV, following single and 3 day multiple ascending oral doses in healthy volunteers and patients with chronic HCV infection. *Hepatology* 2009;50:11A.

29. Lawitz E, Lalezari J, Rodriguez-Torres M, *et al.* High rapid virologic response (RVR) with PSI-7977 daily dosing plus PEG-IFN/RBV in a 28-day phase 2a trial. *Hepatology* 2010; 706A.

30. Pettersen EF, Goddard TD, Huang CC, *et al.* UCSF chimera: a visualization system for exploratory research and analysis. *J Comput Chem* 2004;25:1605–12.

31. Holm L, Park J. DaliLite workbench for protein structure comparison. *Bioinformatics* 2000;16:566–7.

32. Kukolj G, McGibbon GA, McKercher G, *et al.* Binding site characterization and resistance to a class of non-nucleoside inhibitors of the hepatitis C virus NS5B polymerase. *J Biol Chem* 2005;280:39260–67.

33. Beaulieu PL, Gillard J, Bykowski D, *et al.* Improved replicon cellular activity of non-nucleoside allosteric inhibitors of HCVNS5B polymerase: from benzimidazole to indole scaffolds. *Bioorg Med Chem Lett* 2006;16:4987–93.

34. De Francesco R, Paonessa G, Olsen DB, *et al.* Robust antiviral efficacy of a "finger-loop" allosteric inhibitor of the HCV polymerase in HCV infected chimpanzees. HepDart, December 9–13, 2007, Hawai. Available at: www.informedhorizons.com/hepdart2007/pdf/hepdart07_presentations/Tues_07_RDeFrancesco_HepDart_2007export.pdf.

35. Brainard DM, Anderson MS, Petry A, *et al.* Safety and antiviral activity of Ns5B polymerase inhibitor Mk-3281, in treatment-naive genotype 1A, 1B and 3 HCV-infected patients. *Hepatology* 2009;50:1026A–7A.

36. Larrey DG, Benhamou Y, Lohse AW, *et al.* Bi 207127 is a potent HCV RNA polymerase inhibitor during 5 days

monotherapy in patients with chronic hepatitis C. *Hepatology* 2009;50:1044A.

37. Lagace L, Cartier M, Laflamme G, *et al.* Genotypic and phenotypic analysis of the NS5B polymerase region from viral isolates of HCV chronically infected patients treated with BI 207127 for 5-days monotherapy. *Hepatology* 2010;52: 1205A.

38. Larrey D, Lohse A, de Ledinghen V, *et al.* 4 Week therapy with the non-nucleosidic polymerase inhibitor BI 207127 in combination with peginterferon-alfa2a and ribavirin in treatment naive and treatment experienced chronic HCV GT1 patients. *J Hepatol* 2010;52:S466.

39. Zeuzem S, Asselah T, Angus PW, *et al.* Strong antiviral activity and safety of IFN sparing treatment with the protease inhibitor BI201335, the HCV polymerase inhibitor BI207127 and ribavirin in patients with chronic hepatitis C. *Hepatology* 2010;52:876A–7A.

40. Wang M, Ng KK, Cherney MM, *et al.* Non-nucleoside analogue inhibitors bind to an allosteric site on HCV NS5B polymerase. Crystal structures and mechanism of inhibition. *J Biol Chem* 2003;278:9489–95.

41. Biswal BK, Wang M, Cherney MM, *et al.* Non-nucleoside inhibitors binding to hepatitis C virus NS5B polymerase reveal a novel mechanism of inhibition. *J Mol Biol* 2006; 361:33–45.

42. Le Pogam S, Kang H, Harris SF, *et al.* Selection and characterization of replicon variants dually resistant to thumb- and palm-binding nonnucleoside polymerase inhibitors of the hepatitis C virus. *J Virol* 2006;80:6146–54.

43. Rodriguez-Torres M, Lawitz E, Conway B, *et al.* Safety and antiviral activity of the HCV non-nucleoside polymerase inhibitor VX-222 in treatment-naive genotype 1 HCV-infected patients. *J Hepatol* 2010;52:S14.

44. Cooper C, Lawitz EJ, Ghali P, *et al.* Evaluation of VCH-759 monotherapy in hepatitis C infection. *J Hepatol* 2009;51:39–46.

45. Howe AY, Cheng H, Thompson I, *et al.* Molecular mechanism of a thumb domain hepatitis C virus nonnucleoside RNA-dependent RNA polymerase inhibitor. *Antimicrob Agents Chemother* 2006;50:4103–13.

46. Howe AY, Bloom J, Baldick CJ, *et al.* Novel nonnucleoside inhibitor of hepatitis C virus RNA-dependent RNA polymerase. *Antimicrob Agents Chemother* 2004;48:4813–21.

47. Li H, Tatlock J, Linton A, *et al.* Discovery of (R)-6-cyclopentyl-6-(2-(2,6-diethylpyridin-4-yl)ethyl)-3-((5,7-dimethyl-[1, 2, 4]triazolo[1, 5-a]pyrimidin-2-yl)methyl)-4-hydroxy-5,6-dihydropyran-2-one (PF-00868554) as a potent and orally available hepatitis C virus polymerase inhibitor. *J Med Chem* 2009;52:1255–8.

48. Shi ST, Herlihy KJ, Graham JP, *et al.* Preclinical characterization of PF-00868554, a potent nonnucleoside inhibitor of the hepatitis C virus RNA-dependent RNA polymerase. *Antimicrob Agents Chemother* 2009;53:2544–52.

49. Jacobson I, Pockros P, Lalezari J, *et al.* Antiviral activity of filibuvir in combination with pegylated interferon alfa-2a and ribavirin for 28 days in treatment naive patients chronically infected with HCV genotype 1. *J Hepatol* 2009;50:S382–3.

50. Gu BH, Johnston VK, Gutshall LL, *et al.* Arresting initiation of hepatitis C virus RNA synthesis using heterocyclic derivatives. *J Biol Chem* 2003;278:16602–7.

51. Nguyen, T. T., Gates, A. T., Gutshall, L. L., Johnston, V. K., Gu, B., Duffy, K. J., and Sarisky, R. T. 2003. Resistance profile of a hepatitis C virus RNA-dependent RNA polymerase benzothiadiazine inhibitor. *Antimicrob Agents Chemother* 47: 3525–3530.

52. Rodriguez-Torres M, Lawitz E, Cohen D, *et al.* Treatment-naïve, HCV genotype 1-infected subjects show significantly greater HCV RNA decreases when treated with 28 days of ABT-333 plus peginterferon and ribavirin compared to peginterferon and ribavirin alone. *Hepatology* 2009;50: 5A.

53. Thompson P, Patel R, Steffy K, Appleman J. Preclinical studies of ANA598 combined with other anti-HCV agents demonstrate potential of combination treatment. *J Hepatol* 2009;50:S37.

54. Lawitz E, Rodriguez-Torres M, DeMico M, *et al.* Antiviral activity of ANA598, a potent non-nucleoside polymerase inhibitor, in chronic hepatitis C patients. *J Hepatol* 2009;50: S384.

55. Appleman J, Rodriguez-Torres M, Nguyen T, *et al.* Variant genotype 1 HCV viruses observed in treatment-naïve patients following three days of ANA598 administration retain sensitivity to subsequent standard therapy with PEG-IFNalpha and ribavirin. *Global Antiviral J* 2009;5:47.

56. Lawitz E, Rodriguez-Torres M, Rustgi V, *et al.* Safety and antiviral activity of ANA598 in combination with pegylated IFNalpha 2a plus ribavirin in treatment-naïve genotype-1 chronic HCV patients. *Hepatology* 2010;52:334A–5A.

57. Slater MJ, Amphlett EM, Andrews D M, *et al.* Optimization of novel acyl pyrrolidine inhibitors of hepatitis C virus RNA-dependent RNA polymerase leading to a development candidate. *J Med Chem* 2007;50:897–900.

58. Pauwels F, Mostmans W, Quirynen LMM, et al. Binding-site identification and genotypic profiling of hepatitis C virus polymerase inhibitors. *J Virol* 2007;81:6909–19.

59. Gray F, Amphlett E, Bright H, *et al.* GSK625433; a novel and highly potent inhibitor of the HCVNS5B polymerase. *J Hepatol* 2007;46:S225.

60. Gopalsamy A, Aplasca A, Ciszewski G, *et al.* Design and synthesis of 3,4-dihydro-1H-[1]-benzothieno[2, 3-c]pyran and 3,4-dihydro-1H-pyrano[3, 4-b]benzofuran derivatives as non-nucleoside inhibitors of HCV NS5B RNA dependent RNA polymerase. *Bioorg Med Chem Lett* 2006;16:457–60.

61. Howe AY, Cheng H, Johann S, *et al.* Molecular mechanism of hepatitis C virus replicon variants with reduced susceptibility to a benzofuran inhibitor, HCV-796. *Antimicrob Agents Chemother* 2008;52:3327–38.

62. Kneteman NM, Howe AYM, Gao TJ, *et al.* HCV796: a selective nonstructural protein 5B polymerase inhibitor with

potent anti-hepatitis C virus activity in vitro, in mice with chimeric human livers, and in humans infected with hepatitis C virus. *Hepatology* 2009;49:745–52.

63. Hong Z, Cameron CE, Walker MP, *et al.* A novel mechanism to ensure terminal initiation by hepatitis C virus NS5B polymerase. *Virology* 2001;285:6–11.

64. Zeuzem S, Buggisch P, Agarwal K, *et al.* Dual, triple, and quadruple combination treatment with a protease inhibitor (GS-9256) and a polymerase inhibitor (GS-9190) alone and in combination with ribavirin (RBV) or PegIFN/RBV for up to 28 days in treatment naïve, genotype 1 HCV subjects. *Hepatology* 2010;52:400A–401A.

65. Le Pogam S, Kang H, Harris SF, *et al.* Selection and characterization of replicon variants dually resistant to thumb- and palm-binding nonnucleoside polymerase inhibitors of the hepatitis C virus. *J Virol* 2006;80:6146–54.

7 Pharmacology and Mechanisms of Action of Antiviral Drugs: Protease Inhibitors

Laurent Chatel-Chaix,* Martin Baril,* and Daniel Lamarre
Institut de Recherche en Immunologie et en Cancérologie (IRIC), Montréal, Québec, Canada
*These authors contributed equally to this work.

Introduction

Chronic hepatitis C virus (HCV) infection represents a serious public health concern worldwide since it causes progressive fibrosis, and may result in cirrhosis, hepatocellular carcinoma, liver failure, and death. Through its very high genetic variability and several strategies to evade host immunity, chronicity is established in 70–80% of HCV-infected patients. The HCV NS3/4A protein is a membrane-associated serine protease that is responsible for the cleavage at four non-structural (NS) sites within the viral polyprotein to generate mature NS3, NS4A, NS4B, NS5A, and NS5B proteins. HCV replication strictly requires the NS3 protease activity since chimpanzee liver inoculation with an active site mutated HCV molecular clone leads to non-productive infection [1].

Similarly to other chronic infections, HCV have evolved mechanisms to interfere with aspects of pathogen recognition, as recently reported *in vivo* by the existence of NS3-dependent mechanisms that target components of the signaling pathway in dendritic cells [2]. NS3/4A plays a central role in this process by interfering with the pathogen recognition TLR3- and RIG-I/MDA5-mediated signaling pathways, through the cleavage of TRIF and MAVS (also known as Cardif, VISA, or IPS-1) signaling adaptors, respectively. This can result in the loss of pro-inflammatory cytokine expression [2] and downstream transcription of antiviral factors such as type I interferon (IFN) genes and IFN-stimulated genes (ISGs) [3]. For these reasons, the NS3/4A protease is an intensively studied viral protein that represents one of the most attractive targets for drug discovery.

Need for Improved Anti-HCV Therapies

The standard of care (SOC) therapy, presently approved for HCV-infected patients, consists in a weekly administration of pegylated interferon alfa combined with a twice-a-day dose of ribavirin (Peg-IFN/Rib). This treatment is 48 weeks long for HCV genotype 1 infected patients and 24 weeks long for patients infected with genotypes 2 or 3. The therapeutic success is determined by the sustained virologic response (SVR), which is achieved when the levels of plasma HCV RNA are undetectable 24 weeks following the end of the treatment. The rate of SVR is about 50% for genotype 1 and 80% for genotype 2 and 3 [4]. Unfortunately, the combination of two non-specific antiviral agents that were not designed for HCV provides limited efficacy and results in severe and poorly tolerated adverse effects. In addition, the undefined nature of the current IFN-based treatment makes it very difficult to pharmacologically refine combination strategies, especially in treatment of a significant proportion of patients who have experienced drug resistance to SOC and therapeutic failure. Therefore, the HCV treatment paradigm now relies on the design of thoughtful and specific therapeutic strategies elaborated to achieve a high genetic barrier to resistance, to restore HCV-specific immunity, and to ultimately cure HCV infection. Target-based antiviral

Advanced Therapy for Hepatitis C, First Edition. Edited by Geoffrey W. McCaughan, John G. McHutchison and Jean-Michel Pawlotsky.
© 2012 Blackwell Publishing Ltd. Published 2012 by Blackwell Publishing Ltd.

drug discovery that mainly relies on the use of *in vitro* assays has led to the identification of several anti-HCV compounds currently challenged in clinical trials for their therapeutic benefit in HCV-infected patients.

Design of NS3 Protease Inhibitor Ciluprevir/BILN 2061: First Anti-HCV Proof-of-Concept in Humans

Since SVR rates positively correlate with the rapid and significant reduction of plasma HCV RNA during treatment, the combination of specific and potent anti-HCV agents achieving a high genetic barrier, possibly with immunotherapy, offer a strong rationale to eradicate infection in all patients. Many efforts have been made to design compounds that directly and specifically inhibit crucial viral functions (Specifically Targeted Antiviral Therapies for HCV; STAT-C:). The insights gained from the design of human immunodeficiency virus (HIV) protease inhibitors and the discovery of N-terminus product inhibitors of NS3 protease paved the way to the rational design and development of selective active site inhibitors aiming at blocking viral replication in infected patients.

Ciluprevir/BILN 2061 (Boehringer Ingelheim Pharma, Canada) was the first-in-class NS3 protease inhibitor ever clinically challenged for the treatment of HCV infection. Ciluprevir is a non-covalent, specific, and potent competitive inhibitor of the NS3/4A protease, which abrogates HCV polyprotein maturation *in vitro*, consistently with its designed mode of action, and results in a powerful inhibition of viral RNA replication. Furthermore, *in vitro* studies showed that ciluprevir treatment inhibited MAVS cleavage by NS3 protease in primary culture of human hepatocytes overexpressing NS3 [5] and in HCV-infected Huh-7 cells, suggesting a second therapeutic potential of protease inhibitors through the restoration of innate immunity in HCV-infected patients [6]. When orally administered to HCV genotype 1 infected patients, ciluprevir induced up to 4 $\log_{10}$ IU/ml decline of plasma HCV RNA in two days [7]. These very promising results represented the first clinical proof-of-concept of STAT-C efficiency *in vivo*. Although ciluprevir development was halted in phase Ib clinical trials because of toxicity in animals at supra doses, its discovery stimulated the industry to develop new NS3/4A inhibitors. Notably, new macrocyclic inhibitors such as TMC435, danoprevir, and others (Figure 7.1) were designed by exploiting the scaffold of ciluprevir. To date, all developed NS3/4A inhibitors in clinical trials are peptidomimetic compounds derived of

cleavage products, and hence target the serine protease active site (Figure 7.1).

NS3 Protease Inhibitors in Clinical Development

Telaprevir

Telaprevir/VX-950 (Vertex Pharmaceuticals Inc., CA) is a linear peptidomimetic (α-ketoamide) NS3/4A inhibitor forming a covalent but reversible complex with a steady-state inhibition constant (Ki) of 7 nM against the genotype 1 enzyme. Genotype optimization will likely be required since the Ki is 4- to 7-fold and 40-fold higher for genotype 2 and 3 proteases, respectively. Telaprevir demonstrated antiviral activity *in vitro* against genotype 1 with sub-micromolar inhibition of HCV RNA replication. A reduction in viral load (1.3–5.3 $\log_{10}$ IU/mL) was observed in a phase IIa clinical trial of treatment-naïve genotype 1 patients following administration of telaprevir in monotherapy for 15 days at a dose of 750 mg three times a day. Phase II protease inhibitor for viral eradication (PROVE) trials consisted in a 12 weeks lead-in with Peg-IFN/Rib/telaprevir triple therapy regimen followed by 36 (PROVE-1) or 12 (PROVE-2) weeks of Peg-IFN/Rib treatment [8,9]. SVR rate was higher in all telaprevir arms as compared to SOC: 67% versus 41% for PROVE-1 and 69% versus 46% for PROVE-2. Data obtained with these two trials are not substantially different and suggest that Peg-IFN/Rib treatment duration could be shortened to 24 weeks for the majority of treatment naïve patients.

PROVE-3 trials explored the same treatment strategy in previously untreated genotype 1 patients (C208 arm) and in patients who had failed SOC treatment (107 arm). Interestingly, results from the C208 arm showed that a twice-a-day 1125 mg dose yielded similar SVR rates than the three-times-a-day 750 mg dose, conferring a significant advantage in treatment adherence. In the 107 arm, the SVR rate of prior non-responders was 38–39% for patients who received Peg-IFN/Rib/telaprevir triple therapy, compared to 9% for those re-treated with SOC regimen. Additionally, the SVR rate for prior relapsers was 69–76% versus 20% for SOC [10]. These impressive results obtained with HCV genotype 1 treatment-experienced patients suggest that a 48-week treatment period with telaprevir-containing triple therapy regimen is required to maximize SVR rates in this difficult-to-treat group of patients [11]. Additionally, these studies showed that ribavirin was required for the optimal efficacy of the triple therapy by reducing virological breakthrough.

	Inhibitor company	Chemical structure	*In vitro* potency replicon genotype 1b IC$_{50}$(nM)	HCV RNA decline (monotherapy) (Log10 IU/ml)	Half life (hours)	Resistance profile	Current clinical trial stage	% of patients with undetectable HCV RNA
Linear	Telaprevir (VX-950) Vertex Pharmaceuticals	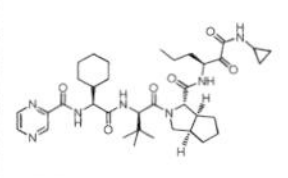	485–560	1.3–5.3	0.8–3.2	V36A/M/L; T54A R155K/Q/T/M/S A156S/T/V	III	81% (RVR) 73% (EVR) 75–79% (SVR)
	Boceprevir (SCH 503034) Merck & Co.	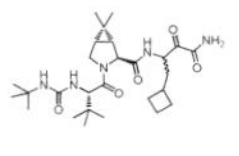	574	1.3–1.6	7–15	V36A/L/M/G F43C/S; T54A/S; V55A R155K/Q/T/M A156S/T; V170A/T	III	60% (RVR) 78% (EVR) 60–65% (SVR)
	Narlaprevir (SCH 900518) Merck & Co.	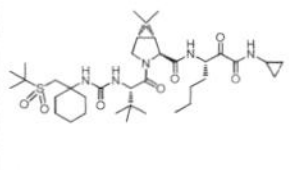	20	4.0–4.5	5 (16 with ritonavir)	V36M/L; T54 A/S R155K; A156 S/T/N	II	58–87% (RVR) 84–87% (EVR)
	BI 201335 Boehringer-Ingelheim	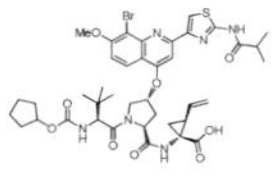	3–6	3.6–4.8	22.3–30.9	R155K/Q A156V/T D168V/A/G V170T	I	84–92% (RVR) 84–91% (EVR)
Macrocyclic	Danoprevir (RG7227 / ITMN-191) InterMune/Roche	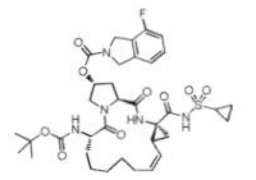	2	1.6–3.9	~2 (~5 with ritonavir)	Q41R; F43S S138T; R155K A156S/V; D168A/V S489L; V23A (NS4A)	II	73–86% (RVR) 89–92% (EVR)
	TMC435 (TMC 435350) Tibotec	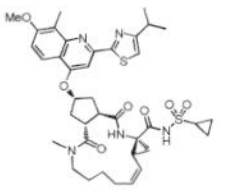	8	2.6–4.1	11.4 (~120 with ritonavir)	D168V	II	89% (RVR)
	Vaniprevir (MK-7009) Merck & Co.	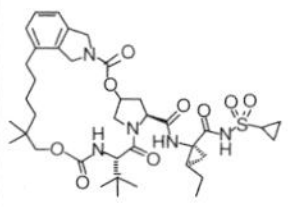	3.5	4.3–5.3	~1	Q41R; F43S; Q80R/K R155K; A156T D168T/V/E/N/I/A/G/Y	II	69–82% (RVR) 77–89% (EVR)
	Ciluprevir (BILN 2061) Boehringer-Ingelheim	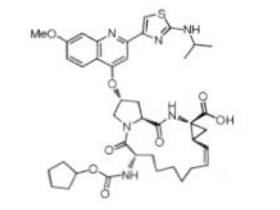	3	2–3	~4	R155Q A156T/V D168A/V	I (discontinued)	—

Figure 7.1 *In vivo* and *in vitro* characteristics and potency of HCV protease inhibitors currently in clinical development. *In vivo* results are from patients chronically infected with HCV genotype 1. RVR, Rapid viral response (4 weeks of treatment); EVR, early viral response (12 weeks of treatment); SVR: sustained viral response (24 weeks after end of treatment).

Unfortunately, the high replication rate of HCV and the poor fidelity of its RNA-dependent RNA polymerase NS5B leads to the emergence of numerous HCV quasispecies, leading to the selection of drug-resistant variants in NS3 within two weeks of telaprevir monotherapy (see Figure 7.1). These NS3 mutations observed *in vivo* were all located in or close to the inhibitor-binding site. These catalytic site mutations of NS3 protease conferred low-level resistance (<25-fold increase in IC$_{50}$: V36M/A, T54A, R155K/T, A156S) or high-level resistance (>50-fold increase in IC$_{50}$: A156V/T, V36M/A + R155K/T, V36M/A + A156V/T). These data clearly support the concept that an IFN/Rib-free treatment will include multiple antiviral drugs independently targeting HCV with no overlapping resistance profile.

Telaprevir is associated with increased rates of gastrointestinal events, anemia, and severe skin rash, when compared to SOC. About half of the patients treated with telaprevir developed skin rash and only 9% of patients stopped treatment due to adverse events.

Telaprevir has been evaluated in phase III clinical trials: ADVANCE, ILLUMINATE (in treatment-naïve patients) and REALIZE (in treatment-experienced patients) to refine the critical determinants of a triple therapy-based strategy in order to maximize the SVR rate. Data from the ADVANCE trials revealed that the addition of telaprevir to the Peg-IFN/Rib regimen during the first 8 or 12 weeks of treatment significantly improved the SVR rate to 69% and 75%, respectively, in treatment-naïve patients as compared to 44% for the SOC control arm [12]. These results are in line with results previously obtained in phase II trials, but treatment discontinuation rate due to adverse effects were notably lower. The FDA Antiviral Drugs Advisory Committee recently reviewed the phase III clinical trials completed in over 2000 patients with chronic hepatitis C genotype 1 infection, and have recommended approval of telaprevir (Incivek) for the treatment of chronic hepatitis C genotype 1 infection in combination with standard therapy.

Boceprevir

Boceprevir/SCH 503034 (Merck & Co., NJ; initially developed by Schering-Plough) is a linear peptidomimetic inhibitor possessing a serine trap forming a covalent bond with the NS3/4A protease (Ki of 14 nM). Following 2 weeks of boceprevir monotherapy in genotype 1 previous non-responders, plasma HCV RNA levels were decreased by $\sim$1.6 $\log_{10}$ IU/ml. This antiviral effect achieved a 2.9 $\log_{10}$ IU/ml when Peg-IFN was co-administered.

After these promising results, Schering-Plough enrolled HCV genotype 1 treatment-naïve patients in the phase II clinical trial SPRINT-1 (serine protease inhibitory therapy) that consisted in a 4-week lead-in with Peg-IFN/Rib followed by a 44- or 24-week Peg-IFN/Rib/boceprevir triple therapy regimen [13]. Results showed that the triple therapy arm was associated with a significant increase in SVR rate (75% and 56% for 44 and 24 weeks triple therapy, respectively) as compared to the SOC arm (38%). Importantly, patients who had a rapid viral response (RVR) following the 4-week lead-in and were further treated for 24 weeks with the boceprevir-based regimen achieved an SVR rate of 82%. Hence, as was shown for telaprevir, these studies suggest that reducing treatment duration from 48 to 28 weeks for treatment-naïve patients who had an RVR can be achieved without decreasing the SVR rate. Results from a phase II clinical trial evaluating the therapeutic potential of a similar strategy in prior non-responders (RESPOND-1) were disappointing as only 7–14% of patients achieved SVR [14]. Two phase III clinical trials, HCV SPRINT-2 (treatment-naïve) and HCV RESPOND-2 (prior non-responders), have been

completed in about 1500 patients with chronic hepatitis C genotype 1 infection. Both clinical trials demonstrated that boceprevir almost doubled the SVR rates compared to standard therapy. The FDA Antiviral Drugs Advisory Committee recently have recommended approval of boceprevir (Victrelis) for the treatment of chronic hepatitis C genotype 1 infection in combination with standard therapy.

Several drug resistance mutations in the NS3 protease emerged upon boceprevir treatment (see Figure 7.1). Boceprevir and telaprevir have an overlapping resistance profile, suggesting that the combination of these two drugs in a putative therapy would not represent a promising therapeutic avenue as it would not increase the genetic barrier to resistance. Adverse effects reported in boceprevir-treated patients were fatigue, anemia, nausea, dysgeusia, and headache.

Danoprevir

Danoprevir/RG7227/ITMN-191 (InterMune Inc., CA and Roche, NJ) is a non-covalent macrocyclic inhibitor of HCV NS3/4A protease. In a phase Ib trial, danoprevir monotherapy for 14 days showed up to 3.9 $\log_{10}$ viral load decrease in treatment-naïve genotype 1 patients and 2.5 $\log_{10}$ viral load decrease in prior non-responders. Co-administration of Peg-IFN/Rib with danoprevir during the two weeks of treatment resulted in a further decrease in viral load (4.7–5.7 $\log_{10}$ IU/ml) [15]. Danoprevir-related adverse effects were generally safe and well tolerated in initial phase I trial. A phase IIb trial is currently ongoing and interim analyses revealed that 88–92% of the patients achieved early viral response (EVR) following a 12-week tri-therapy versus 43% for the SOC control group [16]. Notably, danoprevir is effective at lower doses when boosted with ritonavir, an HIV protease inhibitor allowing some drugs to reach higher concentration through its interference with CYP3A.

Interestingly, co-administration of a NS5B polymerase inhibitor RG7128 (PSI-6130; Roche) with danoprevir significantly increased the antiviral activity in HCV replicon-containing cells *in vitro*. The INFORM-1 clinical trial is currently evaluating the therapeutic potential of this bi-therapy [17]. Interim results showed an increased and sustained antiviral effects of the RG7128/danoprevir combination versus danoprevir monotherapy after 14 days. Adverse effects were mild and, importantly, no treatment-emergent resistance was observed. Patients treated during two weeks with the highest dose of RG7128/danoprevir regimens followed by SOC for 12 weeks achieved 88% RVR and 100% EVR rates [18]. This antiviral strategy represents the first STAT-C-based combination therapy and could eventually lead to the elimination of Peg-IFN/Rib from the therapy regimen.

TMC435

TMC435/TMC 435350 (Tibotec, Belgium and Medivir, Sweden) is a non-covalent cyclopentane-containing NS3/4A protease inhibitor. TMC435 antiviral activity is currently assessed in a phase II clinical trial (OPERA-1) [19]. Naïve, prior relapser, and prior non-responder patients were given once-daily dose of TMC435 (25, 75, 200, or 400 mg) in combination with Peg-IFN/Rib during 4 weeks, followed by a 44-week Peg-IFN/Rib administration. After 28 days, interim results from this study revealed that 89% of the patients achieved RVR and that viral load decreased 4.7–5.4 $\log_{10}$ in all TMC435 arms compared to 3.6 $\log_{10}$ for SOC only, confirming the potent antiviral activity of TMC435 in naïve and treatment-experienced patients. Observed adverse effects consisted mainly of influenza-like illness (nausea, diarrhea, and headache) and never led to treatment discontinuation.

BI 201335

BI 201335 (Boehringer Ingelheim Pharma, Canada) is a linear tripeptide inhibitor of the NS3 protease featuring a C-terminal carboxylic acid. Two weeks of BI 201335 monotherapy resulted in a median HCV RNA decline of 3–4.2 $\log_{10}$ IU/ml, while an additional two weeks of triple therapy increased this decline to 4.8–5.3 $\log_{10}$ IU/ml [20]. Interim results from phase IIb SILEN-C1 trials on HCV genotype 1 treatment naïve patients showed that infected patients who received BI 201335/Peg-IFN/Rib tri-therapy during 12 weeks had RVR and EVR rates of 92% and 91%, respectively, as compared to 16% and 42% in the SOC control arm. This regimen also showed robust antiviral activity in the SILEN-C2 study performed on prior non-responders with RVR and EVR rates of 54–59% and 62–69%, respectively [21]. Reported side effects include skin rash and jaundice, and discontinuation rate was significantly lower in the once-daily arm (4%) compared with the twice-daily arm (24%). If the SVR rate proves to be similar in the once-daily group and the twice-daily group as is the case for EVR, once-daily treatment would be a significant improvement in HCV therapy. The FDA has granted Fast Track designation for BI 201335 phase III trials.

Vaniprevir

Vaniprevir/MK-7009 (Merck & Co., NJ) is a macrocyclic non-covalent NS3/4A protease inhibitor. In a phase IIa trial on HCV genotype 1 treatment-naïve patients, vaniprevir was administered for 4 weeks as part of a triple

therapy with Peg-IFN/Rib, the RVR rate was 69–82% compared to 6% for the SOC arm. An additional 8 weeks of SOC led to an EVR rate of 77–89% versus 60% in the SOC control group [22]. A phase IIb study consisting of the same treatment strategy was initiated with treatment-experienced patients.

Narlaprevir

Narlaprevir/SCH 900518 (Merck & Co., NJ) is a linear NS3/4A protease inhibitor. Eight days of triple therapy led to a 4–4.5 $\log_{10}$ IU/ml viral load reduction in both treatment-experienced and naïve HCV genotype 1 infected patients. Preliminary results of the narlaprevir phase II trial (NEXT-1) showed that treatment-naïve patients receiving a 4-week SOC lead-in followed by a triple therapy regimen had RVR and EVR rates of 58–87% and 84–87%, respectively [23]. However, the addition of narlaprevir to the SOC showed no benefit on prior non-responders, with an SVR of 17%. A phase II trial is currently evaluating SVR rate with and without co-administration of ritonavir as a pharmacokinetic booster.

Presently, numerous pharmaceuticals have NS3 additional protease inhibitors in their pipeline, although limited information is generally available. GS-9256 (Gilead Sciences, CA) has just entered a phase II clinical trial, and other protease inhibitors currently in phase I of clinical development include VX-813, VX-500, and VX-985 (Vertex Pharmaceuticals Inc., CA), VBY-376 (ViroBay, CA), PHX1766 (Phenomix, CA), ABT-450 (Abbott, IL and Enanta Pharmaceuticals, MA), BMS-650032 (Bristol-Myers Squibb, NY), ACH-1625 (Achillion Pharmaceuticals, CT), and MK-5172 (Merck & Co., NJ). Results from long-term treatments with these compounds are still unavailable.

Challenges and Future Directions

In order to significantly impact the unmet medical need and enlarge the treatable population, the HCV protease inhibitors will have to be tested and studied in chronically infected patients who did not previously respond to SOC and also in populations that classically show low response rates (HIV-HCV co-infected individuals, African Americans, patients with kidney failure, cirrhosis, or liver transplant). Moreover, the antiviral activity of these treatments will have to be evaluated in individuals infected with non-genotype 1 HCV. For instance, in contrast to patients infected with both HCV genotype 1 and 2, little or no virological response is achieved following telaprevir-based treatment of HCV genotype

3-infected individuals [24], illustrating the need to design and/or optimize STAT-Cs effective against non-1 or multiple genotypes.Peg-IFN/Rib-based therapy induces severe adverse effects in treated patients whose rate is further increased by co-administrated STAT-C. Therefore, maximizing the tolerability of the patient towards the SOC represents a major challenge in STAT-C development. While ribavirin is one of the major causative agents of adverse symptoms, its removal from the antiviral regimen significantly reduced the SVR rate following telaprevir- and boceprevir-based treatments. Ultimately, it will be important to optimize new Peg-IFN/Rib-free treatments. Meanwhile, a good alternative for enhancing tolerability will probably reside in decreasing STAT-C/Peg-IFN/Rib-based treatment duration from 48 to 24 weeks for treatment-naïve patients.

One of the biggest concerns about a successful anti-HCV therapy is to delay the appearance of drug resistance and virologic breakthrough that were observed after two weeks of STAT-C monotherapy. Interestingly, the NS3/4A inhibitor MK-5172, recently developed by Merck, retains subnanomolar potency against NS3 variants harboring key clinical resistance mutations [25]. This compound is undergoing phase I development and may exhibit a high barrier to the emergence of viral resistance *in vivo*. To limit virus resistance and maintain long-term virus suppression, a drastic selective pressure must be applied on HCV replication. As was done for anti-HIV treatments with antiviral combination regimens, the solution for HCV will similarly reside in a therapy that includes several STAT-Cs with additive or synergistic antiviral efficacies, and more importantly with no overlapping resistance profile. Results from the trials emphasizing the antiviral activity of danoprevir/RG7128-based regimens (see above) are very encouraging and represent the first proof-of-concept of an anti-HCV combination therapy. More recently, Vertex has initiated a phase II clinical trial evaluating the antiviral potency of a treatment that combines telaprevir and VX-222 (an HCV polymerase inhibitor) with or without Peg-IFN/Rib. Hopefully, these treatments will alleviate the need for Peg-IFN/Rib and limit the emergence as well as the severity of adverse effects.

Another challenge resides in the identification of new classes of NS3/4A protease inhibitors. ACH-1095 (Achillion Pharmaceuticals, CT), currently in late-stage pre-clinical assessment, antagonizes NS4A, the NS3 co-factor that is required for its serine protease activity. Furthermore, given that NS3 sub-domains mutually regulate each other [26–28], inhibitors targeting the helicase domain of NS3 could affect its protease activity.

Finally, the identification of conserved and critical NS3/4A protein-host factor interactions could lead to exciting therapeutic avenues and to the discovery of new classes of inhibitors that would hopefully maximize the genetic barrier to resistance.

In conclusion, new promising therapeutic perspectives for the treatment of HCV chronic infection have been highlighted by the identification and development of NS3/4A protease inhibitors. Hopefully, the combination of multiple classes of STAT-C (NS5B polymerase, NS5A, entry or assembly inhibitors) will constitute a new treatment paradigm that will be better tolerated and lead to HCV eradication in infected patients.

Acknowledgments

We thank Daniel Guay for help with the chemical structures in Figure 7.1.

References

1. Kolykhalov AA, Mihalik K, Feinstone SM, Rice CM. Hepatitis C virus-encoded enzymatic activities and conserved RNA elements in the 3′ nontranslated region are essential for virus replication in vivo. *J Virol* 2000; 74(4): 2046–51.

2. Rodrigue-Gervais IG, Rigsby H, Jouan L, *et al.* Dendritic cell inhibition is connected to exhaustion of CD8+ T cell polyfunctionality during chronic hepatitis C virus infection. *J Immunol* 2010; 184(6): 3134–44.

3. Dustin LB, Rice CM. Flying under the radar: the immunobiology of hepatitis C. *Annu Rev Immunol* 2007; 25: 71–99.

4. Hadziyannis SJ, Sette H, Jr., Morgan TR, *et al.* Peginterferon-alpha2a and ribavirin combination therapy in chronic hepatitis C: a randomized study of treatment duration and ribavirin dose. *Ann Intern Med* 2004; 140(5): 346–55.

5. Jouan L, Melancon P, Rodrigue-Gervais IG, *et al.* Distinct antiviral signaling pathways in primary human hepatocytes and their differential disruption by HCV NS3 protease. *J Hepatol* 2010; 52(2): 167–75.

6. Loo YM, Owen DM, Li K, *et al.* Viral and therapeutic control of IFN-beta promoter stimulator 1 during hepatitis C virus infection. *Proc Natl Acad Sci U S A* 2006; 103(15): 6001–6.

7. Lamarre D, Anderson PC, Bailey M, *et al.* An NS3 protease inhibitor with antiviral effects in humans infected with hepatitis C virus. *Nature* 2003; 426(6963): 186–9.

8. Hezode C, Forestier N, Dusheiko G, *et al.* Telaprevir and peginterferon with or without ribavirin for chronic HCV infection. *N Engl J Med* 2009; 360(18): 1839–50.

9. McHutchison JG, Everson GT, Gordon SC, *et al.* Telaprevir with peginterferon and ribavirin for chronic HCV genotype 1 infection. *N Engl J Med* 2009; 360(18): 1827–38.

10. Manns MP, Muir A, Adda N, *et al*. Telaprevir in hepatitis C genotype 1 infected patients with prior non-response, viral breakthrough or relapse to peginterferon-alfa-2a/b and ribavirin therapy: SVR results of the PROVE 3 study. *J Hepatol* 2009; 50: S379.

11. McHutchison JG, Manns MP, Muir AJ, *et al*. Telaprevir for previously treated chronic HCV infection. *N Engl J Med* 2010; 362(14): 1292–303.

12. Vertex Pharmaceuticals Inc. 75% of treatment-naïve patients with chronic hepatitis C achieve SVR (viral cure) with telaprevir-based treatment in phase 3 trial, press release, May 25, 2010 At http://investors.vrtx.com/releasedetail.cfm?ReleaseID=473342.

13. Kwo P, Lawitz EJ, McCone J, *et al*. High sustained virologic response (SVR) in genotype 1 (G1) null responders to PEG-interferon alfa-2b (P) plus ribavirin (R) when treated with boceprevir (BOC) combination therapy. AASLD 60th Annual Meeting, October 29–November 2, 2009, Boston, MA, USA, abstract 62.

14. Schiff ER, Poordad F, Jacobson I, *et al*. Boceprevir (B) combination therapy in null responders (NR): response dependent on interferon responsiveness. *J Hepatol* 2008; 48(Suppl 2): S46.

15. Forestier N, Larrey D, Marcellin P, *et al*. Antiviral activity and safety of ITMN-191 in combination with Peginterferon alfa-2A and ribavirin in patients with chronic hepatitis C virus (HCV). *J Hepatol* 2009; 50(Suppl 1): S35.

16. InterMune (and Roche: phase 2b RG7227/ITMN-191) Reports on Hepatitis C Treatment at EASL, 2010. At www.natap.org/2010/HCV/041510_01.htm.

17. Gane EJ, Roberts SK, Stedman C, *et al*. Combination therapy with a nucleoside polymerase (R7128) and protease (R7227/ITMN-191) inhibitor in HCV: safety, pharmacokinetics, and virologic results from INFORM-1. AASLD 60th Annual Meeting, October 2009, Boston, MA, abstract 193.

18. Gane E, Roberts S, Stedman C, *et al*. Early on-treatment response during pegylated interferon plus ribavirin are increased following 13 days of combination nucleoside polymerase (RG7128) and protease (RG7227) inhibitor therapy (INFORM-1). EASL 45th Annual Meeting, April 2010, Vienna, Austria.

19. Marcellin P, Reesink H, Berg T, *et al*. Antiviral activity and safety of TMC435 combined with peginterferon alpha-2a and ribavirin in patients with genotype-1 hepatitis C infection who failed previous IFN-based therapy.

20. Sulkowski MS, Ferenci P, Emanoil C, *et al*. SILEN-C1: early antiviral activity and safety of BI 201335 combined with peginterferon alfa-2a and ribavirin in treatment-naïve patients with chronic genotype 1 HCV infection. AASLD 60th Annual Meeting, October 29–November 2, 2009, Boston, MA, USA.

21. Sulkowski M, Bourliere M, Bronowicki JP, *et al*. SILEN-C2: early antiviral activity and safety of BI 201335 combined with peginterferon alfa-2a and ribavirin (PegIFN/RBV) in chronic HCV genotype 1 patients with non-response to PegIFN/RBV. EASL 45th Annual Meeting, April 2010, Vienna, Austria.

22. Manns MP, Gane E, Rodriguez-Torres M, *et al*. Early viral response (EVR) rates in treatment-naïve patients with chronic hepatitis C (CHC) genotype 1 infection treated with MK-7009, a novel NS3/4A protease inhibitor, in combination with pegylated interferon alfa-2a and ribavirin for 28 days. AASLD 60th Annual Meeting, October 29–November 2, 2009, Boston, MA, USA.

23. Vierling JM, Poordad F, Lawitz EJ, *et al*. Once daily narlaprevir (SCH 900518) in combination with PEGINTRONTM (peginterferon alfa-2b)/ribavirin for teatment-naïve subjects with genotype-1 CHC: interim results from NEXT-1, a phase 22 study. AASLD 60th Annual Meeting, October 29–November 2, 2009, Boston, MA, USA.

24. Foster GR, Hezode C, Bronowicki JP, *et al*. Activity of telaprevir alone or in combination with peginterferon alfa-2a and ribavirin in treatment-naïve, genotype 2 and 3, hepatitis C patients: final results of study C209. EASL 45th Annual Meeting, April 2010, Vienna, Austria.

25. Liverton L, MK-5172, the 1st HCV protease inhibitor with potent activity against resistance mutations in vitro. EASL 45th Annual Meeting, April 2010, Vienna, Austria.

26. Beran RK, Pyle AM. Hepatitis C viral NS3-4A protease activity is enhanced by the NS3 helicase. *J Biol Chem* 2008; 283(44): 29929–37.

27. Beran RK, Serebrov V, Pyle AM. The serine protease domain of hepatitis C viral NS3 activates RNA helicase activity by promoting the binding of RNA substrate. *J Biol Chem*. 2007; 282(48): 34913–20.

28. Rajagopal V, Gurjar M, Levin MK, Patel SS. The protease domain increases the translocation stepping efficiency of the hepatitis C virus NS3-4A helicase. *J Biol Chem* 2010; 285(23): 17821–32.

EASL 44th Annual Meeting, April 22–26, 2009, Copenhagen, Denmark.

8 Measuring Antiviral Responses

Jean-Michel Pawlotsky and Stéphane Chevaliez

National Reference Center for Viral Hepatitis B, C and delta, Department of Virology and INSERM U955, Hôpital Henri Mondor, Université Paris-Est, Créteil, France

Virologic tools are needed to diagnose acute and chronic hepatitis C virus (HCV) infections, they may be useful to establish their prognosis, but they have found their principal application in assessing the virologic responses to therapy and guiding treatment decisions. The concept of response-guided therapy has been adopted for current treatment with the combination of pegylated interferon (IFN)-α and ribavirin; indeed, treatment duration is tailored to the virologic response at weeks 4 and 12 and the baseline HCV RNA level. Current phase III trials with a triple combination of pegylated IFN-α, ribavirin, and a specific HCV protease inhibitor have integrated this concept, and treatment duration will be based on the virologic response at week 4 when these combinations are approved.

HCV RNA Level Measurement

HCV RNA detection and quantification can be achieved by means of two types of molecular biology-based techniques: target amplification techniques (such as polymerase chain reaction; PCR) and signal amplification methods (such as the "branched DNA" assay). Whatever the technique used, international units per milliliter must be preferred to any other quantitative unit [1].

The classical techniques for viral genome detection and quantification are now progressively replaced by real-time PCR assays in most virology laboratories. Real-time PCR techniques have a broad dynamic range of quantification, well suited to the clinical needs, and they are more sensitive than classical PCR, with lower limits of detection of the order of 10–15 IU/ml. Real-time PCR assays do not yield false-positive results due to carryover contaminations, and they can be fully automated and achieve high throughput. For these reasons, real-time PCR has become the technique of choice to detect and quantify viral genomes in clinical practice.

Two real-time PCR platforms are commercially available for detection and quantification of HCV RNA: the Cobas Taqman® platform, which can be used together with automated sample preparation with the Cobas AmpliPrep® system (CAP-CTM, Roche Molecular Systems, Pleasanton, CA), and the Abbott platform (Abbott Molecular, Des Plaines, IL), which uses the $m2000_{RT}$ amplification platform together with the $m2000_{SP}$ device for sample preparation. Another assay, developed by Siemens Medical Solutions Diagnostics (Tarrytown, NY) will be available soon.

The intrinsic performance of available tests differs. The current version of the Abbott assay has been found to be accurate whatever the HCV genotype [2]. In contrast, HCV RNA levels are substantially underestimated in approximately 15% of HCV genotype 2 and 30% of HCV genotype 4 samples with the first-generation CAP-CTM assay. HCV RNA may occasionally not be detected in patients infected with HCV genotype 4 with high viral levels in other assays. This is due to nucleotide mismatches at the primers or probe level [3,4]. A second-generation CAP-CTM assay will be available soon.

Response-Guided Therapy with Current Standard-of-Care

The current standard treatment for chronic hepatitis C is the combination of pegylated IFN alfa-2a or -2b and ribavirin [5]. The efficacy endpoint of chronic hepatitis C treatment is the sustained virologic response (SVR), defined by an undetectable HCV RNA in serum or plasma with a sensitive assay (lower limit of detection of 10–50 IU/ml) 24 weeks after the end of treatment.

Advanced Therapy for Hepatitis C, First Edition. Edited by Geoffrey W. McCaughan, John G. McHutchison and Jean-Michel Pawlotsky.
© 2012 Blackwell Publishing Ltd. Published 2012 by Blackwell Publishing Ltd.

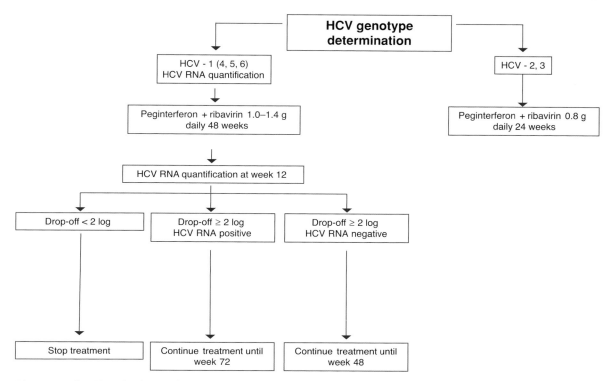

Figure 8.1 Algorithms for the use of HCV virologic tools in the treatment of chronic hepatitis C, according to the HCV genotype.

Indication of Therapy

The decision to treat chronic hepatitis C depends on multiple parameters, including a precise assessment of the severity of liver disease, the presence of absolute or relative contraindications to therapy, and the patient's willingness to be treated.

HCV genotype determination should be systematically performed before treatment, as it determines the indication, the duration of treatment, the dose of ribavirin, and the virologic monitoring procedure (Figure 8.1) [6]. Genotypes 2 and 3 infected patients theoretically require 24 weeks of treatment and a low dose of ribavirin, that is, 800 mg daily. In contrast, genotypes 1, 4, 5, and 6 infected patients require 48 weeks of treatment and a high, body-weight-based, dose of ribavirin, that is, 1000 to 1400 mg daily. However, treatment duration should ideally be tailored to the virologic response to therapy.

Treatment Monitoring

Monitoring of HCV RNA levels is recommended to tailor treatment to the virologic response. A real-time PCR assay should be used. The HCV RNA level should be measured before therapy, and 4 and 12 weeks after its initiation (Fig-

ure 8.1). The HCV RNA level should also be measured at the end of treatment and 24 weeks after treatment withdrawal in order to assess the SVR.

Response-Guided Therapy

Initially, stopping rules based on the virologic response at week 12 were established for patients infected with genotype 1 only. It is now known that the on-treatment virologic response is the best predictor of the SVR and should be used to tailor treatment duration whatever the HCV genotype.

The lack of a 12-week virologic response (i.e., no change or an HCV RNA decrease of less than 2 $\log_{10}$ at week 12) indicates that the patient has virtually no chance to achieve an SVR and should stop treatment. Increasing the dose of pegylated IFN-α and/or ribavirin in these patients may improve the on-treatment antiviral response, but these patients are unlikely to achieve an SVR. Re-treatment with the standard dose of pegylated IFN-α and ribavirin yields low SVR rates, of the order of 15% in patients infected with HCV genotype 1.

Treatment must be continued when a 2 $\log_{10}$ drop in HCV RNA level has been observed at week 12. These patients can be classified into three groups according to their virologic response: the rapid virologic response (RVR) is defined by an undetectable HCV RNA at week 4; the early virologic response (EVR) or complete early virologic response (cEVR) is defined by an HCV RNA that is detectable at week 4 but undetectable at week 12; the slow virologic response or partial early virologic response (pEVR) is defined by an HCV RNA that is still detectable at week 12 but undetectable at week 24.

1 Patients with an RVR (undetectable HCV RNA at week 4) can be treated for 24 weeks only, whatever their infecting genotype [7–12]. However, a recent meta-analysis has suggested that this recommendation should apply to patients infected with genotype 1 only if their baseline HCV RNA level is low, below 400 000–800 000 IU/ml [13]. Thus, in patients with a higher baseline HCV RNA level, treatment should be continued until week 48.

2 Patients with an EVR or cEVR (HCV RNA is detectable at week 4 but undetectable at week 12) should be treated for 48 weeks.

3 In patients with a slow virologic response or pEVR (detectable HCV RNA at week 12), 72 weeks of therapy are recommended as they prevent relapse in a substantial number of patients, provided that HCV RNA is undetectable at week 24 [14,15].

Conflicting results have been reported as to whether patients infected with genotypes 2 or 3 with an RVR could be treated for less than 24 weeks [7–12]. The most recent studies clearly indicate a global benefit in favor of 24 weeks over 12 to 16 weeks [16–18]. In fact, among the patients who achieve an RVR, only those with a low baseline viral load (<400,000 IU/ml) could be treated for less than 24 weeks without losing a chance of achieving a cure [18]. These patients are likely to experience a very rapid virologic response, that is, to lose their HCV RNA days to weeks before week 4. Studies are needed to determine the time point at which HCV RNA must become undetectable to allow for shorter therapy and the ideal treatment duration in these cases.

Response-Guided Therapy with Future Standard-of-Care

Numerous new direct acting antiviral (DAA) drugs are at various stages of pre-clinical and clinical development [19]. The most advanced ones are peptidomimetic inhibitors of HCV protease. Two drugs, telaprevir (Vertex Pharmaceuticals, Cambridge, MA, and Tibotec, Mechelen, Belgium) and boceprevir (Merck, Whitehouse Sta-

tion, NJ), have achieved phase III evaluation in combination with pegylated IFN-α and ribavirin in both treatment-naïve patients and patients who failed on previous therapy with pegylated IFN-α and ribavirin. Both drugs have been approved in Europe and the United States in 2011.

Based on results in the phase II trials [20–22], which have not all been disclosed, it was decided to include response-guided therapy in the design of the phase III trials with both telaprevir and boceprevir. Among treatment-naïve patients, only those who will achieve an extended rapid virological response (eRVR) with telaprevir (undetectable HCV RNA at weeks 4 and 12) or an RVR with boceprevir (undetectable HCV RNA at week 4 of boceprevir administration, i.e., at week 8 of therapy) will be eligible for shorter therapy. Based on the presented results, this represents approximately 60% of treatment-naïve patients who will receive 24 weeks of therapy with telaprevir and 28 weeks with boceprevir. This will also be the case with 46–52% of treatment-experienced patients, who will receive 32 weeks of boceprevir [23–26]. As shorter treatment duration has not been tested in treatment-experienced patients treated with telaprevir, all of them will be retreated with the triple combination of pegylated IFN alfa-2a, ribavirin, and telaprevir for 48 weeks [27].

Response-guided therapy will allow treatment-naïve patients to stop therapy at week 24 or 28 with telaprevir or boceprevir when they achieve an eRVR or an RVR, respectively, eliminating side effects and saving costs while likely improving adherence. It is, however, unclear whether the ideal time points to guide treatment duration have been chosen in the phase III trials, as protease inhibitors potently inhibit HCV replication in the vast majority of patients and less than 20% have not cleared RNA at week 4. Therefore, earlier time points could be more useful to guide therapy. In addition, as many patients clear HCV RNA rapidly on treatment, most of the interesting information brought by the monitoring of HCV RNA levels could happen below the detection limit. Therefore, baseline predictors of treatment outcome could find a better indication to guide therapy in this setting.

References

1. Pawlotsky JM. Use and interpretation of virological tests for hepatitis C. *Hepatology* 2002;36:S65–73.
2. Chevaliez S, Bouvier-Alias M, Pawlotsky JM. Performance of the Abbott real-time PCR assay using $m2000_{SP}$ and $m2000_{RT}$

for hepatitis C virus RNA quantification. *J Clin Microbiol* 2009;47:1726–32.

3. Chevaliez S, Bouvier-Alias M, Brillet R, Pawlotsky JM. Overestimation and underestimation of hepatitis C virus RNA levels in a widely used real-time polymerase chain reaction-based method. *Hepatology* 2007;46:22–31.

4. Chevaliez S, Bouvier-Alias M, Castera L, Pawlotsky JM. The Cobas AmpliPrep-Cobas TaqMan real-time polymerase chain reaction assay fails to detect hepatitis C virus RNA in highly viremic genotype 4 clinical samples. *Hepatology* 2009;49:1397–8.

5. National Institutes of Health. Management of Hepatitis C: 2002. Consensus Conference Statement, June 10–12, 2002. *NIH Consens State Sci Statements* 2002;19(3):1–46.

6. Hadziyannis SJ, Sette H, Jr., Morgan TR, *et al.* Peginterferon-alpha 2a and ribavirin combination therapy in chronic hepatitis C: a randomized study of treatment duration and ribavirin dose. *Ann Intern Med* 2004;140:346–55.

7. Dalgard O, Bjoro K, Hellum KB, *et al.* Treatment with pegylated interferon and ribavarin in HCV infection with genotype 2 or 3 for 14 weeks: a pilot study. *Hepatology* 2004;40:1260–1265.

8. Ferenci P, Bergholz U, Laferl H, *et al.* 24 weeks treatment regimen with peginterferon alpha-2a (40 kDa) (Pegasys) plus ribavirin (Copegus) in HCV genotype 1 or 4 "super-responders". *J Hepatol* 2006;44:S6.

9. Mangia A, Santoro R, Minerva N, *et al.* Peginterferon alfa-2b and ribavirin for 12 vs. 24 weeks in HCV genotype 2 or 3. *N Engl J Med* 2005;352:2609–17.

10. von Wagner M, Huber M, Berg T, *et al.* Peginterferon-alpha-2a (40KD) and ribavirin for 16 or 24 weeks in patients with genotype 2 or 3 chronic hepatitis C. *Gastroenterology* 2005;129:522–7.

11. Zeuzem S, Buti M, Ferenci P, *et al.* Efficacy of 24 weeks treatment with peginterferon alfa-2b plus ribavirin in patients with chronic hepatitis C infected with genotype 1 and low pretreatment viremia. *J Hepatol* 2006;44:97–103.

12. Fried MW, Hadziyannis SJ, Shiffman M, *et al.* Rapid virological response is a more important predictor of sustained virological response (SVR) than genotype in patients with chronic hepatitis C virus infection. *J Hepatol* 2008;48:S5.

13. Moreno C, Deltenre P, Pawlotsky JM, *et al.* Shortened treatment duration in treatment-naive genotype 1 HCV patients with rapid virological response: a meta-analysis. *J Hepatol* 2010;52:25–31.

14. Berg T, von Wagner M, Nasser S, *et al.* Extended treatment duration for hepatitis C virus type 1: comparing 48 versus 72 weeks of peginterferon-alfa-2a plus ribavirin. *Gastroenterology* 2006;130:1086–97.

15. Sanchez-Tapias JM, Diago M, Escartin P, *et al.* Peginterferon-alfa 2a plus ribavirin for 48 versus 72 weeks in patients with detectable hepatitis C virus RNA at week 4 of treatment. *Gastroenterology* 2006;131:451–60.

16. Dalgard O, Bjoro K, Ring-Larsen H, *et al.* Pegylated interferon alfa and ribavirin for 14 versus 24 weeks in patients with hepatitis C virus genotype 2 or 3 and rapid virological response. *Hepatology* 2008;47:35–42.

17. Lagging M, Langeland N, Pedersen C, *et al.* Randomized comparison of 12 or 24 weeks of peginterferon alpha-2a and ribavirin in chronic hepatitis C virus genotype 2/3 infection. *Hepatology* 2008;47:1837–45.

18. Diago M, Shiffman ML, Bronowicki JP, *et al.* Identifying hepatitis C virus genotype 2/3 patients who can receive a 16-week abbreviated course of peginterferon alfa-2a (40KD) plus ribavirin. *Hepatology* 2010;51:1897–1903.

19. Pawlotsky JM, Chevaliez S, McHutchison JG. The hepatitis C virus life cycle as a target for new antiviral therapies. *Gastroenterology* 2007;132:1979–98.

20. McHutchison JG, Everson GT, Gordon SC, *et al.* Telaprevir with peginterferon and ribavirin for chronic HCV genotype 1 infection. *N Engl J Med* 2009;360:1827–38.

21. McHutchison JG, Manns MP, Muir AJ, *et al.* Telaprevir for previously treated chronic HCV infection. *N Engl J Med* 2010;362:1292–1303.

22. Hezode C, Forestier N, Dusheiko G, *et al.* Telaprevir and peginterferon with or without ribavirin for chronic HCV infection. *N Engl J Med* 2009;360:1839–50.

23. Poordad F, McCone J, Bacon BR, *et al.* Boceprevir for untreated chronic HCV genotype 1 infection. *N Engl J Med* 2011: 364:1195–1206.

24. Bacon BR, Gordon SC, Lawitz E, *et al.* Boceprevir for previously treated chronic HCV genotype 1 infection. *N Engl J Med* 2011;364:1207–17.

25. Jacobson IM, McHutchison JG, Dusheiko GM, *et al.* Telaprevir for previously untreated chronic hepatitis C virus infection. *N Engl J Med* 2011;364: 2405–16.

26. Sherman KE, Flamm SL, Afdhal NH, *et al.* Telaprevir in combination with peginterferon alfa2a and ribavirin for 24 or 48 weeks in treatment-naive genotype 1 HCV patients who achieved an extended rapid viral response: final results of phase 3 ILLUMINATE study. *Hepatology* 2010;52 (Suppl): 401A.

27. Zeuzem S, Andreone P, Pol S, *et al.* Telaprevir for retreatment of HCV infection. *N Engl J Med* 2011;364:2417–28.

II   Efficacy and Clinical Use of Antiviral Therapies

9 Genotype 1: Standard Treatment

Rebekah G. Gross and Ira M. Jacobson

Division of Gastroenterology and Hepatology, Weill Cornell Medical College, New York, NY, USA

The current standard of care therapy for patients with chronic hepatitis C who are eligible for treatment involves use of interferon alfa (IFN-α) along with ribavirin. Hoofnagle and colleagues first explored the potential of interferon to treat patients with hepatitis C in 1986 [1]. Noting the activity of this drug against hepatitis B, the group undertook to treat 10 patients with what was then known as chronic non-A, non-B hepatitis using recombinant human alfa interferon. Results were encouraging, and three years later a prospective, randomized, double-blind, placebo-controlled trial followed, investigating the effects of interferon in 41 patients with the disease [2]. The drug was found to be beneficial in reducing disease activity as measured by aminotransferase levels and histologic features of the liver, though responses were often transient. Davis and colleagues obtained similar results in their larger, multicenter, randomized, controlled trial, published in the same journal issue [3]. The group randomly assigned 166 patients with non-A, non-B hepatitis to treatment with interferon, dosed at 3 million or 1 million units three times weekly, or to placebo. Following six months of treatment, 46% of patients in the high-dose interferon group experienced normalization or near-normalization of alanine aminotransferase levels versus 28% in the low-dose group and only 8% in the placebo group. Patients in the treatment arm also experienced regression of lobular and periportal inflammation on biopsy. Contemporaneous with the completion of these clinical trials, the scientific literature announced the identification and cloning of the culprit agent responsible for non-A, non-B hepatitis, a virus designated hepatitis C virus (HCV) [4,5]. The era of interferon treatment for chronic hepatitis C had dawned.

In the interval of 20 years since these groundbreaking discoveries, much has been learned about the nature of HCV, and the treatment has been refined accordingly. Six genotypes of the virus have been elucidated, designated 1 through 6. In the US, genotype 1 is most commonly encountered, comprising 75% of cases [6]. Unfortunately, this genotype has also proven the most challenging to treat, being less likely to become undetectable on therapy and more prone to post-treatment relapse, resulting in lower rates of sustained virologic response (SVR) relative to genotypes 2 and 3, and also requiring longer treatment duration to optimize the chance of SVR. However, certain advances, most notably the addition of ribavirin to the treatment protocol and pegylation of the interferon molecule itself, have enhanced the clinical efficacy of interferon-based therapy, even in the genotype 1 treatment group. This chapter will focus on these developments and the standard treatment algorithm for patients with chronic hepatitis C, genotype 1.

Goals of Therapy

The primary goal of therapy for patients with chronic hepatitis C, regardless of genotype, is achievement of an SVR. Patients whose HCV RNA levels remain undetectable when measured using a sensitive molecular assay 24 weeks after the end of treatment with peginterferon and ribavirin are considered to have attained an SVR [7]. Such patients have a greater than 99% chance of remaining virus-free upon retesting after 5 years of follow-up [8,9], leading many clinicians, in the context of the non-archived life cycle of the virus, to conclude that such patients are truly "cured." This status is associated with important positive clinical outcomes, including regression of fibrosis, decreased incidence of hepatocellular carcinoma in patients with pre-existing cirrhosis, and reductions in overall morbidity and mortality [10].

Advanced Therapy for Hepatitis C, First Edition. Edited by Geoffrey W. McCaughan, John G. McHutchison and Jean-Michel Pawlotsky.
© 2012 Blackwell Publishing Ltd. Published 2012 by Blackwell Publishing Ltd.

Duration of Treatment

Multiple studies have shown that HCV genotype is the main predictor of response to antiviral therapy, critically influencing patients' odds of achieving an SVR. Results of genotype testing dictate duration of treatment with interferon-based regimens and inform strategies for assessment of viral response to therapy. The NIH Consensus Statement on Management of Hepatitis C and various other society position papers assert that patients infected with HCV genotype 1 should receive 48 weeks of treatment with pegylated interferon in combination with ribavirin, whereas genotypes 2 and 3 appear to require only 24 weeks to optimize the chance of SVR [7,11–15].

Deriving the Regimen

A decade following the identification of interferon as a viable therapy for hepatitis C, the treatment algorithm took a quantum leap forward when ribavirin was added to the regimen. As has been discussed in previous chapters, ribavirin is an oral nucleoside analog that is active against viral pathogens, including many flaviviruses. When HCV was identified as a flavivirus, ribavirin was a natural choice as a therapeutic agent [16]. In early studies of ribavirin monotherapy for the treatment of hepatitis C, the drug was found to have little effect on serum HCV RNA levels but did lead to improvements in aminotransferase levels and liver histology [17]. Its exact mechanism of action has yet to be fully elucidated, but multiple functions have been proposed, including direct inhibition of RNA replication, immunomodulation, inhibition of inosine monophosphate dehydrogenase, and enhanced viral mutagenesis [18], as well as augmentation of interferon-response pathways. While ribavirin monotherapy does not induce a significant antiviral response in patients with chronic hepatitis C, its addition to interferon therapy has been found to improve end of treatment response (ETR) rates substantially and also to reduce relapse, markedly improving SVR rates [19–22].

Three major trials support the use of combination therapy with peginterferon and ribavirin as the current standard hepatitis C treatment. The first was a phase III randomized controlled trial published in the *Lancet* in 2001 by Manns and colleagues [23]. The study included 1530 interferon-naïve subjects randomly assigned to three treatment arms for 48 weeks. The first arm received standard interferon alfa-2b 3 million units three times weekly and ribavirin 1000–1200 mg/day, while the second received peginterferon alfa-2b 1.5 mcg/kg/week for a 4-week lead-in period, followed by 0.5 mcg/kg/week for the remainder of the study plus ribavirin 1000–1200 mg/day, and the third received peginterferon alfa-2b 1.5 mcg/kg/week plus ribavirin 800 mg/day. The mean age of the study participants was 43 years, and a majority of the subjects had genotype 1 infection (68%) as well as HCV RNA titers greater than 2 million copies/ml (68%). Advanced histology, defined by bridging fibrosis or cirrhosis, was present in 29%.

The investigators found that the SVR rates were 47%, 47%, and 54% for the standard interferon, low-dose peginterferon, and high-dose peginterferon groups, respectively. The difference between the SVR rate for the high-dose peginterferon group and that for each of the other groups was statistically significant. The presence of advanced histology did appear to influence results; the SVR rate among patients with bridging fibrosis or cirrhosis was 44% as opposed to 57% among those with no or minimal fibrosis. Among patients with genotype 1 infection, the SVR rate was 42% in the high-dose peginterferon group versus 33% in the standard interferon group.

Fried and colleagues published the second major study of peginterferon and ribavirin in the *New England Journal of Medicine* the following year [24]. This was a multicenter trial involving 1121 interferon-naïve patients. This study compared the efficacy of peginterferon alfa-2a 180 mcg administered subcutaneously each week plus ribavirin 1000–1200 mg daily against standard interferon alfa-2b plus ribavirin and peginterferon alfa-2a monotherapy over a 48-week period. Approximately 65% of patients had genotype 1. However, only 12–15% had advanced histology. The mean HCV RNA concentration at baseline was 6 million copies/ml. SVR occurred significantly more often with peginterferon-based therapy than it did with standard combination therapy or with pegylated interferon monotherapy (SVR rates of 56%, 44%, and 29%, respectively). Patients with genotype 1 disease fared worse than did the overall group, with 46%, 36%, and 21% achieving an SVR in the three treatment groups.

The third pivotal trial determining the treatment algorithm for hepatitis C treatment was published by Hadziyannis and colleagues two years later in the *Annals of Internal Medicine* [25]. The trial included 1311 interferon-naïve patients who were randomly assigned to receive peginterferon alfa-2a 180 mcg weekly plus ribavirin 800 mg or 1200 mg daily for 24 weeks or for 48 weeks. Among patients with genotype 1 infection, the highest SVR rate, 52%, was observed after 48 weeks of therapy using the high dose of ribavirin. Among those treated with this dose of ribavirin for 24 weeks, the SVR rate was 42%. Among those who received low-dose ribavirin, 41% of patients treated for 48 weeks achieved an SVR as opposed to 29% of those treated for 24 weeks. Guidelines emerged from these data, recommending 48 weeks of combination therapy as the optimal duration of treatment for genotype 1 infection, with a ribavirin dose of 1000–1200 mg being superior to 800 mg in combination with peginterferon alfa-2a.

Subsequently, a large multicenter trial combining over 200 academic and community sites demonstrated the superiority of weight-based ribavirin 800–1400 mg/day over ribavirin 800 mg/day in combination with peginterferon alfa-2b 1.5 mcg/kg/week for patients with HCV genotype 1 [26]. The WIN-R study group randomly assigned 5027 patients with chronic hepatitis C to receive peginterferon alfa-2b plus ribavirin at a fixed dose of 800 mg daily or to receive peginterferon alfa-2b plus ribavirin according to a sliding scale determined by weight (800 mg/day for those weighing less than 65 kg, 1000 mg/day for those 65–85 kg, 1200 mg/day for those greater than 85 but less than 105 kg, and 1400 mg/day for those 105–125 kg). SVR rates were found to be higher for the group dosed by weight (34% versus 29% among patients with genotype 1 disease). Serious adverse events were similar in all study arms.

A large comparative study of peginterferon alfa-2b 1.5 mcg/kg/week and ribavirin 800–1400 mg/day, peginterferon alfa-2b 1.0 mcg/kg/week plus ribavirin 800–1400 mg/day, peginterferon alfa-2a 180 mcg/kg/week and ribavirin 1000–1200 mg/day was completed recently [27]. The study, containing about 1000 patients in each group, showed similar rates of SVR in the three groups: 40%, 38%, and 41%, respectively. ETR rates were somewhat higher in the peginterferon alfa-2a group (64% versus 53% for peginterferon alfa-2b 1.5mcg/kg/week), but relapse rates were higher as well (32% versus 24%), accounting for the similar rates of SVR.

Monitoring Treatment Response

For patients with genotype 1 infection, current recommendations outline critical time points at which to measure viral load during treatment. These data points are understood to be predictive of SVR and therefore influence decisions regarding whether to pursue a full course of therapy for a given patient or to terminate early, in advance of the 48-week mark. Monitoring of the viral load during the course of treatment is important not only for prognosticating regarding the success of therapy, but ultimately for documenting it.

The first milestone sought in treatment is a rapid virologic response (RVR), defined by an undetectable viral load at week 4 using a highly sensitive assay (limit of detection $\leq$50 IU/ml) and measuring between the fourth and fifth dose of peginterferon, as close to day 28 as possible [20,28]. Studies suggest that attaining an RVR is the strongest independent positive predictor of achieving an SVR for all genotypes [29]. Ferenci and colleagues found that among 1121 patients participating in a mutinational trial of pegylated interferon plus placebo or ribavirin versus standard interferon plus ribavirin, those with genotype 1 whose viral load became undetectable by week 4 had an SVR of over 90%, regardless of their treatment group [30]. By contrast, among patients treated with peginterferon plus ribavirin, those who had detectable HCV RNA at week 4 but then went on to become undetectable at weeks 12 or 24 had SVR rates of 60–72% and 43–48%, respectively. This study, among others, suggests that rapidity of HCV RNA suppression plays an important role in treatment outcomes. Other studies have suggested that for genotype 1 patients with low viral load (<400 000–600 000 IU/ml) who have an RVR, 24 weeks of total treatment may provide an optimized chance of SVR [31–33]. Based on such data, in the EU the option of a shortened course (24 weeks) of pegylated interferon and ribavirin has been approved for patients with genotype 1 with low viral load who achieve an RVR. The concept of individualizing treatment length based on viral response patterns is addressed in depth elsewhere in this book.

The second important data point that informs the course of treatment in the standard protocol for patients with genotype 1 disease is viral load measurement at week 12. As in week 4 monitoring, week 12 viral load assessments should be performed as close as possible to the week 12 dose of interferon, using a test with high sensitivity [20]. If the viral load is undetectable at this point or has declined by $\geq$2 log(10) from baseline values (i.e., at least 100-fold), the patient is classified as having attained an early virologic response (EVR). Such patients are encouraged to press on with therapy toward a goal of reaching 48 weeks. Those with undetectable RNA at week 12 (a complete EVR) are better poised to attain an SVR than are those who have a 2 log(10) reduction but whose HCV RNA remains detectable at this time (a partial EVR). Of those with a complete EVR, 83% will achieve an SVR as opposed to 21% of those with a partial EVR [34]. In fact, those who meet the 2 log(10) decline mark, but still have detectable HCV RNA at week 12, with subsequent clearance of HCV RNA by week 24, may consider going on to 72 weeks of therapy to enhance their chances of achieving an SVR [33,35,36] (a full discussion of extended therapy for slow responders appears later in this book). By contrast, patients who fail to meet criteria for an EVR (i.e., those who do not achieve a 2 log(10) decline) are advised to discontinue therapy altogether. For these patients, the likelihood of attaining an SVR is negligible, that is, the negative predictive value approaches 100% [30,34]. The week 12 "stopping rule" is intended to protect patients from ongoing exposure to toxic side effects from futile treatment. Unfortunately, 15–29% of patients with genotype 1 fall into this category.

If the HCV RNA level has declined by at least 2 log(10) from baseline at week 12, patients are counseled to continue treatment with the goal of reaching 48 weeks. However, another critical reassessment is performed at week 24. Patients who meet EVR criteria but whose RNA remains detectable at week 24 have a minimal likelihood of achieving an SVR (the negative predictive value is 98–100%) [23,34,37]. Given the toxicity associated with therapy and the low SVR rate predicted, it is most appropriate to recommend termination of treatment at this time. Such patients may be best served at this point by referral for future participation in clinical trials of novel agents for non-responders, if available, or deferral of re-treatment until such agents become available. Later chapters focus on therapeutic options for non-responders and relapsers, including agents under investigation that have been reported to increase response rates when combined with standard therapy.

For patients with genotype 1 virus who do complete 48 weeks of treatment, viral load should be measured at week 48 to document an ETR. Patients whose RNA is undetectable at end of treatment must then follow up at 72 weeks to confirm an SVR.

Medication Dosing

Two formulations of pegylated interferon have been licensed for use with ribavirin for the treatment of chronic hepatitis C in the United States, regardless of genotype. These are peginterferon alfa-2a (Pegasys, Genentech, San Francisco, CA) and peginterferon alfa-2b (PegIntron, Schering Corporation, Kenilworth, NJ) [6]. The drugs consist of molecules of standard IFN-α covalently linked to polyethylene glycol (PEG) of variable sizes (40 kDa for peginterferon alfa-2a, 12 kDa for peginter-

feron alfa-2b). Pegylation produces a biologically active molecule of interferon with a longer half-life and more favorable pharmacokinetics, allowing for once weekly dosing [38].

The indicated dose for peginterferon alfa-2a is 180 mcg/kg delivered subcutaneously on a weekly basis [24]. That for peginterferon alfa-2b is weight-based, at 1.5 mcg/kg weekly [23]. While the two forms of peginterferon differ in pharmacokinetics, the response rates in trials evaluating the two forms of the drug alone and in combination with ribavirin have been similar [27]. Side effect profiles of the two formulations have also been found to be similar [27,39–41].

Side Effects and Dose Adjustments

Virtually every patient treated with interferon and ribavirin therapy experiences side effects, including, but not limited to, flu-like symptoms, anemia, rash, and depression. Serious adverse effects of combination therapy with peginterferon and ribavirin are seen in up to 10% of patients, and irreversible injury and fatality can occur [24,25]. Before treatment is initiated, patients should be counseled extensively regarding medication-related toxicity and arrangements for symptom and blood count monitoring should be made, with visits scheduled at routine intervals.

Among patients with genotype 1, dose reduction of medication, primarily ribavirin, is necessary in 30–40% of patients, and early discontinuation is deemed necessary in up to 20% [23–25,42]. Of note, however, discontinuation for adverse events has been noted in as few as 5% of patients in more recent trials with standard peginterferon and ribavirin therapy [43–45]. In cases of anemia, with a hemoglobin level <10 g/dl or a drop by up to 2 g/dl in patients with stable cardiac disease, ribavirin can be reduced by 200–600 mg decrements, depending on the starting dose and degree of anemia, and it can be temporarily withheld. Particularly during the first several months of therapy, keeping ribavirin dose reductions to the minimal degree consistent with patient safety is advisable (see below). Peginterferon alfa-2a doses can be reduced from 180 to 135 mcg/week, then to 90 mcg/week; and peginterferon alfa-2b from 1.5 to 1.0, to 0.5 mcg/kg/week as needed.

Though at times necessary, dose reduction does generally compromise response rates. A retrospective analysis of two large phase III clinical trials found that dose reductions of interferon and/or ribavirin to less than 80% of the standard prescription resulted in a significant decrease in SVR rates [46]. Further review of these data revealed that SVR rates were similarly diminished if the drugs were discontinued before 80% of the treatment course had been completed. While decreases in either of the two medications can impact response rates, the effect is most pronounced when both medications are reduced. Data examining the impact of dose reduction on EVR rates showed that decreases in the dose of interferon by greater than 20% in the first 12 weeks of treatment led to a decline in EVR rates from 80% to 70%, whereas the same degree of decrease in the doses of both interferon and ribavirin in this time period caused the EVR rate to plummet to 33% [34]. Of the two medications, dose reduction of ribavirin appears to be the more impactful, especially for patients who do not achieve an RVR [22].

Identifying Candidates for Therapy

Given the duration of treatment and potential toxicity of combination therapy, not to mention medication and monitoring costs, the standard treatment as outlined above may not be appropriate for every patient with genotype 1. It is generally accepted that a liver biopsy is useful to identify patients with moderate or advanced fibrosis who are at higher risk for development of liver-related complications, including liver failure and hepatocellular carcinoma, for whom treatment is most urgent. At the opposite end of the spectrum, the biopsy can identify patients with mild disease who may reasonably defer treatment, awaiting the development of agents that promise higher response rates and/or a more tolerable side effect profile. At present, therapy is usually recommended for patients whose biopsies show changes beyond portal fibrosis alone (an Ishak score ≥ 3 or a Metavir score ≥ 2) [7]. Biopsy is costly and invasive, and the procedure is inherently flawed by sampling error. Nevertheless, it remains the gold standard by which disease is staged, helping to prioritize treatment for those most in need.

The Future

Despite the hope that combination therapy offers to patients with genotype 1 disease, the treatment is far from ideal. At best, 40–50% of those undergoing treatment will achieve an SVR, and certain groups are even less responsive. African Americans, for example, appear to be particularly resistant to interferon, with only 28% of those with genotype 1 infection attaining SVR after 48 weeks of combination therapy [42]. Other factors associated with lower response rate include higher initial viral load, increased body weight, and advanced fibrosis or significant steatosis on biopsy. Furthermore, as we have seen, for most patients with genotype 1 the road to cure is a long one, and the side effects of the medications are not trivial. Already, attention is being focused on ways to tailor standard therapy, adjusting treatment length based on viral response profiles in an effort to spare patients drug toxicity without compromising their SVR rates. At the same time, investigations are under way focusing on novel, rationally designed, and specifically targeted agents that promise greater antiviral potency and increased rates of SVR when used as adjuncts to interferon and ribavirin therapy, as covered elsewhere in this volume. It remains to be seen whether combinations of these newer agents might one day be tolerable and effective enough to replace interferon-based regimens entirely; excitingly, such studies have been initiated but are still in their infancy [47]. For now, pegylated interferon and ribavirin remain the cornerstones of treatment for genotype 1 disease, and the standard treatment protocol is likely to be amended rather than abandoned as therapies evolve. Thus, it is imperative that practitioners remain familiar with this regimen, its toxicities, and the recommended timeline for assessing treatment response.

References

1. Hoofnagle JH, Mullen KD, Jones DB, Rustgi V, Di Bisceglie A, Peters M, et al. Treatment of chronic non-A, non-B hepatitis with recombinant human alpha interferon. A preliminary report. N Engl J Med 1986;315(25):1575–8.
2. Di Bisceglie AM, Martin P, Kassianides C, et al. Recombinant interferon alfa therapy for chronic hepatitis C. A randomized, double-blind, placebo-controlled trial. N Engl J Med 1989;321(22):1506–10.
3. Davis GL, Balart LA, Schiff ER, et al. Treatment of chronic hepatitis C with recombinant interferon alfa. A multicenter randomized, controlled trial. Hepatitis Interventional Therapy Group. N Engl J Med 1989;321(22):1501–6.
4. Choo QL, Kuo G, Weiner AJ, et al. Isolation of a cDNA clone derived from a blood-borne non-A, non-B viral hepatitis genome. Science 1989;244(4902):359–62.
5. Kuo G, Choo QL, Alter HJ, et al. An assay for circulating antibodies to a major etiologic virus of human non-A, non-B hepatitis. Science 1989;244(4902):362–4.
6. Hoofnagle JH, Seeff LB. Peginterferon and ribavirin for chronic hepatitis C. N Engl J Med 2006;355(23):2444–51.

7. National Institutes of Health. Management of Hepatitis C: 2002. Consensus Conference Statement, June 10–12, 2002. *NIH Consens State Sci Statements* 2002;19(3):1–46.

8. Swain MG, Lai M-Y, Shiffman ML, *et al.* Durable sustained virological response after treatment with peginterferon alfa-2a (PEGASYS) alone or in combination with riabvirin (COPEGUS): 5-year follow-up and the criteria of a cure. *J Hepatol* 2006;46(Suppl 1):S3.

9. Lindsay K, Manns MP, Gordon SC, *et al.* Clearance of HCV at 5 year follow-up for peginterferon alfa-2b + ribavirin is predicted by sustained virologic response at 24 weeks post treatment. *Gastroenterology* 2008;134(4) Suppl 1: A-772.

10. Veldt BJ, Heathcote EJ, Wedemeyer H, *et al.* Sustained virologic response and clinical outcomes in patients with chronic hepatitis C and advanced fibrosis. *Ann Intern Med* 2007;147(10):677–84.

11. Strader DB, Wright T, Thomas DL, Seeff LB. Diagnosis, management, and treatment of hepatitis C. *Hepatology* 2004;39(4):1147–71.

12. Yee HS, Currie SL, Darling JM, Wright TL. Management and treatment of hepatitis C viral infection: recommendations from the Department of Veterans Affairs Hepatitis C Resource Center program and the National Hepatitis C Program office. *Am J Gastroenterol* 2006;101(10):2360–78.

13. Dienstag JL, McHutchison JG. American Gastroenterological Association technical review on the management of hepatitis C. *Gastroenterology* 2006;130(1):231–64; quiz 14–7.

14. Farrell GC. New hepatitis C guidelines for the Asia-Pacific region: APASL consensus statements on the diagnosis, management and treatment of hepatitis C virus infection. *J Gastroenterol Hepatol* 2007;22(5):607–10.

15. Ghany MG, Strader DB, Thomas DL, Seeff LB. Diagnosis, management, and treatment of hepatitis C: an update. *Hepatology* 2009;49(4):1335–74.

16. Hoofnagle JH. A step forward in therapy for hepatitis C. *N Engl J Med* 2009;360(18):1899–901.

17. Di Bisceglie AM, Conjeevaram HS, Fried MW, *et al.* Ribavirin as therapy for chronic hepatitis C. A randomized, double-blind, placebo-controlled trial. *Ann Intern Med* 1995;123(12):897–903.

18. Dixit NM, Perelson AS. The metabolism, pharmacokinetics and mechanisms of antiviral activity of ribavirin against hepatitis C virus. *Cell Mol Life Sci* 2006;63(7–8):832–42.

19. Davis GL, Esteban-Mur R, Rustgi V, *et al.* Interferon alfa-2b alone or in combination with ribavirin for the treatment of relapse of chronic hepatitis C. International Hepatitis Interventional Therapy Group. *N Engl J Med* 1998;339(21):1493–9.

20. Zeuzem S, Berg T, Moeller B, *et al.* Expert opinion on the treatment of patients with chronic hepatitis C. *J Viral Hepat* 2009;16(2):75–90.

21. McHutchison JG, Gordon SC, Schiff ER, *et al.* Interferon alfa-2b alone or in combination with ribavirin as initial treatment for chronic hepatitis C. Hepatitis Interventional Therapy Group. *N Engl J Med* 1998;339(21):1485–92.

22. Reddy KR, Shiffman ML, Morgan TR, *et al.* Impact of ribavirin dose reductions in hepatitis C virus genotype 1 patients completing peginterferon alfa-2a/ribavirin treatment. *Clin Gastroenterol Hepatol* 2007;5(1):124–9.

23. Manns MP, McHutchison JG, Gordon SC, *et al.* Peginterferon alfa-2b plus ribavirin compared with interferon alfa-2b plus ribavirin for initial treatment of chronic hepatitis C: a randomised trial. *Lancet* 2001;358(9286):958–65.

24. Fried MW, Shiffman ML, Reddy KR, *et al.* Peginterferon alfa-2a plus ribavirin for chronic hepatitis C virus infection. *N Engl J Med* 2002;347(13):975–82.

25. Hadziyannis SJ, Sette H, Jr., Morgan TR, *et al.* Peginterferon-alpha2a and ribavirin combination therapy in chronic hepatitis C: a randomized study of treatment duration and ribavirin dose. *Ann Intern Med* 2004;140(5):346–55.

26. Jacobson IM, Brown RS, Jr., Freilich B, *et al.* Peginterferon alfa-2b and weight-based or flat-dose ribavirin in chronic hepatitis C patients: a randomized trial. *Hepatology* 2007;46(4):971–81.

27. McHutchison JG, Lawitz EJ, Shiffman ML, *et al.* Peginterferon alfa-2b or alfa-2a with ribavirin for treatment of hepatitis C infection. *N Engl J Med* 2009;361(6):580–93.

28. Sarrazin C, Gartner BC, Sizmann D, *et al.* Comparison of conventional PCR with real-time PCR and branched DNA-based assays for hepatitis C virus RNA quantification and clinical significance for genotypes 1 to 5. *J Clin Microbiol* 2006;44(3):729–37.

29. Mihm U, Herrmann E, Sarrazin C, Zeuzem S. Review article: Predicting response in hepatitis C virus therapy. *Aliment Pharmacol Ther* 2006;23(8):1043–54.

30. Ferenci P, Fried MW, Shiffman ML, *et al.* Predicting sustained virological responses in chronic hepatitis C patients treated with peginterferon alfa-2a (40 KD)/ribavirin. *J Hepatol* 2005;43(3):425–33.

31. Jensen DM, Morgan TR, Marcellin P, *et al.* Early identification of HCV genotype 1 patients responding to 24 weeks peginterferon alpha-2a (40 kd)/ribavirin therapy. *Hepatology* 2006;43(5):954–60.

32. Zeuzem S, Buti M, Ferenci P, *et al.* Efficacy of 24 weeks treatment with peginterferon alfa-2b plus ribavirin in patients with chronic hepatitis C infected with genotype 1 and low pretreatment viremia. *J Hepatol* 2006;44(1):97–103.

33. Mangia A, Minerva N, Bacca D, *et al.* Individualized treatment duration for hepatitis C genotype 1 patients: a randomized controlled trial. *Hepatology* 2008;47(1):43–50.

34. Davis GL, Wong JB, McHutchison JG, *et al.* Early virologic response to treatment with peginterferon alfa-2b plus ribavirin in patients with chronic hepatitis C. *Hepatology* 2003;38(3):645–52.

35. Berg T, von Wagner M, Nasser S, *et al.* Extended treatment duration for hepatitis C virus type 1: comparing 48 versus 72 weeks of peginterferon-alfa-2a plus ribavirin. *Gastroenterology* 2006;130(4):1086–97.

36. Pearlman BL, Ehleben C, Saifee S. Treatment extension to 72 weeks of peginterferon and ribavirin in hepatitis C genotype 1-infected slow responders. *Hepatology* 2007;46(6):1688–94.

37. Berg T, Sarrazin C, Herrmann E, *et al.* Prediction of treatment outcome in patients with chronic hepatitis C: significance of baseline parameters and viral dynamics during therapy. *Hepatology* 2003;37(3):600–9.

38. Zeuzem S, Welsch C, Herrmann E. Pharmacokinetics of peginterferons. *Semin Liver Dis* 2003;23(Suppl 1):23–8.

39. Silva M, Poo J, Wagner F, *et al.* A randomised trial to compare the pharmacokinetic, pharmacodynamic, and antiviral effects of peginterferon alfa-2b and peginterferon alfa-2a in patients with chronic hepatitis C (COMPARE). *J Hepatol* 2006;45(2):204–13.

40. Di Bisceglie AM, Ghalib RH, Hamzeh FM, Rustgi VK. Early virologic response after peginterferon alpha-2a plus ribavirin or peginterferon alpha-2b plus ribavirin treatment in patients with chronic hepatitis C. *J Viral Hepat* 2007;14(10):721–9.

41. Laguno M, Cifuentes C, Murillas J, *et al.* Randomized trial comparing pegylated interferon alpha-2b versus pegylated interferon alpha-2a, both plus ribavirin, to treat chronic hepatitis C in human immunodeficiency virus patients. *Hepatology* 2009;49(1):22–31.

42. Conjeevaram HS, Fried MW, Jeffers LJ, *et al.* Peginterferon and ribavirin treatment in African American and Caucasian American patients with hepatitis C genotype 1. *Gastroenterology* 2006;131(2):470–77.

43. McHutchison JG, Everson GT, Gordon SC, *et al.* Telaprevir with peginterferon and ribavirin for chronic HCV genotype 1 infection. *N Engl J Med* 2009;360(18):1827–38.

44. Hezode C, Forestier N, Dusheiko G, *et al.* Telaprevir and peginterferon with or without ribavirin for chronic HCV infection. *N Engl J Med* 2009;360(18):1839–50.

45. Zeuzem S, Sulkowski M, Lawitz E, *et al.* Efficacy and safety of albinterferon alfa 2b in combination with ribavirin in treatment-naive patients with chronic hepatitis C genotype 1. *J Hepatol* 2009;50(Suppl 1):S380.

46. McHutchison JG, Manns M, Patel K, *et al.* Adherence to combination therapy enhances sustained response in genotype-1-infected patients with chronic hepatitis C. *Gastroenterology* 2002;123(4):1061–9.

47. Gane E, Roberts S, Stedman C, *et al.* First-in-man demonstration of potent antiviral activity with a nucleoside polymerase (R7128) and protease (R7227/ITMN-191) inhibitor combination in hepatitis C virus: safety, pharmacokinetics, and virologic results from INFORM-1. *J Hepatol* 2009;50(Suppl 1):S377.

10 Individually Tailored Treatment Strategies in Treatment-naïve Chronic Hepatitis C Genotype 1 Patients

Johannes Wiegand and Thomas Berg
Department of Gastroenterology and Rheumatology, Division of Hepatology, University of Leipzig, Leipzig, Germany

Introduction

Pegylated interferon alfa (IFN-α) plus ribavirin has become therapeutic standard of care for chronic hepatitis C during the past decade, but treatment response has been shown to depend upon several factors. For instance, genotype 1 infected individuals could only be successfully treated in 40–50% of cases after 48–52 weeks of therapy [1,2], while in genotype 2 and 3 infected patients high sustained virologic response (SVR) rates around 80% were observed.

Today highly sensitive HCV-RNA assays and detailed investigation of viral kinetics during therapy enabled the development of individually tailored strategies that are based on two major parameters: baseline viral load and viral decline at weeks 4, 12, and 24 of therapy. Approximately 15% of patients can benefit from shorter treatment duration without impairing SVR rates, whereas 20% of cases are slow responders who should be treated for up to 72 weeks.

In addition, ribavirin dosage and host determinants like presence of liver cirrhosis or IL28B genotype have been shown to influence the efficacy of antiviral therapy.

This chapter focuses on the concept of individually tailored treatment approaches and provides clear recommendations for the management of HCV-genotype 1 patients in daily practice.

Assessment of Baseline Viral Load

A thorough differentiation between low and high viral loads at baseline in treatment-naïve HCV-genotype 1 patients is still a matter of debate. Established thresholds were defined on the basis of standard real-time polymerase chain reaction (RT-PCR) and branched DNA (bDNA) assays and are not yet confirmed by modern RT-PCR-based test systems (Table 10.1). Moreover, it has not been elucidated whether determination of baseline viral load should rely on a single measurement or on repeated evaluations at serial time points.

The basic principle is the lower HCV-RNA prior to treatment initiation, the higher are the chances to shorten treatment duration without compromising efficacy. So far, a threshold of 800 000 IU/ml is accepted to define high-baseline viremia [3]. However, other trials observed highest SVR rates if HCV-RNA levels were below 400 000 IU/ml or even <250 000 IU/ml [4].

Current guidelines recommend a shortened treatment duration of 24 weeks in treatment-naïve cases with baseline HCV-RNA <800 000 IU/ml and loss of viremia after four weeks of therapy [5,6]. HCV-RNA should be determined with modern quantitative assays with a wide dynamic range of linear quantification from approximately 10^1 to 10^{7-8} IU/ml and a very sensitive lower detection limit around 10 IU/ml (Table 10.1).

Advanced Therapy for Hepatitis C, First Edition. Edited by Geoffrey W. McCaughan, John G. McHutchison and Jean-Michel Pawlotsky.
© 2012 Blackwell Publishing Ltd. Published 2012 by Blackwell Publishing Ltd.

Table 10.1 Interpretation of commercially available HCV-RNA assays.

Test system	HCV-RNA (IU/ml)		
	Quantifiable	Not quantifiable	Not detectable
Cobas Amplicor HCV Qualitative, Version 2.0	NA	>50	<50
Cobas Amplicor Monitor HCV Quantitative, Version 2.0	>500	NA	<500
Cobas TaqMan (Cobas Ampliprep/Cobas TaqMan or Cobas HPS Vs 2/Cobas TaqMan)	>15	<15 (but detectable)	<10
RealTime HCV	>12	<12 (but detectable)	<10
Versant HCV Qualitative (TMA)	NA	>5–10	<5–10
Versant HCV Quantitative (bDNA)	>615	NA	<615

For shortening treatment duration to 24 weeks in case of an RVR HCV-RNA assays with a detection limit of 30–50 IU/ml were used in the past, because real-time PCRs were not yet available. If highly sensitive real-time PCR assays are applied, retrospective data indicate that HCV-RNA results <12 or <15 IU/ml are sufficient to shorten therapy in HCV-genotype 1 patients from 48 to 24 weeks [8]. If HCV-RNA is <12 or <15 IU/ml at week 4, patients should be re-tested at week 8.
However, definitions of RVR and cEVR on the basis of real-time PCR-based assays have to be confirmed in prospective trials in the future.

Viral Kinetics during Therapy: When to Measure HCV-RNA in Serum

It is well established that the rate of SVR is inversely correlated with the time on treatment that is necessary to clear HCV-RNA from serum. Rational background of any individualized therapy is based on the concept that rapid responders need less therapy compared to those patients who are slow responders. The sooner HCV-RNA becomes undetectable in serum, the higher is the chance for SVR. However, an undetectable on treatment viremia, even if evaluated by standard qualitative HCV-RNA tests (detection limit 50 IU/ml) does not per se indicate that

the virus is completely eliminated from serum. There is emerging evidence that by applying more sensitive assays, such as transcription-mediated amplification (TMA) or RT-PCR assays with a detection limit <10 IU/ml (Table 10.1), a proportion of patients who were shown to have undetectable HCV RNA levels by standard assays, are still viremic (Figure 10.1) [7,8]. This implies that many patients considered so far to have suffered from a relapse might have been in fact non-responders with minimal residual viremia.

During therapy, HCV-RNA quantification should be performed at least at weeks 4, 12, and 24. Assessment of viral kinetics will not only allow prediction of treatment

Figure 10.1 Percentage of HCV-RNA negative samples by the Amplicor assay (Roche Diagnostics, detection limit <50 IU/ml) in which minimal residual viremia could be detected by the transcription mediated amplification (TMA) assay (Siemens, detection limit <5.3 IU/ml) at various time points during antiviral combination therapy. Reproduced with permission from [7].

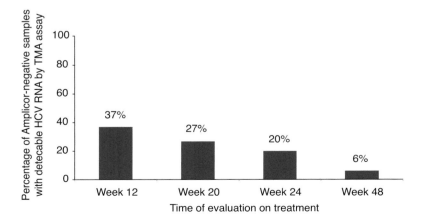

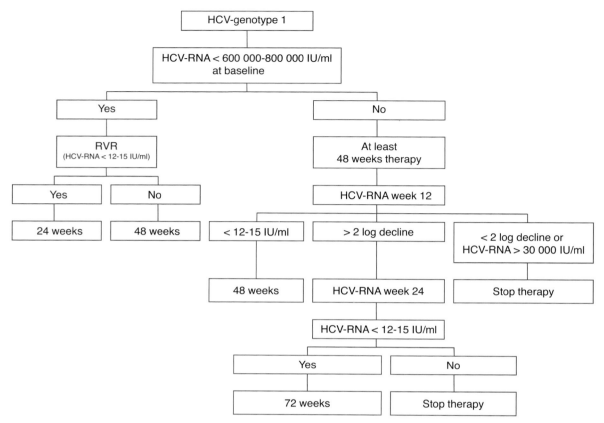

Figure 10.2 Flow-chart for treatment individualization with pegylated interferon alfa plus ribavirin in naïve chronic hepatitis C genotype 1 patients.

duration and success of therapy, it can serve as a tool to ensure therapeutic adherence and to keep patients motivated during the treatment course.

Week 4: Rapid Virologic Response

A rapid virologic response (RVR) is defined by HCV-RNA negativity after four weeks of therapy. It should be assessed between the forth and fifth peginterferon injection with a highly sensitive assay (detection limit <15–50 IU/ml) [8]. Patients with low baseline viral load (<600 000–800 000 IU/ml) and RVR can be considered for shortened treatment duration of 24 weeks only (Table 10.2, Figure 10.2) [5,6]. They should be tested again at week 12.

Patients without assessment of RVR or cases who fail to achieve RVR should not be considered for abbreviated treatment duration.

Week 12: Early Virologic Response

Early virologic response (EVR) is analyzed at week 12 and can be subdivided into complete (cEVR) and partial (pEVR) virologic response. In the case of cEVR, HCV-RNA is undetectable at week 12. Patients with positive HCV-RNA at week 4 and HCV-RNA negativity at week 12 should be considered for 48 weeks of therapy (Figure 10.2) [5,6]. A pEVR is defined as a ≥2 log drop in viral load compared to baseline. A 2 log drop at week 12 is crucial for further treatment decisions, because patients who fail this criterion or show an absolute HCV-RNA concentration >30 000 IU/ml have an almost 100% risk of missing SVR and should therefore discontinue therapy [12–14]. Thus, there is a week 12 stopping rule that should avoid unnecessary treatment (Figure 10.2). Whether the 2 log drop stopping rule at week 12 represents the most accurate cut-off level for the decision on treatment termination or continuation remains to be further investigated

Table 10.2 Randomized controlled trials evaluating a shortened treatment duration of 24 weeks versus 48 weeks in naïve HCV genotype 1 patients.

Study	HCV-genotype 1 (n)	Treatment duration (weeks)	PEG-IFNa (µg/week)	Ribavirin (mg/d)	Baseline viral load (IU/ml)	Definition of RVR (decline of HCV-RNA concentration)	SVR (Relapse) in RVR patients	
							24 weeks	48 weeks
Zeuzem et al. [9]	70	24 versus 48	180	1000–1200	24 weeks: 1.9 Mio. 48 weeks: 1.1 Mio	≥2log week 4 and >0.09 log/day (Cobas Amplicor v2.0, Roche)	65% (22%)	83% (6%)
Zeuzem et al. [10]	237	24 versus 48 (historical control group (1))	1.5/kg	800–1400	< 600 000	HCV-RNA negative (<29 IU/ml) at week 4	89% (8%)	85% (8%)
Jensen et al. [11]	389	24 versus 48	180	1000–1200	NA	HCV-RNA negative (<50 IU/ml) at week 4	88% (NA)	91% (NA)

in the future. Mathematical and post hoc analysis of multicenter trials indicate that the relapse risk may be already predicted at week 8 [15,16]. Importantly, accurate relapse prediction is only possible with sensitive assays with a broad range of linear quantification (i.e., RT-PCR).

Week 24: Slow Response

If treatment-naïve HCV-genotype 1 individuals achieve pEVR at week 12 and become HCV-RNA negative at week 24, therapy should be extended to 72 weeks (Table 10.3, Figure 10.2) [5,6]. A recent meta-analysis pooled data of six studies comparing 48 weeks treatment duration against up to 72 weeks. Extended treatment regimes significantly improved SVR rates in slow responders (14.7% increase in overall SVR; 95% CI: 4–25.5%; $p = 0.0072$), because relapse rates were lowered from 33.3% to 17.2% (95% CI: -22.2 to -8.3%; $p< 0.001$) [17].

Patients who benefit most from treatment extension are cases with <2 log HCV-RNA decline at week 8, 2–3 log decline at week 12, and negative HCV-RNA at week 24. However, individuals with a >2 log decline at week 8 and >3 log decline at week 12 do not profit from 72 weeks of therapy [23].

If patients remain HCV-RNA positive at week 24, they should prematurely discontinue treatment, because they will not achieve SVR (negative predictive value 98–100%) [5,6]. Thus, evaluation of viremia at week 24 is especially indicated in cases with a 2-log drop of HCV-RNA at week 12 (Figure 10.2).

Is it Possible to Further Individualize Treatment Beyond the Time Points of Weeks 4, 12, and 24?

Recent studies tried to further individualize treatment duration beyond the three intervals of 24, 48, and 72 weeks. Based on weekly HCV-RNA measurements during the first eight weeks of therapy, treatment was individually tailored to 18–48 weeks [24]. Initially, this therapeutic approach was not equally effective compared to a 48-week standard control arm. Significantly lower SVR rates (34% versus 48%) were mainly caused by high relapse rates in the individualized treatment arms (33% versus 14%). However, in this pilot trial HCV-RNA kinetics were based on the bDNA assay with a detection limit of 615 IU/ml. In addition, patients were not stratified according to high or low baseline viral load and were not planed for a 72-week treatment extension in case of slow response. Thus, a second multicenter trial was performed which stratified treatment duration on a highly sensitive TMA assay (limit of quantification 50 IU/ml), baseline viral load (>800 000 or <800 000 IU/ml), and prolonged therapy in slow responders [25]. Respecting these important prognostic variables, individualized treatment durations between 24 and 72 weeks were not inferior to a fixed 48-week treatment course (Figure 10.3).

In conclusion, the two INDIV-trials proof the major milestones, baseline viral load and early viral kinetics analyzed with a highly sensitive HCV-RNA assay, as a

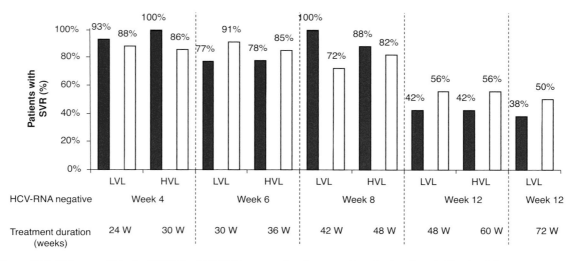

Figure 10.3 SVR rates within the INDIV-2 trial [25]. Treatment duration was adjusted to baseline viral load and the time point HCV-RNA became undetectable during therapy. LVL, low viral load; HVL, high viral load.

Table 10.3 Randomized controlled trials evaluating treatment extension beyond 48 weeks in treatment-naïve HCV-genotype 1 patients.

Study	HCV-genotype 1/4 (n)	Treatment duration (weeks)	PEG-IFNa (µg/week)	Ribavirin (mg/d)	Baseline viral load (IU/ml)	Fibrosis stage (%)	Definition of slow response (HCV-RNA concentration)	SVR (relapse) in slow-responders (%)		Premature stop of therapy (%)	
								48 weeks	72 weeks	48 weeks	72 weeks
Sanchez-Tapias et al. [14]	291	48 versus 72	180	800	>800 000: 44% <800 000: 56%	NA	>50 IU/ml week 4 ≥2 log week 12	28 (53) 16	44 (17) 44	18	36
Berg et al. [13]	455	48 versus 72	180	800	577 000	0–2 (92%)	>50 IU/ml week 12 >50 IU/ml week 4 and <50 IU/ml week 24 ≥2 log week 12	17 (NA) NA (64) 33	29 (NA) NA (40) 46	24	41
Pearlman et al. [18]	361	48 versus 72	1.5/kg	800–1400	>800 000: 78% <800 000: 22%	0–2 (74%)	≥2 log week 12 and <10 IU/ml week 24	18 (59)	38 (20)	14	15
Mangia et al. [19]	696	48 versus 72	180 or 1.5/kg	1000–1200	>400 000: 76% <400 000: 24%	0–2 (63%)	<50 IU/ml week 12 ≥2 log week 12	38 (43) 0 (100)	64 (15) 8 (60)	10	13
Buti et al. [20]	159	48 versus 72	1.5/kg	800–1400	>800 000: 80% <800 000: 20%	NA	≥2 log week 12	43 (47)	48 (33)	11	23
Ide et al. [21]	113	48 versus 52–68	1.5/kg	800–1000	2 133 000	0–2 (76%)	Variable	9 (NA)	78 (NA)	11	12
Ferenci et al. [22]	289	48 versus 72	180	1000–1200	>800 000: 34% <400 000: 66%	0–2 (79%)	≥2 log week 12	29 (34)	35 (19)	12	6

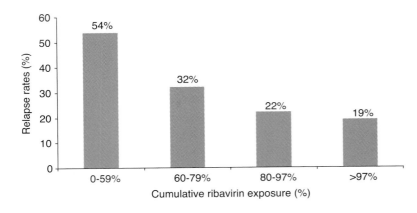

Figure 10.4 Importance of the overall cumulative ribavirin exposure for the prevention of viral relapse in chronic hepatitis C genotype 1 patients treated with pegylated interferon alfa-2a plus ribavirin. Relapse rates increase with reduced cumulative ribavirin exposure. Reproduced from [30]. Copyright (2007), with permission from Elsevier.

prerequisite of treatment individualization in naïve HCV-genotype 1 patients. Individually tailored therapy offers the possibility to improve patients' adherence, to lower the rate of treatment-related side effects, and to enhance cost efficacy. However, repetitive HCV-RNA measurements may not always be possible in clinical routine and may be restricted to specialized centers.

Impact of Ribavirin in Individualized Treatment Strategies for Chronic Hepatitis C Genotype 1 Infection

Hadziyannis *et al.* proved the beneficial outcome of weight-based ribavirin in HCV-genotype 1 patients treated with pegylated interferon alfa-2a [26]. Similar results were obtained with pegylated interferon alfa-2b, which was significantly more effective with weight-based ribavirin (800–1400 mg/d) compared to a low 800 mg/d ribavirin dosage (34% versus 29%) [27]. Thus, ribavirin should always be administered weight based in a dosage of approximately 15 mg/kg/d to ensure optimal SVR rates and to offer the opportunity of shortened treatment duration in the case of low-level pre-treatment viremia [28,29].

Difficult-to-treat HCV genotype 1 patients with high viral load (HCV-RNA >800 000 IU/ml) and a body weight >85 kg can be treated with ribavirin dosages of up to 1600 mg/d.

Two recent studies demonstrated the close relationship between cumulative ribavirin exposure and the risk of virologic relapse [30,31]. Viral relapse occurred in 19% of patients with 97% of the planned ribavirin dosage, but in 54% of cases with <60% drug exposure [30] (Figure 10.4). SVR rates between individuals with less than or equal to

60% of the ribavirin target dose were significantly different (64% versus 33%, $p < 0.0001$). Importantly, loss of efficacy was also observed in patients with 97% of the planned ribavirin dosage who reduced exposure during weeks 13–48. Thus, maintaining patients on the starting dose as long as possible is crucial in order to maximize antiviral efficacy [30,31]. If dose reductions should become necessary, stepwise 200 mg decrements with stepping back up to the starting dose after resolution of side effects as soon as possible might be preferable to maintain exposure during treatment. In contrast, immediate ribavirin reduction to 600 mg/d as suggested by the manufacturer's instructions may result in an effective 50–60% reduction in the ribavirin dose per kilogram and can therefore no longer be recommended [30].

Patients in Whom Shorter Treatment Durations May Not Be Considered

Individuals with advanced fibrosis, liver cirrhosis, metabolic syndrome, insulin resistance, gGT-levels above the upper limit of normal, platelets <150 000/μl, or age >40 years may not be candidates for abbreviated treatment regimens, although the impact of these baseline host factors should be further evaluated in prospective trials [32,33]. Recent data indicate that the extent of liver fibrosis negatively correlates with SVR, because patients with advanced fibrosis and liver cirrhosis showed slower virological responses at weeks 4 (21% versus 34%) and 8 (19% versus 26%) and high relapse rates (16–26% versus 50–80%) compared to individuals with F0–F2 fibrosis despite adequate dosage of peginterferon alfa-2a plus ribavirin [34].

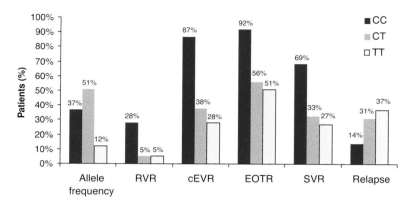

Figure 10.5 Treatment response according to IL28B genotype in Caucasian HCV-genotype 1 patients. Reproduced from [41]. Copyright (2010), with permission from Elsevier.

Impact of IL28B Genotype on Treatment Individualization

In 2009 several research groups identified variants in the *IL28B* gene as prognostic markers for spontaneous clearance of HCV infection and for SVR after peginterferon alfa therapy. The favorable CC genotype exists in 39% of Caucasian patients, whereas 12% of cases harbor the less favorable TT genotype [35–40]. Consequently, *IL28B* variants also impact early viral kinetics and can be used for treatment individualization (Figure 10.5) [41]. Caucasian individuals with CC genotype experience a greater HCV-RNA decline already during the first 24 weeks after start of peginterferon alfa therapy and during phase 1 (days 0–2) and phase 2 (days 7–28), which results in higher RVR and SVR rates compared to patients with CT or TT genotypes [42,43]. In contrast, homozygous TT patients are at risk for null-response (<1 log HCV-RNA decline during the first 12 weeks of therapy) [44,45]. Thus, analysis of different host (i.e., baseline viral load, platelets) and genetic variables may help to identify patients who will not benefit from peginterferon alfa therapy and may prefer to wait for more effective therapies [46]. Ongoing and future studies on treatment individualization with peginterferon alfa as well as trials with modern protease and polymerase inhibitors already prospectively include *IL28B* genotypes as prognostic markers for viral kinetics and SVR.

Summary

Individually tailored treatment concepts with pegylated interferon alfa plus ribavirin in naïve chronic hepatitis C genotype 1 patients are standard of care until directly antiviral protease and polymerase inhibitors become available in daily clinical practice. The most important parameters to individualize treatment duration are baseline viral load and viral kinetics during therapy (Figure 10.2). Viral load should be assessed at least prior to therapy and at weeks 4, 12, and 24. According to the INDIV-2 data [25], additional weekly HCV-RNA analysis may allow further treatment adjustment in individual cases. If frequent HCV-RNA quantification should not be possible in clinical practice, additive viral load assessment at week 8 may be helpful to define the relapse risk after the end of therapy [15,16].

IL28B genotypes will be further evaluated as host genetic factors in prospective clinical trials and will allow treatment stratification already prior to treatment initiation.

References

1. Manns MP, McHutchison JG, Gordon SC, *et al.* Peginterferon alfa-2b plus ribavirin compared with interferon alfa-2b plus ribavirin for initial treatment of chronic hepatitis C: a randomised trial. *Lancet* 2001 Sep 22; 358(9286):958–65.
2. Fried MW, Shiffman ML, Reddy KR, *et al.* Peginterferon alfa-2a plus ribavirin for chronic hepatitis C virus infection. *N Engl J Med* 2002;347(13):975–82.
3. Pawlotsky JM, Bouvier-Alias M, Hezode C, *et al.* Standardization of hepatitis C virus RNA quantification. *Hepatology* 2000;32(3):654–9.
4. Zeuzem S, Berg T, Moeller B, *et al.* Expert opinion on the treatment of patients with chronic hepatitis C. *J Viral Hepatitis* 2009;16(2):75–90.
5. Sarrazin C, Berg T, Ross RS, *et al.* [Prophylaxis, diagnosis and therapy of hepatitis C virus (HCV) infection: the German guidelines on the management of HCV infection]. *Z Gastroenterol* 2010;48(2):289–351.

6. Ghany MG, Strader DB, Thomas DL, Seeff LB. Diagnosis, management, and treatment of hepatitis C: an update. *Hepatology* 2009;49(4):1335–74.

7. Morishima C, Morgan TR, Everhart JE, *et al.* HCV RNA detection by TMA during the hepatitis C antiviral long-term treatment against cirrhosis (Halt-C) trial. *Hepatology* 2006;44(2):360–67.

8. Sarrazin C, Shiffman ML, Hadziyannis SJ, *et al.* Definition of rapid virologic response with a highly sensitive real-time PCR-based HCV RNA assay in peginterferon alfa-2a plus ribavirin response-guided therapy. *J Hepatol* 2010;52(6): 832–8.

9. Zeuzem S, Pawlotsky JM, Lukasiewicz E, *et al.* International, multicenter, randomized, controlled study comparing dynamically individualized versus standard treatment in patients with chronic hepatitis C. *J Hepatol* 2005;43(2): 250–57.

10. Zeuzem S, Buti M, Ferenci P, *et al.* Efficacy of 24 weeks treatment with peginterferon alfa-2b plus ribavirin in patients with chronic hepatitis C infected with genotype 1 and low pretreatment viremia. *J Hepatol* 2006;44(1):97–103.

11. Jensen DM, Morgan TR, Marcellin P, *et al.* Early identification of HCV genotype 1 patients responding to 24 weeks peginterferon alpha-2a (40 kd)/ribavirin therapy. *Hepatology* 2006;43(5):954–60.

12. Berg T, Sarrazin C, Herrmann E, *et al.* Prediction of treatment outcome in patients with chronic hepatitis C: significance of baseline parameters and viral dynamics during therapy. *Hepatology* 2003;37(3):600–609.

13. Berg T, von Wagner M, Nasser S, *et al.* Extended treatment duration for hepatitis C virus type 1: comparing 48 versus 72 weeks of peginterferon-alfa-2a plus ribavirin. *Gastroenterology* 2006;130(4):1086–97.

14. Sanchez-Tapias JM, Diago M, Escartin P, *et al.* Peginterferon-alfa2a plus ribavirin for 48 versus 72 weeks in patients with detectable hepatitis C virus RNA at week 4 of treatment. *Gastroenterology* 2006;131(2):451–60.

15. Scherzer TM, Kerschner H, Beinhardt S, *et al.* Week 8 HCV-RNA is the optimal predictor of relapse in non-RVR patients with genotype 1/4 randomized to 48 or 72 weeks PEG-IFN alfa-2a plus RBV. *J Hepatol* 2009;50(Suppl 1): S225.

16. Lukasiewicz E, Gorfine M, Freedman LS, *et al.* Prediction of nonSVR to therapy with pegylated interferon-alpha2a and ribavirin in chronic hepatitis C genotype 1 patients after 4, 8 and 12 weeks of treatment. *J Viral Hepatitis* 2010;17(5): 345–51.

17. Farnik H, Lange CM, Sarrazin C, *et al.* Meta-analysis shows extended therapy improves response of patients with chronic hepatitis C virus genotype 1 infection. *Clin Gastroenterol Hepatol* 2010;8(10):884–90.

18. Pearlman BL, Ehleben C, Saifee S. Treatment extension to 72 weeks of peginterferon and ribavirin in hepatitis c geno-type 1-infected slow responders. *Hepatology* 2007;46(6): 1688–94.

19. Mangia A, Minerva N, Bacca D, *et al.* Individualized treatment duration for hepatitis C genotype 1 patients: a randomized controlled trial. *Hepatology* 2008;47(1):43–50.

20. Buti M, Lurie Y, Zakharova NG, *et al.* Randomized trial of peginterferon alfa-2b and ribavirin for 48 or 72 weeks in patients with hepatitis C virus genotype 1 and slow virologic response. *Hepatology* 2010;52(4):1201–7.

21. Ide T, Hino T, Ogata K, *et al.* A randomized study of extended treatment with peginterferon alpha-2b plus ribavirin based on time to HCV RNA negative-status in patients with genotype 1b chronic hepatitis C. *Am J Gastroenterol* 2009;104(1): 70–75.

22. Ferenci P, Laferl H, Scherzer TM, *et al.* Peginterferon alfa-2a/ribavirin for 48 or 72 weeks in hepatitis C genotypes 1 and 4 patients with slow virologic response. *Gastroenterology* 2010;138(2):503–12.

23. Buti M, Morozov VG, Rafalskiy VV, *et al.* Predicting treatment outcome among slow responders: a retrospective analysis of the success study. *J Hepatol* 2010;52(S1):S104.

24. Berg T, Weich V, Teuber G, *et al.* Individualized treatment strategy according to early viral kinetics in hepatitis C virus type 1-infected patients. *Hepatology* 2009;50(2):369–77.

25. Sarrazin C, Schwendy S, Möller B, *et al.* Individualized treatment duration with peginterferon alfa-2b and ribavirin for 24, 30 or 36 weeks in HCV genotype 1 infected patients with undetectable HCV-RNA early during therapy (INDIV-2 Study). *J Hepatol* 2009;50(Suppl 1):S236.

26. Hadziyannis SJ, Sette H, Jr., Morgan TR, *et al.* Peginterferon-alpha2a and ribavirin combination therapy in chronic hepatitis C: a randomized study of treatment duration and ribavirin dose. *Ann Intern Med* 2004;140(5):346–55.

27. Jacobson IM, Brown RS, Jr., Freilich B, *et al.* Peginterferon alfa-2b and weight-based or flat-dose ribavirin in chronic hepatitis C patients: a randomized trial. *Hepatology* 2007; 46(4):971–81.

28. Snoeck E, Wade JR, Duff F, *et al.* Predicting sustained virological response and anaemia in chronic hepatitis C patients treated with peginterferon alfa-2a (40KD) plus ribavirin. *Br J Clin Pharmacol* 2006;62(6):699–709.

29. Shiffman ML, Fried MW, Hadziyannis SJ, *et al.* Probability of virological relapse during follow-up varies with the rapidity of the on-treatment virological response in HCV genotype 1 patients treated with peginterferon alfa-2a (40 KD) and ribavirin, *Hepatology* 2008;4(Suppl):879A.

30. Reddy KR, Shiffman ML, Morgan TR, *et al.* Impact of ribavirin dose reductions in hepatitis C virus genotype 1 patients completing peginterferon alfa-2a/ribavirin treatment. *Clin Gastroenterol Hepatol* 2007;5(1):124–9.

31. Hiramatsu N, Oze T, Yakushijin T, *et al.* Ribavirin dose reduction raises relapse rate dose-dependently in genotype 1

patients with hepatitis C responding to pegylated interferon alpha-2b plus ribavirin. *J Viral Hepatitis* 2009;16(8):586–94.

32. Mauss S, Hueppe D, John C, *et al.* Estimating the likelihood of sustained virological response in chronic hepatitis C therapy. *J Viral Hepatitis* 2010; 18(4):e81–90.

33. Kau A, Vermehren J, Sarrazin C. Treatment predictors of a sustained virologic response in hepatitis B and C. *J Hepatol* 2008;49(4):634–51.

34. Cheng WS, Roberts SK, McCaughan G, *et al.* Low virological response and high relapse rates in hepatitis C genotype 1 patients with advanced fibrosis despite adequate therapeutic dosing. *J Hepatol* 2010;53(4):616–23.

35. Suppiah V, Moldovan M, Ahlenstiel G, *et al.* IL28B is associated with response to chronic hepatitis C interferon-alpha and ribavirin therapy. *Nat Genet* 2009;41(10):1100–104.

36. Ge D, Fellay J, Thompson AJ, *et al.* Genetic variation in IL28B predicts hepatitis C treatment-induced viral clearance. *Nature* 2009;;461(7262):399–401.

37. Tanaka Y, Nishida N, Sugiyama M, *et al.* Genome-wide association of IL28B with response to pegylated interferon-alpha and ribavirin therapy for chronic hepatitis C. *Nat Genet* 2009;41(10):1105–109.

38. Rauch A, Kutalik Z, Descombes P, *et al.* Genetic variation in IL28B Is associated with chronic hepatitis C and treatment failure: a genome-wide association study. *Gastroenterology* 2010;138(4):1338–45 .

39. McCarthy JJ, Li JH, Thompson A, *et al.* Replicated association between an interleukin-28B gene variant and a sustained response to pegylated interferon and ribavirin. *Gastroenterology* 2010;138(7):2307–14.

40. Thomas DL, Thio CL, Martin MP, *et al.* Genetic variation in IL28B and spontaneous clearance of hepatitis C virus. *Nature* 2009;461(7265):798–801.

41. Thompson AJ, Muir AJ, Sulkowski MS, *et al.* Interleukin-28B polymorphism improves viral kinetics and is the strongest pretreatment predictor of sustained virologic response in genotype 1 hepatitis C virus. *Gastroenterology* 2010;139(1): 120–29.

42. Stattermayer AF, Stauber R, Hofer H, *et al.* Impact of IL28B genotype on the early and sustained virologic response in treatment-naive patients with chronic hepatitis C. *Clin Gastroenterol Hepatol* 2010; 9(4):344–50.e2.

43. Howell C, Thompson AJ, Ryan K, *et al.* IL28B genetic variation associated with early viral kinetics and SVR in HCV genotype 1 in the VIRAHEP-C study. *J Hepatol* 2010;52(S1): S451.

44. O'Brien TO, Bonkovsky HL, Pfeiffer R, *et al.* Association of IL28B genotype with virological response to pegylated interferon plus ribavirin in patients with advanced chronic hepatitis C enrolled in the HALT-C trial. *J Hepatol* 2010; 52(S1):S454.

45. Maekawa S, Kanayama A, Omori T, *et al.* Analysis of the response to pegylated interferon plus ribavirin therapy in chronic HCV-1b infection using comprehensive information of viral and host factors. *J Hepatol* 2010;52(S1): S256.

46. Kurosaki M, Tanaka Y, Nishida N, *et al.* Genetic polymorphism in IL28B predicts null virological response to pegylated interferon plus ribavirin therapy for chronic hepatitis C. *J Hepatol* 2010;52(S1):S451.

11 | Genotype 1 Relapsers and Non-responders

Salvatore Petta and Antonio Craxì
University of Palermo, Palermo, Italy

The Burden of Failures of Anti-HCV Therapy

Over the past 15–20 years different evolving therapeutic approaches have been used, increasing the rate of viral eradication from 10% using standard interferon (IFN), to about 30% using standard IFN plus ribavirin (RBV), and to about 50% using pegylated (Peg) IFN plus RBV. However, also using standard of care (SOC) (Peg-IFN plus RBV), about 50% of patients failed to achieve a sustained virologic response (SVR) [1–4], identifying, according to the virologic kinetic, two major group of patients: relapsers (RR) and non-responders (NR). In the registration trial of Manns *et al.* [1] on Peg-IFN alfa-2b the authors showed rates of NR and RR of 28% and 18%, respectively, observing a higher rate of therapy failure (58%) in genotype 1 (G1) chronic hepatitis C (CHC) patients. Similar results have been found in the non-sponsored trial of Bruno *et al.* [2] that, using also Peg-IFN alfa-2b, showed in G1 CHC patients RR and NR rates of 13% and 46%, respectively, observing also an increase in RR and NR rates in difficult to treat patients, namely G1 with fibrosis ≥3 by Ishak (22% and 61%), G1 with fibrosis ≥5 by Ishak (14% and 75%), and G1 with high viral load (HVL; 10% and 52%). Registration trials on Peg-IFN alfa-2a [3,4] highlighted a therapy failure rate of 37–44%, increasing to 48–54%, 53–59%, and 65–70%, in patients with G1 CHC, HVL G1 CHC, and G1 cirrhotic, respectively. In particular Hadziyannis *et al.* [4] found RR and NR rates of 17% and 31% in G1 patients, 18% and 35% in HVL G1 subjects, and 18% and 41% in G1 patients with fibrosis 3–4.

Interestingly, considering the favorable effect of viral eradication on natural history of hepatitis C, the clinical course of the disease can be more severe in these patients, with an accelerated progression toward end-stage liver disease and development of hepatocellular carcinoma (HCC) [5], leading to the final consideration that treatment failure is associated with a higher long-term mortality.

Management of Patients Who Failed to Respond to Antiviral Therapy

Several factors must be considered when deciding how to manage patients who have failed to respond to a course of therapy for chronic hepatitis C virus (HCV) infection. Three important considerations are the pattern of response to the previous treatment (RR versus NR), the specific type of previous therapy (i.e., standard versus Peg-IFN; with or without RBV) they received, and the adherence on Peg-IFN/RBV therapy doses and duration. Other factors to consider include the presence of advanced liver disease or an unfavorable HCV genotype, high HCV viral load, black race, ongoing alcohol abuse, HIV/HBV co-infection, steatosis, obesity, and insulin resistance. Tolerability to the initial therapeutic regimen should also be assessed when deciding whether to re-treat. There is no standardized approach to the management of patients who fail to respond to conventional therapy. However, there are a number of options, such as re-treatment with Peg-IFN/RBV-based regimens, maintenance therapy, and considering emerging treatments.

Re-treatment of Non-responders
Several recent trials have investigated whether patients who have failed to respond to standard IFN-based or Peg-IFN-based treatments may benefit from re-treatment

Advanced Therapy for Hepatitis C, First Edition. Edited by Geoffrey W. McCaughan, John G. McHutchison and Jean-Michel Pawlotsky.
© 2012 Blackwell Publishing Ltd. Published 2012 by Blackwell Publishing Ltd.

with Peg-IFN/RBV. According to the available data, the AASLD 2009 [6] guideline recommended that re-treatment with Peg-IFN plus RBV can be considered for NR who have previously been treated with standard IFN with or without RBV, or with Peg-IFN monotherapy, while it is not recommended in NR to Peg-IFN plus RBV.

Re-treatment of Non-responders to Standard IFN ± RBV

The largest studies evaluating the efficacy or re-treatment of patients NR to IFN-based therapies are the HALT-C [7] and the EPIC 3 [8] trials. In the HALT-C trial 604 patients with CHC (89% with G1) and advanced fibrosis NR to prior treatment with IFN alone (218 patients) or in combination with RBV (386 patients) were re-treated with Peg-IFN alfa-2a plus RBV, and 18% achieved an SVR. The response rate was higher for those patients who had previously been treated with IFN alone (28%) than for those previously treated with IFN plus RBV (12%). Interestingly, the subgroup of 82 difficult-to-treat patients with G1 HVL cirrhosis NR to a previous course of IFN and RBV showed an SVR rate of 6% only. The EPIC 3 trial evaluated the use of Peg-IFN alfa-2b (1.5 μg/kg/week) and weight-based dosing of RBV in patients who failed to respond to a previous trial of IFN or Peg-IFN and RBV. The SVR rates among G1 patients, NR to a previous course of standard IFN plus RBV, were 13% only. Other studies have shown similarly disappointing rates of SVR in these patients. In particular, considering data about G1 patients NR to combined therapy with standard IFN and RBV, SVR rates have been reported ranging from 5% to 21.7%. Also in this setting, patients with a lower likelihood to achieve SVR were G1 NR with high viral load (11%) and G1 NR with cirrhosis (0–7%). Nevertheless, these different studies evaluated the efficacy or re-treatment in patients NR to standard IFN-RBV based protocols, the results are inconclusive or conflicting, and important questions still remain unanswered. To increase statistical power and to resolve uncertainty, a recent meta-analysis [9], including all these papers, has been performed, showing that re-treatment with a course of 48 weeks of Peg-IFN plus RBV achieves an SVR in 16% of patients with a 12% withdrawal rate due to adverse reactions or intolerance to drugs, showing also a significant improvement in SVR rate only in patients not overweight and non G1 infected. These data, together with clinical evidences from all the above presented studies, therefore identified, in the setting of NR patients, baseline factors able to influence SVR rate. Interestingly, these factors, together with the type of

previous course of therapy, are not different to those that negatively influence viral eradication in naïve patients, namely G1 infection, HVL, severe fibrosis/cirrhosis, race, high BMI, and low RBV doses. These results, therefore, do not support an indiscriminate re-treatment of all NR to combination therapy. Given the relatively poor response to re-treatment with standard regimens of Peg-IFN and RBV among previous NR to conventional IFN ± RBV, several studies have been conducted to evaluate the utility of a higher dose or an extended course of Peg-IFN/RBV in these patients. The RENEW trial [10] showed that NR to a previous course of IFN plus RBV had higher rates of SVR upon re-treatment with high-dose Peg-IFN (3.0 μg/week) and weight-based RBV. Similar positive results have been observed by Diago and colleagues [11] using escalating doses of Peg-IFN alfa-2a and RBV in NR to IFN and RBV. However, other studies have reported conflicting findings. Bergmann and colleagues [12], in fact, found no significant difference in SVR rates comparing SOC to high-dose induction regimen with an extended course with Peg-IFN in patients who previously failed to respond to treatment with conventional IFN ± RBV. Another option is to address the issue of whether extending the length of therapy with Peg-IFN/RBV may improve SVR rates. This approach showed encouraging results in slow responder G1 naïve patients, and has been proposed for use in NRs as well.

Re-treatment of Non-responders to Peg-IFN plus RBV

The most important study that first evaluated the efficacy of re-treatment with Peg-IFN/RBV in previous NR to SOC was EPIC 3 [8]. In this study, considering the 476 patients NR to Peg-IFN plus RBV, the authors reported an SVR rate of 6% only, confirming this very poor result in the group of 431 G1 patients (SVR 4%), compared to the encouraging data observed in G2 and G3 subjects (36% SVR). Similarly to patients NR to standard IFN/RBV, it should be interesting to evaluate if increasing the dose of Peg-IFN and/or extending the length of therapy may improve SVR rates in NR to Peg-IFN plus RBV. The REPEAT study [7] assessed the efficacy of these two strategies as well as the utility of switching to Peg-IFN alfa-2a in 950 patients (91% G1) who had previously failed to respond to therapy with Peg-IFN alfa-2b plus RBV. Patients were treated with higher-dose Peg-IFN alfa-2a (360 μg/week) plus RBV, given as an induction dose for 12 weeks followed by standard treatment for an additional 36 or 60 weeks, or standard-dose Peg-IFN alfa-2a (180 μg/week) plus RBV given for 48 or 72 weeks. The SVR rates for the 72-week arms were

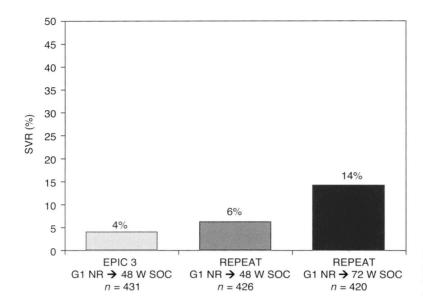

Figure 11.1 SVR rates in patients with genotype 1 chronic hepatitis C non-reponsive to standard of therapy, re-treated for 48 [8] or 72 [7,8] weeks.

16% and 14%, respectively, for those who received the induction dosing and those who did not. By contrast, the SVR rates for the 48-week arms were 7% for those who received the induction dosing versus 9% for those who did not, confirming the poor efficacy of a standard course of Peg-IFN/RBV in patients previously NR to Peg-IFN/RBV reported in EPIC 3. Stratifying the data for genotype, it was possible to observe an SVR rate of about 14% for G1 in 72-week arms, compared to about 30% for other genotypes. Furthermore, considering difficult-to-treat G1 cirrhotic patients, we observed an SVR rate in the 72-week arm of 5% only, compared to 17% observed in G1 non-cirrhotic subjects. On the basis of these results, it appears that switching to Peg-IFN alfa-2a in NRs to Peg-IFN alfa-2b does not greatly affect the SVR rate, and that extending the duration of treatment has a greater impact on SVR than induction dosing. Interestingly, also in this setting of patients, G1, severe fibrosis/cirrhosis, older age, high body weight, and HVL were negative predictors of SVR. Figure 11.1 summarizes SVR rates in G1 CHC patients NR to SOC, obtained in EPIC 3 and REPEAT studies according to treatment duration.

Re-treatment of Relapsers

Re-treatment of RR is more likely to give favorable results than re-treatment of NR. In fact, patients who have relapsed following treatment with standard IFN-based regimens often respond to re-treatment with Peg-IFN plus RBV. Accordingly, the AASLD 2009 guideline [6] recommended that re-treatment with Peg-IFN plus RBV can be considered for RR who have previously been treated with non-Peg-IFN with or without RBV, or with Peg-IFN monotherapy. In particular, different studies on patients RR to standard IFN/RBV reported, in G1 infected subjects, SVR rates ranging from 20% to 55%. Interestingly, also in the setting of RR patients, G1, HVL, and sever fibrosis/cirrhosis were reported as factors independently associated with a lower SVR rate. All these data have been recently confirmed in the EPIC 3 study [8], where, among G1 patients RR after a previous course of IFN/RBV or Peg-IFN/RBR, SVR rates of 32% and 23%, respectively, have been reported. Finally, considering the data on naïve and NR patients about a possible advantage in increased drug doses or prolongation of therapy, recent papers evaluated these issues also in RR. Bergmann and colleagues [12], as mentioned above, failed to document an advantage of higher Peg-IFN doses in a group of NR and RR patients. Instead, positive results have been found in a recent paper [13], evaluating the effect of 72-week SOC treatment in patients (81% G1) who were previously RR after a course of Peg-IFN plus RBV. This study, in fact, found that about 50% of patients achieved an SVR, confirming also in RR the positive effect on SVR of extending the duration of treatment. Figure 11.2 shows the SVR rates obtained in G1 CHC patients RR to SOC, according to treatment duration.

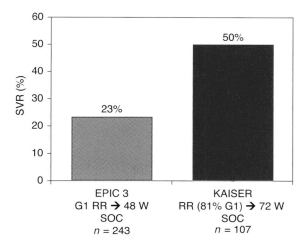

Figure 11.2 SVR rates in patients with genotype 1 chronic hepatitis C relapser to standard of therapy, re-treated for 48 [8] or 72 weeks [13].

On-treatment Evaluation According to Virologic Response in Patients Who Failed Viral Eradication

Early virologic response (EVR) and rapid virologic response (RVR) are two important instruments to evaluate the response on treatment in naïve patients. According to these data different studies evaluated also the effect of EVR and RVR in patients who failed a previous course of antiviral therapy. In patients NR (prevalently G1) to a course of standard IFN-based treatment, different studies reported an EVR rate ranging from 24% to 60%. Interestingly, about 35–70% of these subjects achieving an EVR had an SVR, compared to an SVR rate of less than 5% in patients without EVR. Considering subjects who relapsed to a previous course of standard IFN-based therapy, it is possible to observe a prevalence of EVR of about 70–80%, with an SVR rate of 40–50% in these subjects. All these data on RR and NR have been recently confirmed in a large-scale study (EPIC 3) [8] that, in a population of patients RR and NR to IFN or Peg-IFN plus RBV therapy, observed, in G1 individuals, an EVR rate of 36.7%, showing that about 39% of these patients achieved SVR. It is noteworthy to underline that considering G1 patients with undetectable HCV RNA at week 12 (28%), 48% of them achieved SVR, compared to 12% only of subjects with detectable HCV RNA but ≥2log decrease at week 12, and compared to no SVR in subjects without EVR. The determinant role of EVR in the management or the re-

treatment of NR patients has been underlined in the REPEAT study [7], also in a population of patients NR to Peg-IFN plus RBV. In this work the frequency of EVR was 52.5%. Although complete viral suppression (HCV RNA <50 IU/ml) at week 12 was less frequent (about 17%), this variable was a stronger on-treatment predictor of SVR than EVR. In particular, among patients with complete viral suppression at week 12, the rate of SVR was 57% in the pooled 72-week treatment group and 35% in the pooled 48-week treatment group. In contrast, the rate of SVR among patients with detectable HCV RNA at week 12 was 4% in both pooled 72- and 48-week treatment groups. A recent paper [13] also evaluated the effect of EVR in RR (81% G1) after a course of Peg-IFN plus RBV re-treated with 72 weeks of SOC. This study found that HCV RNA was undetectable at week 12 in 43% of patients, and that 93% of them achieved an SVR.

Nevertheless, despite the growing interest on RVR in SVR prediction, only few data are available on this issue in NR and RR patients. Moucary et al. [14], in a cohort of 45 patients NR or RR to standard IFN plus RBV and retreated with SOC, showed that at week 4 60% of patients had ≥2 log decline in HCV RNA level or undetectable HCV RNA in serum, and 52% of them achieved SVR. In contrast, among the 18 patients without ≥2 log decline in HCV RNA, only one developed SVR. Furthermore, in the same study, all patients with undetectable HCV RNA at week 4 achieved SVR, compared to 23% of those with detectable HCV RNA at week 4. Similar data have been proposed by Bergmann et al. [12], who, in a population of prior RR and NR to standard IFN-based therapy, found an RVR rate of 38%, showing that 80% of these subjects achieved SVR, compared to 15% only of subjects without RVR. However, they also highlighted that only 18% of patients with difficult-to-treat genotypes obtained an RVR. Another recent paper [15], evaluating also CHC patients of all genotypes, RR and NR to Peg-IFN or Peg-IFN plus RBV, showed that RVR was obtained in 31% and 7% of RR and NR patients, respectively, with a positive predictive value of 100% in both groups. Finally, in the above mentioned paper of Kaiser et al. [13] on patients RR to Peg-IFN plus RBV, an RVR was present in 27% of patients, and 97% of them achieved a SVR.

Maintenance Therapy

Several recent trials [16–19] have investigated whether long-term viral suppression with maintenance therapy may be of benefit in RR and NR patients, not by helping

Table 11.1 Characteristics and results of studies evaluating maintenance therapy in patients with chronic hepatitis C.

	HALT-C [16]	EPIC 3 [8,19]	COPILOT [20]
Patients (all genotypes)	604	2333 (two studies)	537
Stage of fibrosis	Ishak 4–6	Metavir 2–4	Ishak 3–6
Endpoint	Fibrosis/clinical	Fibrosis/clinical	Clinical
Run-in phase with Peg-IFN + RBV	Yes	Yes	No
NR: SVR to (Peg-)IFN + RBV	12%	10%	n.a.
Arm 1	Peg-IFN alfa-2a, 90 μg	Peg-IFN alfa-2b, 0.5 μg/kg	Peg-IFN alfa-2b, 0.5 μg/kg
Arm 2	Observation	Observation	Colchicine
Years of Peg-IFN maintenance therapy	3.5	5	4
Status	Complete, no difference	Complete, difference in portal hypertension	Complete, difference in portal hypertension

them achieve an SVR, but by slowing the progression of liver disease in the absence of SVR. However, these large studies failed to show an overall improvement in significant endpoints, such as progression of fibrosis, HCC, or death, showing only a slight effect in the subset of patients with portal hypertension (Table 11.1). In this setting, in fact, maintenance therapy might delay variceal bleeding and disease progression, at the expense of more infections.

Emerging Treatments

Different basic and clinical research efforts are ongoing to develop efficacious approaches to treat RR and NR patients, and different data are available on newer formulations of interferon and on agents that directly target viral enzymes required for HCV replication, namely protease and polymerase inhibitors (STAT-C agents). Novel IFN-based formulations included IFN alfacon-1 ("consensus IFN") and albumin IFN alfa-2b (albIFN), which, however, showed only minimal efficacy in the treatment of NRs to prior combination therapy with Peg-IFN or standard IFN and RBV. Considering STAT-C agents, more data are now available for two protease inhibitors, namely boceprevir and telaprevir. Boceprevir, in addition to SOC in the re-treatment of G1 patients who were null responders to IFN-based plus RBV treatment, showed an SVR rate of only 7–14% [21]. By contrast, telaprevir for 12 weeks, in addition to Peg-IFN alfa2a and RBV for 24 weeks, achieved encouraging results, showing an SVR rate of 39% in prior NR and of 69% in prior RR [22].

Conclusion

In summary, the options involving re-treatment with Peg-IFN and RBV for patients who have failed to respond to initial therapy with the SOC regimen are limited, and better results have been obtained in RR subjects. Re-treatment with higher doses or extended duration of therapy, switching Peg-IFN products, or the use of maintenance therapy with low-dose Peg-IFN have not demonstrated sufficient benefit to support the routine implementation of these strategies. In fact, none of these strategies can be recommended. Patients who have failed to respond to treatment with Peg-IFN plus RBV may benefit from enrolling in a clinical trial of an emerging treatment option. If the patient is not eligible for a clinical trial, a watch-and-wait approach may be the best option.

References

1. Manns MP, McHutchison JG, Gordon SC, *et al.* PegIFN alfa-2b plus RBV compared with IFN alfa-2b plus RBV for initial treatment of CHC: a randomised trial. *Lancet* 2001;358: 958–65.
2. Bruno S, Cammà C, Di Marco V, *et al.* Peginterferon alfa-2b plus ribavirin for naïve patients with genotype 1 chronic hepatitis C: a randomized controlled trial. *J Hepatol* 2004; 41:474–81.
3. Fried MW, Shiffman ML, Reddy KR, *et al.* PegIFN alfa-2a plus RBV for CHC virus infection. *N Engl J Med* 2002;347: 975–82.
4. Hadziyannis SJ, Sette H, Morgan TR, *et al.* PegIFN-alpha2a and RBV combination therapy in CHC: a randomized study

of treatment duration and RBV dose. *Ann Intern Med* 2004; 140:346–55.

5. Veldt BJ, Heathcote EJ, Wedemeyer H, *et al.* Sustained virologic response and clinical outcomes in patients with chronic hepatitis C and advanced fibrosis. *Ann Intern Med* 2007;147: 677–84.

6. Ghany MG, Strader DB, Thomas DL, Seeff LB. Diagnosis, management, and treatment of hepatitis C: an update. *Hepatology* 2009;49:1335–1374.

7. Jensen DM, Marcellin P, Freilich B, *et al.* Re-treatment of patients with chronic hepatitis C who do not respond to peginterferon-alpha2b: a randomized trial. *Ann Intern Med* 2009;150:528–40.

8. Poynard T, Colombo M, Bruix J, *et al.* Epic Study Group. Peginterferon alfa-2b and ribavirin: effective in patients with hepatitis C who failed interferon alfa/ribavirin therapy. *Gastroenterology* 2009;136:1618–28.

9. Cammà C, Cabibbo G, Bronte F, *et al.* Retreatment with pegylated interferon plus ribavirin of chronic hepatitis C non-responders to interferon plus ribavirin: a meta-analysis. *J Hepatol* 2009;51:675–81.

10. Gross J, Johnson S, Kwo P, *et al.* Double-dose peginterferon alfa-2b with weight-based ribavirin improves response for interferon/ribavirin non-responders with hepatitis C: final results of "RENEW". *Hepatology* 2005;42:219A.

11. Diago M, Crespo J, Olveira A, *et al.* Clinical trial: pharmacodynamics and pharmacokinetics of re-treatment with fixed-dose induction of peginterferon alpha-2a in hepatitis C virus genotype 1 true non-responder patients. *Aliment Pharmacol Ther* 2007;26:1131–8.

12. Bergmann JF, Vrolijk JM, van der Schaar P, *et al.* Gammaglutamyltransferase and rapid virological response as predictors of successful treatment with experimental or standard peginterferon-alpha-2b in chronic hepatitis C non-responders. *Liver Int* 2007;27:1217–25.

13. Kaiser S, Lutze B, Hass HG, *et al.* High sustained virologic response rates in HCV genotype 1 relapser patients retreated with peginterferon alfa-2a (40kd) plus ribavirin for 72 weeks. *Hepatology* 2008;48(Suppl 4);1140A.

14. Moucari R, Ripault M, Oulès V, *et al.* High predictive value of early viral kinetics in retreatment with peginterferon and ribavirin of chronic hepatitis C patients non-responders to standard combination therapy. *J Hepatol* 2007;46:596–604.

15. Martinot-Peignoux M, Maylin S, Moucari R, *et al.* Virological response at 4 weeks to predict outcome of hepatitis C treatment with pegylated interferon and ribavirin. *Antivir Ther* 2009;14:501–11.

16. Di Bisceglie AM, Shiffman ML, Everson GT, *et al.* HALT-C Trial Investigators. Prolonged therapy of advanced chronic hepatitis C with low-dose peginterferon. *N Engl J Med* 2008; 359:2429–41.

17. Afdhal N, Freilich, B, Levine R, *et al.* Colchicine versus PEG-Intron long term (COPILOT) trial: interim analysis of clinical outcomes at year 2. *Hepatology* 2004;38:239A.

18. Kaiser S, Lutzer B, Werner CR, Hass HG. Long-term low dose treatment with pegylated interferon alpha 2b for 6 years leads to a significant reduction in fibrosis and inflammatory score in a subgroup of chronic hepatitis C nonresponder patients with fibrosis or cirrhosis. *Hepatology* 2008;48: 357A.

19. Bruix J, Poynard T, Colombo M *et al.* PEGINTRON manteinance therapy in cirrhotic (Metavir 4) HCV patients, who failed to respond to interferon/ribavirin (IR) therapy: final results of the EPIC 3 cirrhosis maintenance trial. *J Hepatol* 2009;50:S22.

20. Afdhal, NH, Levine R, Brown R, *et al.* Colchicine versus peg-interferon alfa 2b long term therapy: results of the 4 year COPILOT trial. *J Hepatol* 2008;48(Suppl 2): S4.

21. Schiff E, Poordad F, Jacobson I, *et al.* Boceprevir (B) combination therapy in null responders (NR): response dependent on interferon responsiveness. *J Hepatol* 2008;48(Suppl 2): S46.

22. McHutchison J, Shiffman ML, Terrault N, *et al.* A phase 2b study of telaprevir with pegIFN-alfa-2a and RBV in hepatitis C G1 null and partial responders and RRs following a prior course of pegIFN-alfa-2a/b and RBV therapy: PROVE 3 interim results. *Hepatology* 2008;48:269.

Standard Therapy for Genotypes 2/3

Kenneth Yan and Amany Zekry

Department of Gastroenterology and Hepatology, Clinical School of Medicine, St George Hospital, Sydney, NSW, Australia

Introduction

Over the past decade, significant advances have been made in the clinical management of patients with chronic hepatitis C virus (HCV) infection. Sustained virologic response (SVR) rates (defined as undetectable serum HCV RNA levels <50 IU per milliliter at 24 weeks after completing treatment) have progressively increased with the use of interferon (IFN) monotherapy (6–12%), to conventional IFN and ribavirin (RBV) (38–42%), and further more recently with pegylated interferon (Peg-IFN) and RBV (55–80%). Moreover, studies involving Peg-IFN and RBV therapy have shown SVR rates of 75–80% among people infected with HCV genotypes 2 or 3, whereas those with genotype 1 had response rates of only 40–45%. This has led to the development of standard treatment regimens for HCV genotype 1 which differ to those used for genotypes 2 or 3. However, emerging data are now necessitating that other viral, host, and drug-related factors be considered when treating patients with chronic HCV, and in this setting a recommendation adopting a fixed treatment strategy may not be applicable to all infected subjects. This chapter will discuss standard treatment regimens for genotype 2 and 3 HCV infections, and data on other emerging therapeutic approaches aimed at optimizing outcomes for these individuals.

Peginterferon Alfa and Ribavirin for Genotype 2 or 3

In the 1990s, several international multicenter randomized controlled trials used combination Peg-IFN and RBV

to treat HCV-infected subjects [1,2]. The study of Manns *et al.* included 448 subjects infected with genotypes 2 or 3 treated for 48 weeks. The three treatment groups were: IFN alfa-2b 3 million units thrice weekly plus weight-based RBV; Peg-IFN alfa-2b 1.5 mcg/kg weekly plus daily RBV 800 mg; and Peg-IFN alfa-2b 1.5 mcg/kg weekly for four weeks then 0.5 mcg/kg weekly plus weight-based RBV. The authors found comparable SVR rates of approximately 80% among the three treatment arms for HCV genotypes 2 or 3 infected subjects. The second study of Fried *et al.* included 152 patients infected with HCV genotype 2 and 202 infected with genotype 3. All patients received 48 weeks of treatment and were randomly assigned to three groups: Peg-IFN alfa-2a 180 mcg weekly plus daily weight-based RBV (1000 mg or 1200 mg); Peg-IFN alfa-2a 180 mcg weekly with placebo; or IFN alfa-2b 3 million units thrice weekly plus daily weight-based RBV (1000 mg or 1200 mg). The SVR rate for subjects treated with Peg-IFN alfa-2a and RBV was significantly higher than the other two treatment arms. Thus, the SVR rate for Peg-IFN alfa-2a and RBV was 76% compared to 61% for IFN alfa-2b plus RBV and 45% for Peg-IFN alfa-2a alone. Thus, these two large studies demonstrated that for patients infected with HCV genotypes 2 or 3, the combination of RBV with either Peg-IFN alfa-2a or Peg-IFN alfa-2b produced comparable, if not better, virologic response rates compared to either standard IFN plus RBV or Peg-IFN alone.

The study of Hadziyannis *et al.* [3] was designed to examine the effect of different treatment durations in HCV infection. Included in the study were 204 subjects infected with HCV genotype 2 and 288 infected with HCV genotype 3. Patients were randomly assigned to four groups. Subjects received either Peg-IFN alfa-2a 180 mcg weekly for either 24 or 48 weeks, plus either a flat dose

Advanced Therapy for Hepatitis C, First Edition. Edited by Geoffrey W. McCaughan, John G. McHutchison and Jean-Michel Pawlotsky.
© 2012 Blackwell Publishing Ltd. Published 2012 by Blackwell Publishing Ltd.

of RBV (800 mg) daily or a weight-based dose of RBV (1000 mg or 1200 mg) daily. The authors found comparable SVR rates in HCV genotype 2 or 3 infected subjects of approximately 80% in all four treatment arms. Therefore, this study suggested that 24 weeks of combination Peg-IFN with fixed-dose RBV is sufficient for treating HCV genotype 2 or 3 infected patients.

These initial results were confirmed by two further large clinical trials. In a phase IV, multicenter, single-arm, open-label, historical-control study [4], 224 patients infected with genotypes 2 or 3 were treated with Peg-IFN alfa-2b 1.5 mcg weekly plus weight based daily RBV (800 mg or 1400 mg) for 24 weeks. The overall SVR was 81%, which was comparable to the response rates reported in the previous pivotal studies where patients were treated for 24–48 weeks [1–3]. Another multicenter randomized trial conducted at 236 United States sites reported 476 patients infected with HCV genotype 2 or 3 [5]. Study subjects were assigned in four groups to receive either 24 or 48 weeks of Peg-IFN alfa-2b 1.5 mcg/kg weekly plus either a flat dose of RBV (800 mg) daily or a weight-based dose of RBV (800–1400 mg) daily. The authors again found comparable SVR rates between HCV genotype 2 or 3 infected subjects treated for 48 weeks (58.6%) and 24 weeks (66.2%). In addition, for those subjects treated for 24 weeks, there was also no difference in SVR rates between those who received weight-based RBV (67.7%) compared to those who received flat-dose RBV (65.0%). Hence, these later studies again confirmed that in HCV genotype 2 or 3 infections, 24 weeks of treatment with Peg-IFN and RBV is sufficient and that weight-based RBV dosing offers no added advantage over a fixed daily RBV dose of 800 mg.

Based on these findings, the current HCV treatment guidelines, including recommendations from both AASLD [6] and APASL [7], recommend that for HCV genotype 2 or 3 infections, a 24-week regimen with Peg-IFN in combination with RBV represents the current standard of care with SVR rates ranging from 70% to 80%. There is evidence, however, that these recommended guidelines can in clinical practice be modified to facilitate the management of individual patients without compromising the SVR rates [8].

Differences in Response to Treatment between HCV Genotype 2 and 3 Infections

HCV genotypes 2 and 3 are often grouped together for analysis in most clinical trials, as they are considered to

be the most favorable genotypes to treat in comparison to the others. There is, however, ample evidence to suggest that genotypes 2 and 3 behave differently in the host and respond differently to antiviral therapy. For instance, genotype 3 (but not genotype 2) has long been known to be associated with hepatic steatosis, which resolves with successful antiviral therapy. Moreover, there is evidence that genotype 3 is associated with accelerated fibrosis progression compared to genotype 2 [9,10].

Several studies have now reported significantly higher SVR rates in patients with genotype 2 compared to patients with genotype 3 infections [4,11,12]. This data was further confirmed in a subsequent meta-analysis [13], including data on 2275 treated patients from eight different trials. Hence, Andriulli *et al.* estimated overall SVR rates of 74% in patients infected with HCV genotype 2 versus 69% in patients with genotype 3 [13]. Further, the difference in response rates between the two genotypes was most significant among those patients with advanced fibrosis [13]. In patients with cirrhosis (fibrosis score of 4), the SVR rates of genotypes 2 and 3 were 78% and 17%, respectively. It therefore appears that the negative effect on treatment response of advanced fibrosis, especially cirrhosis, is limited to genotype 3 infections with no demonstrable effect on genotype 2. Thus, different treatment strategies may be required to treat the two genotypes. In particular, genotype 3 infected patients with advanced fibrosis may benefit from more intensive therapy.

Relevance of a Rapid Virological Response in HCV Genotype 2 or 3

Early virologic response (EVR), defined as a non-detectable HCV RNA level at week 12 of antiviral therapy, was shown to be associated with an SVR in genotype 1 HCV infections [14,15]. In contrast, in HCV genotype 2 or 3 infections, since almost 95% of patients achieve an EVR, this parameter is not useful in predicting long-term SVR rates. Rapid virologic response (RVR), defined as a non-detectable HCV RNA level at week 4, was found to be more useful clinically. The antiviral mechanism that leads to RVR has been best described by the biphasic pattern of HCV RNA decline, due to IFN's effect of blocking virion production or release (first-phase viral decline), followed by loss of infected cells (second-phase slope of viral decline) [16]. Further, with IFN therapy, the viral decline among genotype 2 patients is significantly more rapid than that for genotype 1 patients [17]. Thus, emerging evidence has characterized RVR (determined by sensitive assays) as a reliable predictor for SVR in HCV treated patients. For genotypes 2 and 3, an earlier study [4] treating 224 patients with Peg-IFN alfa-2b plus weight-based RBV for 24 weeks identified RVR as a strong predictor of SVR in this cohort. Thus, the SVR in genotype 1 or 3 infected patients who had undetectable serum HCV RNA levels by 4 weeks of combination therapy was 94% (31 of 33 patients) and 85% (117 of 137 patients), respectively. Further, in the same study in patients with genotype 3, but not genotype 2, RVR rates were higher for those with a low baseline HCV RNA level compared to those with a high baseline HCV RNA level (90% with baseline HCV RNA <600 000 IU/ml versus 79% HCV RNA >600 000 IU/ml) [4].

Subsequent randomized studies [12,18–21] comparing shorter treatment durations for genotype 2 or 3 infections (12–16 weeks) versus standard 24 weeks have confirmed the importance of RVR in guiding the duration of therapy for this group without compromising the SVR.

Peg-IFN Formulations, Ribavirin Dose, and Response to Treatment

Presently, there are two formulations of Peg-IFN commercially available, namely Peg-IFN alfa-2a (Pegasys™, Hoffmann-La Roche) and Peg-IFN alfa-2b (PEGINTRON™, Schering-Plough). The two available forms of Peg-IFN differ at a molecular level and whether they differ in clinical efficacy prompts an important issue. Peg-IFN alfa-2b is bound to a single linear 12 kDa polyethylene glycol molecule while Peg-IFN alfa-2a is covalently attached to a 40 kDa branched chain polyethylene glycol moiety. The difference in molecular structure between the two formulations of Peg-IFN leads to differences in both pharmacodynamics and pharmacokinetics. With respect to their effect on treatment outcomes, however, several studies have shown no differences in SVR rates between the two Peg-IFN formulations [22,23]. The latter data include the IDEAL trial [23], a randomized study comparing the two Peg-IFN regimens in 3070 patients infected with HCV genotype 1. Patients were randomized to receive a weekly injection of either Peg-IFN alfa-2b at the standard dose of 1.5 mcg/kg body weight, or at a lower dose of 1.0 mcg/kg, in combination with daily weight-based oral ribavirin (800–1400 mg). In the third arm of the study, patients received Peg-IFN alfa-2a at a dose of 180 mcg/week, plus oral ribavirin at a dose of 1000–1200 mg/day, according to body weight. The investigators found the SVR rates

did not differ significantly among the three treatment groups [23].

Very recently however, two investigator-initiated, randomized trials suggested superiority of the Peg-IFN alfa-2a preparation over Peg-IFN alfa-2b in the treatment of chronic HCV infections [24,25]. In this regard, Ascione et al. [24] enrolled 320 HCV-infected patients. An overall SVR was obtained in 68.8% with Peg-IFN alfa-2a versus 54.3% with the Peg-IFN alfa-2b regimen ($p = 0.008$). Among 186 patients infected with genotypes 1 or 4, an overall SVR was obtained in 47.3%, including 54.8% treated with Peg-IFN alfa-2a and 39.8% with Peg-IFN alfa-2b ($p = 0.04$). Similarly, in the 134 patients infected with genotypes 2 or 3, a SVR was achieved in 91.8% with Peg-IFN alfa-2a and 76% with Peg-IFN alfa-2b ($p = 0.06$). Specifically, patients infected with HCV genotype 2 demonstrated a superior response to Peg-IFN alfa-2a compared to those receiving Peg-IFN alfa-2b (SVR 91.8% versus 76%, respectively) while no difference in SVR rates was observed between the formulations for genotype 3 infections. Irrespective of genotype, SVR rates were not statistically different with either Peg-IFN formulation among patients with either baseline HCV RNA levels ≤500 000 IU/ml or in patients with cirrhosis [24]. In another comparative study, Rumi et al. [25] randomized 447 patients to receive either Peg-IFN alfa-2a or Peg-IFN alfa-2b. Again, overall SVR rates were higher in those receiving Peg-IFN alfa-2a compared to Peg-IFN alfa-2b (66% versus 54%, respectively, $p = 0.02$). Of the 222 patients infected with genotypes 1 or 4, the response to Peg-IFN alfa-2a was 48% versus 32% for Peg-IFN alfa-2b ($p = 0.04$). In 143 patients with genotype 2 infections, 96% treated with Peg-IFN alfa-2a achieved an SVR compared to 82% receiving Peg-IFN alfa-2b ($p = 0.01$). Consistent with Ascione et al.'s findings in genotype 3 infected patients, there was no difference in SVRs between the two Peg-IFN formulations. Additionally in both of these Italian studies, the use of Peg-IFN alfa-2a was independently predictive of an SVR. Overall, the results from the IDEAL and the two Italian studies are not comparable as these trials were designed differently with varying treatment strategies (different ribavirin dosing and dose-reduction protocols) and were conducted in very different populations (African American and Latinos versus European).

With respect to RBV dose, several studies in patients with HCV genotype 2 or 3 have clearly shown that 24-week treatment regimens containing an RBV dose higher than 800 mg per day does not achieve higher SVR rates [1–3]. Others, however, investigated the efficacy of combination therapy in patients with genotype 2 or 3 infections using a lower dose of RBV and concluded that in patients infected with HCV genotype 3, daily RBV 400 mg achieved comparable SVR rates to standard RBV 800 mg (SVR: 64% versus 68%, respectively) [26]. In contrast, in patients with HCV genotype 2, reducing the daily RBV dose to 400 mg resulted in significantly lower SVR rates compared to the standard RBV 800 mg regimen (55.6% versus 77.8%, respectively).

In contrast, patients receiving truncated RBV treatment regimens (14–16 weeks) seem to achieve higher SVR rates with weight-based rather than fixed or reduced RBV dosing. In this setting, several studies have shown relapse rates to be significantly lower with weight-based RBV compared to standard fixed-dose regimens [12,18,19,27,28]. Other data in support of higher RBV dosing comes from the ACCELERATE study [29], in which the effect of the cumulative exposure to RBV dose on the probability of achieving an SVR was assessed in over 1000 HCV patients with genotype 2 or 3 infection, while simultaneously controlling for other potential variables that could influence an SVR. The authors found that the highest SVR rate (87%) was observed in patients who received the longest duration and the highest mean dose of RBV based upon body weight. Despite this data, there have been no prospective randomized trials comparing weight-based and fixed RBV dosing in the setting of shortened treatment regimens.

Albinterferon in the Treatment of Hepatitis C Genotype 2 or 3

Albinterferon-α2b (albIFN) is a long-acting fusion polypeptide composed of albumin and IFN alfa-2b, exhibiting a prolonged half-life and duration of antiviral activity. This allows IFN dosing intervals of between 2 and 4 weeks [30]. In a phase II study of patients with genotype 2 or 3 HCV, albIFN 1500 mcg was administered either every 2 weeks or 4 weeks with daily RBV 800 mg for 24 weeks. Combination albIFN therapy achieved SVR rates of 62–77% [31]. RVR rates were 68.2% and 76.2% for the 4 weekly and 2 weekly dosage protocols, respectively, with corresponding SVR of 77.3% and 61.9%. Adverse events were not seen more frequently with albIFN than with Peg-IFN. Interestingly, the presence of insulin resistance at baseline was shown to influence viral decline with albIFN, independent of body mass index [31,32]. AlbIFN phase III trials in genotype 2 or 3 HCV infection are presently under way.

Duration of Treatment in Hepatitis C Genotype 2 or 3

The earlier data on high RVR rates in HCV genotype 2 or 3 infections has promoted interest in whether treatment duration can be individualized (i.e., either shortened or extended) in some patients (for full discussion of this topic, see Chapter 13). Thus, emerging data suggest that a subgroup of patients with genotype 2 or 3 infection may respond to a shorter duration of combination therapy to 12–16 weeks without compromising SVR rates [8,12,19]. Suitable patients are those who have a low baseline viral load, a BMI < 30 kg/m^2, and minimal hepatic fibrosis, who subsequently achieve an RVR [19,21].

Similarly, there may be other patient subgroups with genotype 2 or 3 HCV infection who would benefit from extended treatment duration to reduce relapse rates. Hence, a post hoc analysis of three large trials [2,3,29] found evidence for reduced relapse rates in genotype 2 and 3 patients with advanced liver disease as well as high baseline viral load when treated for 48 weeks compared to standard 24-week therapy [33]. Similarly, in patients without an RVR, the lowest relapse rates and the highest SVR rates were achieved with 48 weeks rather than 24 weeks of therapy. Despite these data, prospective comparative studies addressing the issue of extended therapy in these "difficult-to-treat" groups is still lacking and hence no definite recommendations can be made in this regard.

Treatment of Patients with Advanced Liver Disease

The use of Peg-IFN and RBV among patients with bridging fibrosis or compensated cirrhosis has been reported to achieve SVR rates of 13–41% for genotype 1 HCV infection and 70–80% for genotypes 2 and 3 [34,35]. In these patients, the baseline platelet count, RVR rate, and EVR rate were predictors of an SVR [36].

In the setting of compensated cirrhosis and portal hypertension, a study in 102 patients using Peg-IFN alfa-2b (1.0 μg/kg/week) and daily RBV 800 mg for 52 weeks achieved, as expected, improved SVR rates in patients with genotype 2 or 3 compared to genotype 1 (66.6% versus 11.3%, respectively) [37]. However, in the latter trial, the majority of patients were infected with genotype 1 (86%) while 9% had genotype 2 or 3 infection. Additionally, one third of the patients stopped treatment due to a variety of side effects.

Another challenging group to treat is patients with hepatic decompensation. In managing these patients, a low-accelerating dosage of weekly Peg-IFN alfa-2b 0.5 mcg/kg or Peg-IFN alfa-2a 90 mcg, given alone or in combination with daily RBV 400 mg is recommended. Subsequent drug doses are adjusted every 2 weeks based on treatment tolerance [38]. In this setting, SVR rates of 13% in patients infected with genotype 1 and 50% in patients infected with non-1 genotypes ($p < 0.0001$) have been reported. Another study went further by examining whether standard (rather than low accelerating) doses of antiviral therapy could be safely tolerated in decompensated cirrhotic patients [39]. In this study, 94 subjects with Child-Turcotte-Pughe score classes A or B, who had recovered from a previous episode of hepatic decompensation, received standard doses of Peg-IFN alfa-2b (1.5 mcg/kg) and RBV (800–1000 mg/day for genotypes 2 and 3 or 1000–1200 mg/day for genotypes 1 and 4) for the standard treatment durations (either 24 or 48 weeks). For the entire cohort the overall SVR rate was 35% with the majority of responders (56.8%) being in the genotype 2 or 3 groups. Erythropoietin and granulocyte growth factors were administered to 13% of treated subjects to manage cytopenias. Encouragingly, almost 60% of patients were able to tolerate full dosage and duration of treatment. However, 19% of patients discontinued treatment, including 4 who developed severe infections. Collectively, the data indicate that although response rates appear to be lower in cirrhotic patients with and without previous hepatic decompensation, successful antiviral therapy is still feasible in this subgroup, provided that subjects are carefully selected and followed (discussed in Chapter 17).

Predictors of Treatment Response: Other Factors to Consider

Adherence to therapy is undoubtedly an important factor in success of antiviral therapy. One study that pooled data from three previous clinical trials [40] found that patients who received more than 80% of Peg-IFN and RBV for more than 80% of the expected treatment duration had a higher chance of achieving a SVR than those who did not (63% versus 52%). Of interest, however, this observed difference in response rate was not observed in the subgroup of patients infected with genotypes 2 or 3, who were

found to have an SVR rate of around 90% regardless of treatment adherence. These surprising results were likely secondary to the excellent RVR rates observed with genotype 2 and 3 HCV infections, and so to find significant incremental virologic response rates with improved treatment adherence is likely to require larger study numbers. However, clearly these observations should not lessen the importance of emphasizing treatment adherence in these patients.

Several baseline host and virologic factors in genotype 2 and 3 HCV infections have also been identified to predict treatment responses. Factors associated with a lower SVR rate included older age, male gender, higher body weight, the presence of steatosis on liver biopsy, insulin resistance, higher fibrosis scores, and higher baseline viral loads [1–4]. These factors, however, have not yet led to modifications of current recommendations for standard of antiviral therapies.

Long-Term Outcome of Peg-IFN Alfa and RBV Treatment

An undetectable HCV RNA level at 6 months after antiviral therapy, namely SVR, is routinely regarded as the endpoint in all anti-HCV therapy trials. It is seen as a surrogate marker for long-term viral clearance, and has been shown in a number of previous treatment studies using either IFN monotherapy or combination standard IFN and RBV therapy to lead to improved fibrosis stage, reduced fibrosis progression rates, and better long-term clinical outcomes [41–46]. A study pooled the data from four previous randomized controlled trials containing ten different treatment regimens including 3010 patients (28% infected with genotypes 2 or 3) and compared subjects' pre-treatment and post-treatment liver biopsies [44]. The authors found that for patients treated with Peg-IFN alfa-2b and RBV, only 8% had worsened necroinflammatory scores while 73% had improved fibrosis scores; these findings were superior to the historical treatment regimens. Similarly, in patients with HCV-related, histologically proven cirrhosis, achievement of an SVR after antiviral therapy is associated with a reduction of liver-related mortality, lowering the risk of both hepatic decompensation and hepatocellular carcinoma (HCC) development [34]. However, irrespective of treatment-induced SVR, patients with cirrhosis should continue regular surveillance because the risk of subsequent development of HCC was not entirely avoided [34].

Summary and Conclusions

With present antiviral regimens we are able to achieve viral clearance in 70–80% of those patients infected with HCV genotype 2 or 3. There have been several studies suggesting different treatment strategies (shorter or longer treatment duration, higher ribavirin doses) aiming at further optimizing therapy in these patients. The data might not be conclusive as yet, but it is highly suggestive that we heading toward individualizing management and therapeutic regimens for patients with chronic HCV, even in patients with HCV genotype 2 or 3, and excellent overall results.

References

1. Manns MP, McHutchison JG, Gordon SC, *et al.* Peginterferon alfa-2b plus ribavirin compared with interferon alfa-2b plus ribavirin for initial treatment of chronic hepatitis C: a randomised trial. *Lancet* 2001;358:958–65.
2. Fried MW, Shiffman ML, Reddy KR, *et al.* Peginterferon alfa-2a plus ribavirin for chronic hepatitis C virus infection. *N Engl J Med* 2002;347:975–82.
3. Hadziyannis SJ, Sette H, Jr., Morgan TR, *et al.* Peginterferon-alpha2a and ribavirin combination therapy in chronic hepatitis C: a randomized study of treatment duration and ribavirin dose. *Ann Intern Med* 2004;140:346–55.
4. Zeuzem S, Hultcrantz R, Bourliere M, *et al.* Peginterferon alfa-2b plus ribavirin for treatment of chronic hepatitis C in previously untreated patients infected with HCV genotypes 2 or 3. *J Hepatol* 2004;40:993–9.
5. Jacobson IM, Brown RS, Jr., Freilich B, *et al.* Peginterferon alfa-2b and weight-based or flat-dose ribavirin in chronic hepatitis C patients: a randomized trial. *Hepatology* 2007;46:971–81.
6. Ghany MG, Strader DB, Thomas DL, Seeff LB. Diagnosis, management, and treatment of hepatitis C: an update. *Hepatology* 2009;49:1335–74.
7. McCaughan GW, Omata M, Amarapurkar D, *et al.* Asian Pacific Association for the Study of the Liver consensus statements on the diagnosis, management and treatment of hepatitis C virus infection. *J Gastroenterol Hepatol* 2007;22:615–33.
8. Dalgard O, Mangia A. Management of patients with hepatitis C virus genotype 2 or 3: comments on updated American Association for the Study of Liver Diseases practice guidelines. *Hepatology* 2009;50:323; author reply 4–5.
9. Poynard T, Ratziu V, Charlotte F, *et al.* Rates and risk factors of liver fibrosis progression in patients with chronic hepatitis C. *J Hepatol* 2001;34:730–39.
10. Bochud PY, Cai T, Overbeck K, *et al.* Genotype 3 is associated with accelerated fibrosis progression in chronic hepatitis C. *J Hepatol* 2009;51:655–66.
11. Powis J, Peltekian KM, Lee SS, *et al.* Exploring differences in response to treatment with peginterferon alpha 2a (40kD) and ribavirin in chronic hepatitis C between genotypes 2 and 3. *J Viral Hepatitis* 2008;15:52–7.
12. Mangia A, Santoro R, Minerva N, *et al.* Peginterferon alfa-2b and ribavirin for 12 vs. 24 weeks in HCV genotype 2 or 3. *N Engl J Med* 2005;352:2609–17.
13. Andriulli A, Mangia A, Iacobellis A, *et al.* Meta-analysis: the outcome of anti-viral therapy in HCV genotype 2 and genotype 3 infected patients with chronic hepatitis. *Aliment Pharmacol Ther* 2008;28:397–404.
14. Ferenci P, Fried MW, Shiffman ML, *et al.* Predicting sustained virological responses in chronic hepatitis C patients treated with peginterferon alfa-2a (40 KD)/ribavirin. *J Hepatol* 2005;43:425–33.
15. Di Bisceglie AM, Ghalib RH, Hamzeh FM, Rustgi VK. Early virologic response after peginterferon alpha-2a plus ribavirin or peginterferon alpha-2b plus ribavirin treatment in patients with chronic hepatitis C. *J Viral Hepatitis* 2007;14:721–9.
16. Neumann AU, Lam NP, Dahari H, *et al.* Hepatitis C viral dynamics in vivo and the antiviral efficacy of interferon-alpha therapy. *Science* 1998;282:103–7.
17. Neumann AU, Lam NP, Dahari H, *et al.* Differences in viral dynamics between genotypes 1 and 2 of hepatitis C virus. *J Infect Dis* 2000;182:28–35.
18. von Wagner M, Huber M, Berg T, *et al.* Peginterferon-alpha-2a (40KD) and ribavirin for 16 or 24 weeks in patients with genotype 2 or 3 chronic hepatitis C. *Gastroenterology* 2005;129:522–7.
19. Dalgard O, Bjoro K, Ring-Larsen H, *et al.* Pegylated interferon alfa and ribavirin for 14 versus 24 weeks in patients with hepatitis C virus genotype 2 or 3 and rapid virological response. *Hepatology* 2008;47:35–42.
20. Yu ML, Dai CY, Huang JF, *et al.* A randomised study of peginterferon and ribavirin for 16 versus 24 weeks in patients with genotype 2 chronic hepatitis C. *Gut* 2007;56:553–9.
21. Mangia A, Minerva N, Bacca D, *et al.* Determinants of relapse after a short (12 weeks) course of antiviral therapy and re-treatment efficacy of a prolonged course in patients with chronic hepatitis C virus genotype 2 or 3 infection. *Hepatology* 2009;49:358–63.
22. Escudero A, Rodriguez F, Serra MA, *et al.* Pegylated alpha-interferon-2a plus ribavirin compared with pegylated alpha-interferon-2b plus ribavirin for initial treatment of chronic hepatitis C virus: prospective, non-randomized study. *J Gastroenterol Hepatol* 2008;23:861–6.
23. McHutchison JG, Lawitz EJ, Shiffman ML, *et al.* Peginterferon alfa-2b or alfa-2a with ribavirin for treatment of hepatitis C infection. *N Engl J Med* 2009;361:580–93.

24. Ascione A, Luca MD, Tartaglione MT, *et al.* Peginterferon alfa-2a plus ribavirin is more effective than peginterferon alfa-2b plus ribavirin for treating chronic hepatitis C virus infection. *Gastroenterology* 2010;138(1):116–22.

25. Rumi M, Aghemo A, Prati GM, *et al.* Randomized study of peginterferon-alpha2a plus ribavirin vs peginterferon-alpha2b plus ribavirin in chronic hepatitis C. *Gastroenterology* 2010;138 (1): 108–15.

26. Ferenci P, Brunner H, Laferl H, *et al.* A randomized, prospective trial of ribavirin 400 mg/day versus 800 mg/day in combination with peginterferon alfa-2a in hepatitis C virus genotypes 2 and 3. *Hepatology* 2008;47:1816–23.

27. Lagging M, Langeland N, Pedersen C, *et al.* Randomized comparison of 12 or 24 weeks of peginterferon alpha-2a and ribavirin in chronic hepatitis C virus genotype 2/3 infection. *Hepatology* 2008;47:1837–45.

28. Shiffman ML, Ghany MG, Morgan TR, *et al.* Impact of reducing peginterferon alfa-2a and ribavirin dose during retreatment in patients with chronic hepatitis C. *Gastroenterology* 2007;132:103–12.

29. Shiffman ML, Suter F, Bacon BR, *et al.* Peginterferon alfa-2a and ribavirin for 16 or 24 weeks in HCV genotype 2 or 3. *N Engl J Med* 2007;357:124–34.

30. Subramanian GM, Fiscella M, Lamouse-Smith A, *et al.* Albinterferon alpha-2b: a genetic fusion protein for the treatment of chronic hepatitis C. *Nat Biotechnol* 2007;25: 1411–19.

31. Bain VG, Kaita KD, Marotta P, *et al.* Safety and antiviral activity of albinterferon alfa-2b dosed every four weeks in genotype 2/3 chronic hepatitis C patients. *Clin Gastroenterol Hepatol* 2008;6:701–6.

32. Neumann AU, Bain VG, Yoshida EM, *et al.* Early prediction of sustained virological response at day 3 of treatment with albinterferon-alpha-2b in patients with genotype 2/3 chronic hepatitis C. *Liver Int* 2009;29:1350–55.

33. Willems B, Hadziyannis S, Morgan TR, *et al.* Should treatment with peginterferon plus ribavirin be intensified in patients with HCV genotype 2/3 without a rapid virological response? *J Hepatol* 2007;46:S6.

34. Bruno S, Stroffolini T, Colombo M, *et al.* Sustained virological response to interferon-alpha is associated with improved outcome in HCV-related cirrhosis: a retrospective study. *Hepatology* 2007;45:579–87.

35. Heathcote EJ, Shiffman ML, Cooksley WG, *et al.* Peginterferon alfa-2a in patients with chronic hepatitis C and cirrhosis. *N Engl J Med* 2000;343:1673–80.

36. Roffi L, Colloredo G, Pioltelli P, *et al.* Pegylated interferon-alpha2b plus ribavirin: an efficacious and well-tolerated treatment regimen for patients with hepatitis C virus related histologically proven cirrhosis. *Antivir Ther* 2008;13: 663–73.

37. Di Marco V, Almasio PL, Ferraro D, *et al.* Peg-interferon alone or combined with ribavirin in HCV cirrhosis with portal hypertension: a randomized controlled trial. *J Hepatol* 2007;47:484–91.

38. Everson GT, Trotter J, Forman L, *et al.* Treatment of advanced hepatitis C with a low accelerating dosage regimen of antiviral therapy. *Hepatology* 2005;42:255–62.

39. Iacobellis A, Siciliano M, Annicchiarico BE, *et al.* Sustained virological responses following standard anti-viral therapy in decompensated HCV-infected cirrhotic patients. *Aliment Pharmacol Ther* 2009;30:146–53.

40. McHutchison JG, Manns M, Patel K, *et al.* Adherence to combination therapy enhances sustained response in genotype-1-infected patients with chronic hepatitis C. *Gastroenterology* 2002;123:1061–9.

41. Marcellin P, Boyer N, Gervais A, *et al.* Long-term histologic improvement and loss of detectable intrahepatic HCV RNA in patients with chronic hepatitis C and sustained response to interferon-alpha therapy. *Ann Intern Med* 1997;127: 875–81.

42. Lau DT, Kleiner DE, Ghany MG, *et al.* 10-Year follow-up after interferon-alpha therapy for chronic hepatitis C. *Hepatology* 1998;28:1121–7.

43. Shiratori Y, Imazeki F, Moriyama M, *et al.* Histologic improvement of fibrosis in patients with hepatitis C who have sustained response to interferon therapy. *Ann Intern Med* 2000;132:517–24.

44. Poynard T, McHutchison J, Manns M, *et al.* Impact of pegylated interferon alfa-2b and ribavirin on liver fibrosis in patients with chronic hepatitis C. *Gastroenterology* 2002;122:1303–13.

45. Veldt BJ, Heathcote EJ, Wedemeyer H, *et al.* Sustained virologic response and clinical outcomes in patients with chronic hepatitis C and advanced fibrosis. *Ann Intern Med* 2007;147:677–84.

46. George SL, Bacon BR, Brunt EM, *et al.* Clinical, virologic, histologic, and biochemical outcomes after successful HCV therapy: a 5-year follow-up of 150 patients. *Hepatology* 2009;49:729–38.

13

Altered Dosage or Durations of Current Antiviral Therapy for HCV Genotypes 2 and 3

Alessandra Mangia, Leonardo Mottola and Angelo Andriulli

IRCCS Casa Sollievo della Sofferenza, San Giovanni Rotondo, Italy

Background

Current guidelines for treating patients with genotype 2 or 3 chronic hepatitis C infection recommend pegylated interferon (Peg-IFN) and ribavirin to be administered for 24 weeks. Following this regimen, up to 80% of patients will be expected to ultimately clear HCV RNA [1,2]. Because therapy is expensive and commonly associated with frequent and at time serious side effects, treatment paradigms for these patients continue to evolve.

A number of clinical trials have recently reported that a substantial proportion of genotype 2 and 3 patients can experience a favorable outcome after abbreviated courses of therapy [3–6]. Because of substantial differences in the results achieved in these studies, the physician perception of the benefit of this innovative schedule of therapy has been hampered by the intrinsic variability of the design of available trials. It is of the utmost importance to fully understand these differences. Indeed, following the pivotal trial by Dalgard *et al.* in 2004 that proved the benefit of short therapy [3], some randomized studies explored the efficacy of a variable duration of therapy based on the treatment week 4 response: shortened duration was reserved to patients who had undetectable HCV RNA at week 4, whereas patients still viremic at this time point evaluation were kept on treatment for the standard 24 weeks [4–6]. By contrast, other studies evaluated the feasibility of reducing duration of therapy independently of an on-treatment response and assessed the therapeutic outcome after short or standard duration by randomizing patients at baseline [7–9].

We shall make a brief survey of therapeutic responses reported in trials on patients with chronic genotype 2 and 3 infection. We will separately consider the outcome of trials that adopted a variable length of treatment in accordance with on-treatment response at week 4, and of those that reported a direct comparison of standard or shortened duration in the whole population of patients.

Variable Length of Antiviral Therapy

The initial study that evaluated the benefit of a treatment shorter than 24 weeks for patients with genotype 2 and 3 was a non-randomized trial in which 122 patients, most of them bearing a genotype 3 infection, were treated with 1.5 μg/kg/week Peg-IFN alfa-2b and ribavirin at a dosage of 800–1400 mg/day [3]. In the trial design, patients with undetectable HCV RNA at week 4 (labeled as rapid virologic responders, RVR) had to stop therapy at week 14, whereas those without RVR were kept on treatment until week 24: 78% of patients attained an RVR, and 90% of them had a sustained virologic response (SVR) [3]. This proof-of concept study ascertained the feasibility of treating RVR patients with only 14 weeks of therapy.

Three randomized studies confirmed with an appropriate design the benefit of short therapy. We enrolled 283 Italian patients, the majority of them with genotype 2, to receive combination therapy of 1.0 μg/kg/week Peg-IFN alfa-2b with ribavirin at the dose of 1000–1200 mg/day [4]. Treatment duration had, per protocol, to be given for 24 weeks (control group) or could vary in accordance

Advanced Therapy for Hepatitis C, First Edition. Edited by Geoffrey W. McCaughan, John G. McHutchison and Jean-Michel Pawlotsky.
© 2012 Blackwell Publishing Ltd. Published 2012 by Blackwell Publishing Ltd.

Table 13.1 Features of patients and schedules of treatment in the studies evaluating the efficacy of short treatment in patients with RVR.

Authors	Mangia *et al.* [4]	von Wagner *et al.* [5]	Dalgard *et al.* [6]
Year of publication	2005	2005	2008
Total number of patients	283	153	428
Genotype 2 (*n*)	213	40	85
Genotype 3 (*n*)	70	123	343
Mean age (yr)	48.1	40.0	39.6
Male gender	56%	68%	63%
Mean body weight (kg)	69.4	76.6	78.0
Mean body mass index	26	—	25.3
Bridging fibrosis/cirrhosis (%)	24	n.a.	15
Viremia cut-off level (IU/ml)	800 000	800 000	400 000
Low viremic patients (%)	35	—	28.3
Patients with RVR (*n*)	178	142	298
Type of Peg-INF	2b	2a	2b
Dosage of Peg-INF	1.0 µg/kg/week	180 µg/week	1.5 µg/kg/week
Dosage of ribavirin (mg/day)	1000–1200	1000–1200	1000–1400

to the HCV RNA status at treatment week 4: patients with undetectable (≤ 50 IU/ml) HCV RNA at week 4 were allocated to therapy for 12 weeks, while individuals still viremic received treatment for 24 weeks. The RVR status was attained by two thirds of patients, and SVR was observed in 85% and 91% of patients allocated to the variable and standard duration groups, respectively. Among genotype 2 patients the respective SVR rates were 76% versus 82%, and 62% versus 76% among genotype 3 [4]. In a successive study by von Wagner *et al.* the RVR was defined as an undetectable viremia by a quantitative assay, with a threshold level of 600 IU/ml [5]. The trial enrolled 153 German patients, the majority of them infected with genotype 3, and randomized 142 RVR patients to a 16-week course or to standard duration: the SVR was reported in 82% and 80% of patients in the treatment arms, respectively [5]. The recent North-C study enrolled a total of 428 patients, 80% of them with genotype 3. The RVR status, assessed by an assay with a sensitivity of 50 IU/ml, was reported in 71.1% of patients, who were then randomized to 14 or 24 weeks of treatment: respective SVR rates were marginally better after standard treatment than after an abbreviated course (91% versus 81%) [6].

Summary data from the three randomized trials are presented in Table 13.1. After a careful reading of the data,

one encouraging and one cautionary note can be made: genotype 2 and 3 infected patients with viral clearance at treatment week 4 may efficaciously undergo therapy for ≤ 16 weeks, as they will clear the infection in about 85% of cases; on the cautionary side, patients with advanced fibrosis were under-represented in these trials and, until further data are available, they should continue to receive standard length of therapy.

Studies Randomizing Patients at Baseline to Short or Standard Treatment Duration

At variance with previous studies that reserved short therapy to the subset of patients with RVR, three other trials randomized at baseline all patients with genotype 2 and 3 infection to an abbreviated or a standard course of therapy [7–9]. It is important to keep in mind this difference in the design of these trials in order to appreciate or disprove the benefit of the innovative treatment schedule. Characteristics of patients enrolled in these new trials are shown in Table 13.2.

Shiffman *et al.* randomized patients at baseline to short (16 weeks) or standard (24 weeks) duration of Peg-IFN alfa-2a given in combination with a flat ribavirin dose

Table 13.2 Features of patients and schedules of treatment in the studies comparing head-to-head short versus standard treatment duration after randomization at baseline.

Authors	Shiffman et al. [7]	Yu et al. [8]	Lagging et al. [9]
Year of publication	2007	2007	2008
Total number of patients	1469	150	382
HCV genotype 2, n (%)	437 (30)	150 (100)	104 (27)
HCV genotype 3, n (%)	1026 (70)	—	276 (73)
Mean age (yr)	46.6	50.0	42.0
Male gender, n (%)	909 (62)	90 (60)	228 (62)
Mean body weight (kg)	81.6	65.8	78.0
Mean body mass index	27.7	25.0	26.0
Bridging fibrosis/cirrhosis, n (%)	350 (24)	31 (21)	140 (37)
Viremia cut off levels (IU/ml)	400 000	800 000	400 000
Low viremic patients, n (%)	307 (21)	126 (84)	102 (27)
Type of Peg-IFN	2a	2b	2a
Dosage of Peg-IFN μg/week	180	180	180
Dosage of ribavirin (mg/day)	800	1000–1200	800

(800 mg/day): the overall SVR rate was significantly lower in patients treated for 16 weeks than in those treated for 24 weeks (62% versus 70%), and this difference appeared totally secondary to the higher relapse rate registered in the short therapy arm (31% versus 18%) [7]. Although the authors advised against treating patients for less than 24 weeks, they reserved little attention to the finding that more patients in the 24-week arm were unable to tolerate the full course of therapy. Additionally, at a closer scrutiny of the trial data, genotype 2 patients attained SVR in 62% or 75% of cases after the abbreviated or the standard duration, respectively, a difference that could have been secondary to differences in viral load at baseline. Indeed, SVR rates were, respectively, 83% and 82% in low viremic (≤400 000 IU/ml) genotype 2 patients treated for the standard or the abbreviated therapy, and 73% versus 58% in high viremic individuals. Among genotype 3 patients, the overall SVR rates were 62% versus 66% after a short or standard therapy, 81% versus 81% in the subset of patients with low viremia, and 52% versus 59% in those with high viremia [7]. In addition, at a post hoc analysis of trial data 82% of patients with RVR attained an SVR, whereas this relevant outcome was achieved by only 27% of those without an RVR. Among RVR patients, 14% of individuals relapsed after 16 weeks of treatment, and 7% after 24 weeks. A more appropriate reading of the trial

data would indicate short treatment to be both sufficient and advantageous for genotype 2 and 3 patients with RVR.

Two subsequent, investigator-driven studies also randomized patients at baseline [8,9]. In a study from Taiwan, 150 HCV genotype 2 infected patients were treated with Peg-IFN alfa-2a and weight-based dosing of ribavirin (1000–1200 mg per day) for either 16 or 24 weeks: the overall SVR rates were not different between the two treatment schedules (94% versus 95%). Moreover, excellent rates were attained in both low viremic (<800 000 IU/ml) patients (95% versus 95%) and in high viremic individuals (89% versus 93%) [8]. However, the number of high viremic individuals in the study was very limited. In a Scandinavian study, Peg-IFN alfa-2a and a fixed dose of ribavirin (800 mg per day) given for 12 weeks proved inferior to 24 weeks either in the overall population of patients (SVR 59% versus 78%), and in the subgroup of patients with genotype 2 (SVR 56% versus 82%) or genotype 3 infection (SVR 58% versus 78%) [9]. This study was flawed, as 8.25% and 6.1% of patients in the two treatment arms failed to have a plasma sample drawn 24 weeks after completion of therapy and were classified on the basis of whether or not HCV RNA was detectable at the end of treatment.

Collectively in these studies, 707 of 963 patients (73%) attained an SVR after 24 weeks of treatment, and 658 of 1022 patients (64%) after 14–16 weeks. Therefore, for patients with genotypes 2 or 3 the response to current antiviral therapy was higher after 24 weeks treatment duration than after 12–16 weeks duration. Consequently, uncritical shortening of the treatment duration to less than 24 weeks in all genotype 2 and 3 patients should not be recommended as it may lead to unacceptably high rates of relapse. However, in the subset of patients with RVR, three randomized studies have reported similar rates after treating these patients with a short or a standard duration course. Therefore, we would advise short therapy to genotype 2 and 3 infected patients who are capable of attaining viral clearance at treatment week 4.

Conquering HCV Clearance in All Patients

The appreciation that after short therapy SVR rates were not higher than 85% would suggest that other factors, besides RVR, might be further delineated to push up these rates. Moreover, the higher relapse observed in the abbreviated regimen should be taken into consideration (Table 13.1). Consequently, two treatment strategies for RVR patients could be implemented. The first one would advise standard treatment duration for all patients, whereas the second would implement short therapy only for patients at low risk of relapse. The problem is now to better refine features of patients with lower likelihood of relapse. In our ongoing protocol, all RVR patients receive a 12-week course of Peg-IFN alfa-2b (1.5 μg/kg/week) and weight-based dose of ribavirin: of 496 individuals entered so far into the protocol, 96% attained an end-of-treatment response, but 14% of them relapsed after stopping therapy [10] (Table 13.3). By comparing baseline features of RVR patients with or without relapse, we found platelet counts and body mass index as the only two independent predictors of a favorable outcome: lean patients (BMI <30) with

normal (>140 000 cells) platelet count were the best candidates for short treatment as they experienced an SVR in 91.8% of case, whereas those with BMI >30 and/or low platelet count (<140 000) achieve after short therapy SVR rates not higher than 72.5% with a relapse rate of 27.5% [10].

It is of reassurance that the occurrence of relapse after short therapy did not impact negatively on the outcome of a repeat 24-week treatment. Indeed, of 43 RVR patients who relapsed after short therapy, 70% achieved an SVR after being re-treated for the standard 24-week duration [10]. On balance, the option to treat with a ≤16 week regimen lean patients without advanced fibrosis who attain an RVR, and reserve longer treatment for the minority of relapsers appears to benefit the great majority of patients with either genotype 2 and 3.

Optimal Treatment Duration for Non-RVR Patients

A third of patients with genotype 2 and 3 infection are still viremic at treatment week 4: this subset of patients has been recently delineated as difficult to treat with current treatment regimens. No formal investigations on longer length and higher dosage of drugs to be administered in these patients are yet available. Data from two studies [7,8] shown in Figure 13.1 demonstrated that in non-RVR patients the length of treatment seems of paramount relevance for achieving SVR. Indeed, in non-RVR patients the SVR rate ranged from 26% after short therapy to 46% after standard therapy in the Shiffman *et al.* trial [7], and from 41% to 62%, respectively, in the Lagging *et al.* study [9]. These data raise the question of whether such patients might benefit from more intensive treatments than the current 24-week regimen. In a retrospective analysis of data from five different trials [4,6,7,11,12], Willems

Table 13.3 Rates of relapse after short or standard duration treatment in the subset of patients infected with genotypes 2 and 3.

Study	SVR 12–16 weeks (%)	Relapse rate (%)	SVR 24 weeks (%)	Relapse rate (%)
Mangia *et al.* 2005 [4]	85	10	91	2
von Wagner *et al.* 2005 [5]	82	12	80	5
Yu *et al.* 2007 [8]	94	6	95	3
Dalgard *et al.* 2008 [6]	81	14	91	7
Shiffman *et al.* 2007 [7]	79	14	85	7

Figure 13.1 Summary of the different design of the studies on short treatment duration for patients with genotypes 2 and 3 HCV. Patients were directly randomized to treatment of different durations at baseline [7–9] or after achievement of RVR [6,10]. In the study by Mangia *et al.* [10], patients enrolled into the control arm received fixed 24 weeks of treatment irrespective of RVR; in the study by Dalgard *et al.* [6] patients with RVR were randomized to 14 or 24 weeks of treatment. In both studies patients without RVR received 24 weeks of treatment.

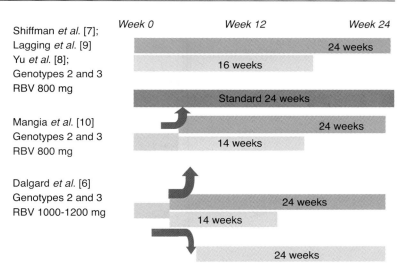

et al. have reported that, among patients without an RVR, the SVR rate was higher for patients receiving 48-week treatment than for those receiving 24-week (76% versus 65%) [13]. This difference was seen in both genotype 2 (75% versus 56%) and 3 (76% versus 68%) patients. These findings indicate that duration of therapy could be essential in improving the outcome for patients without RVR. Prospective data investigating the role of an intensified treatment in patients with genotype 3 have been published recently by our group. The results do not support the advantage of a course of treatment extended up to 36 weeks in patients without RVR [14]. The evaluation of the recently discovered *IL28B* genetic polymorphism as a major predictor of SVR in patients with genotype 2 and 3 suggests also that in patients without RVR the "good" CC-type of *IL28B* identifies patients with likelihood of achieving SVR [15]. Future studies are needed to confirm the predictive role in a large cohort of genotype 3 patients.

Dosages of Peginterferon Alfa

In two studies on variable treatment duration, Peg-IFN alfa-2b was administered at the dose of 1.5 μg/kg/week in combination with ribavirin [3,6], whereas a third study used a dose of 1.0 μg/kg/week [4]: the reported rates of either RVR and SVR did not differ. The lack of a dose-response effect for Peg-IFN alfa-2b raises the question of the optimal dose to be used in patients with genotypes 2 or 3. A formal trial addressing this point is lacking and we have to refer to the post hoc analysis of data

from the registration trial by Manns *et al.*: the dose of Peg-IFN correlated with the SVR rates among patients with genotype 1, but among those with genotypes 2 and 3 infection higher doses were equally effective as the 1.0 μg/kg dose [16].

The efficacy of 135 mcg/weekly dosage of Peg-IFN alfa-2a in combination with ribavirin in patients with non-1 genotype was investigated by Weiland *et al.*: Peg-IFN alfa-2a at a dose of 135 μg/weekly plus weight-based ribavirin for 24 weeks in 100 patients [17]. With this lower dose of Peg-IFN alfa 2a, SVR rates were attained in 85% and 86% of genotypes 2 and 3, respectively [17]. These rates appear to be comparable to those reported in the Hadziyannis *et al.* trial in patients treated for 24 weeks with standard 180 μg/weekly doses of Peg-IFN alfa-2a and either 800 mg or 1000–1200 mg of ribavirin (84% and 81%, respectively) [11]. Remarkably, RVR rate in this study was 70% for genotype 2 and 71% for genotype 3 patients.

Therefore, for treatment of genotype 2 and 3 infected patients, lower doses of either Peg-IFN alfa-2b and -2a may be used, when given in combination with ribavirin, although a formal trial addressing the issue is needed.

Dosages of Ribavirin

Ribavirin increases the initial viral kinetic response to interferon, potentially improving early virologic response and overall efficacy of treatment. The relationship between SVR and ribavirin dose depends on HCV genotype: in patients with genotype 1, but not in non-1 genotypes, the likelihood of achieving an SVR increases as a function of the ribavirin dose [18]. These observations suggest that a dose of 800 mg/day of ribavirin might be enough to maximize the likelihood of SVR in patients with genotype 2 or 3. However, these threshold doses were derived from two randomized studies that administered therapy for 24 or 48 weeks [11,12], and may not necessarily apply to studies on shorter duration of treatment. As a matter of fact, all the studies that established the benefit of a variable duration treatment in RVR patients administered ribavirin at a weight-based dosage and all reported low relapse rates [3–6]. By contrast, two out of three studies administered a flat dose (800 mg) of ribavirin in combination with Peg-IFN alfa-2a [7,8] and came out with higher relapse rates in the short therapy arms. These results suggest that the 800 mg dose of ribavirin attains optimal SVR rates after 24 weeks of therapy, while higher doses of the drug might be needed after shorter treatment.

Conclusions

A number of incremental advances have been made to improve therapeutic outcomes in chronic hepatitis C. For genotype 2 and 3 infection, the approved regimen includes Peg-IFN and ribavirin for 24 weeks, but several modifications of this regimen have been directed at reducing side effects and costs, and increasing tolerability and compliance. Currently, two strategies are contrasting each other: the first one would recommend standard 24-week duration for all genotype 2 and 3 infected patients without considering the on-treatment viral clearance; the second strategy would restrict short therapy to those who lack signs of advanced liver fibrosis at baseline and clear the virus at treatment week 4. Both strategies are expected to attain an SVR in about 90% of patients, but the second one offers the benefit of considerable economic savings and fewer side effects. Prolongation of treatment in patients with cirrhosis and in those without an RVR may improve the overall outcome, but needs confirmation in future trials.

References

1. Strader DB, Wright T, Thomas DL, Seeff LB. American Association for the Study of Liver Diseases. Diagnosis, management, and treatment of hepatitis C. *Hepatology* 2004;39(4):1147–71.

2. Ghany MG, Strader DB, Seef LB. Diagnosis, management, and treatment of hepatitis C: an update. *Hepatology* 2009;49:1335–74.

3. Dalgard O, Bjøro K, Hellum KB, et al. Treatment with pegylated interferon and ribavarin in HCV infection with genotype 2 or 3 for 14 weeks: a pilot study. *Hepatology* 2004;40:1260–65.

4. Mangia A, Santoro R, Minerva N et al. Peginterferon alpha-2b and RBV for 12 vs 24 weeks in HCV genotype 2 and 3. *N Engl J Med* 2005;35:2609–17

5. von Wagner H, Huber H, Berg T et al. Peginterferon-alpha-2a (40KD) and ribavirin for 16 or 24 weeks in patients with genotype 2 or 3 chronic hepatitis C. *Gastroenterology* 2005;129(2):522–7.

6. Dalgard O, Bjøro K, Ring-Larsen H, et al. Pegylated interferon alfa and ribavirin for 14 versus 24 weeks in patients with hepatitis C virus genotype 2 or 3 and rapid virological response. *Hepatology* 2008;47(1):35–42.

7. Shiffman ML, Suter F, Bacon BR, et al. Peginterferon alfa-2a and RBV for 16 or 24 weeks in HCV genotype 2 or 3. *N Engl J Med* 2007;357:124–34.

8. Yu ML, Dai CY, Huang JF, et al. A randomised study on PegInterferon and ribavirin for 16 versus 24 weeks in patients with genotype 2 chronic hepatitis C. *Gut* 2007;56:553–9.

9. Lagging M, Langeland N, Pedersen C, et al. Randomized comparison of 12 or 24 weeks of peginterferon alpha-2a and ribavirin in chronic hepatitis C virus genotype 2/3 infection. *Hepatology* 2008;47:1837–45.

10. Mangia A, Minerva N, Bacca D, et al. Determinants of relapse after a short (12 weeks) course of antiviral therapy and re-treatment efficacy of a prolonged course in patients with chronic HCV genotype 2 or 3 infection. *Hepatology* 2009;49:358–63

11. Hadziyannis SJ, Sette H, Jr., Morgan TR, et al. Peginterferon-alpha2a and ribavirin combination therapy in chronic hepatitis C: a randomized study of treatment duration and ribavirin dose. *Ann Intern Med* 2004;140:346–55.

12. Fried MW, Schiffman ML, Reddy KR, et al. Peginterferon alfa2a plus ribavirin for chronic hepatitis C virus infection. *N Engl J Med* 2002;347:975–82.

13. Willems B, Hadziyanni SJ, Morgan TR, et al. Should treatment with peginterferon plus ribavirin be intensified in patients with HCV genotype 2/3 without a rapid virologic response? *J Hepatol* 2007;46(Suppl 1): S6.

14. Mangia A, Bandiera F, Montalto G, et al. Individualized treatment with combination of Peg-interferon alpha 2b and ribavirin in patients infected with HCV genotype 3. *J Hepatol* 2010;53(6):1000–1005.

15. Mangia A, Thompson AJ, Santoro R, et al. Interleukin-28B polymorphism determines treatment response of patients with hepatitis C genotypes 2 and 3 who do not achieve a rapid virologic response. *Gastroenterology* 2010;139: 821–7.

16. Manns MP, McHutchinson JG, Gordon SC, *et al.* Peginterferon alfa-2b plus ribavirin compared with interferon alfa-2b plus ribavirin for initial treatment of chronic hepatitis C: a randomized trial. *Lancet* 2001;358:958–56.

17. Weiland O, Hollander A, Mattson L, *et al.* Lower tan standard dose of peg-IFN alfa-2a for chronic hepatitis C caused by genotype 2 and 3 is sufficient when given in combination with weight-based ribavirin. *J Viral Hepatitis* 2008;15:641–5.

18. Snoeck E, Wade JR, Duff F, *et al.* Predicting sustained virological response and anaemia in chronic hepatitis C patients treated with peginterferon alfa-2a plus ribavirin. *Br J Clin Pharmacol* 2006;62:699–709.

14 Genotypes 2 and 3 Relapse and Non-response

Stella Martínez, Jose María Sánchez-Tapias and Xavier Forns

Liver Unit, Hospital Clinic, IDIBAPS, and Ciberehd (Centro de Investigación en Red de Enfermedades Hepáticas y Digestivas), Barcelona, Spain

Background

In patients with chronic hepatitis C who undergo antiviral therapy the most important prognostic factor at baseline is the infecting genotype. Patients with chronic hepatitis C infected with genotypes 2 or 3 (G2/G3) have a significantly better response as compared to those infected with genotype 1. These patients are currently treated with pegylated interferon and ribavirin for 24 weeks. The doses of ribavirin (800 mg/day) and the duration of therapy (24 weeks) are based on the results obtained by the study of Hadziyannis et al. [1]. In this study, patients were randomized to receive peginterferon alfa-2a and ribavirin (800 mg/d versus 1000–1200 mg/d) with two different treatment durations (24 weeks versus 48 weeks). Sustained virologic response (SVR) rates were similar in patients treated with either dose of ribavirin and with either treatment duration, ranging from 84% in the 24-week low-dose ribavirin group to 79% in the 48-week low-dose ribavirin group [1].

Probably because of the high rate of success, there has been little effort to find out better strategies for G2/G3 non-responders. In fact, most of the clinical trials in G2/G3 infected patients have focused on shortening treatment regimens for those individuals with a good virologic profile [2–7]. Thus, the information on antiviral therapy in G2/G3 relapsers or non-responders is scarce. Similarly, the development of new antiviral components (mainly protease and polymerase inhibitors) is focused on individuals infected with genotype 1. The latter underscores the relevance of improving the efficacy of current antiviral therapy in G2/G3 infected patients.

Why Do Patients Infected with Genotypes 2 and 3 Not Have SVR?

There are three different situations that can prevent SVR in HCV-infected patients: (i) non-response (lack of HCV RNA clearance during therapy); (ii) virologic breakthrough (HCV RNA clearance during therapy but reappearance before treatment withdrawal); and (iii) relapse (HCV RNA clearance during therapy but reappearance after treatment withdrawal). Treatment failure in patients with chronic hepatitis C infected with genotypes 2 or 3 is largely due to virologic relapse after treatment withdrawal (Table 14.1) [1,3,4,6–9]. Data on the end of treatment (EOT) response in large clinical trials show that around 90% of these patients achieve HCV RNA clearance by the end of treatment. In fact, a per protocol analysis of the data shows that the figure can be even better: in the largest clinical trial performed in patients with chronic hepatitis C infected with G2/G3 almost 95% of individuals who completed therapy achieved EOT response [6]. Thus, true non-responders to therapy represent only a small subset of patients, whereas relapse is largely the main reason explaining treatment failure in patients.

Preventing Treatment Failure in G2/G3 Patients

Identification of naïve G2/G3 infected patients with a high probability of relapse or non-response is important before starting antiviral therapy. Most of the studies identify the same predictors of treatment failure. In the

Advanced Therapy for Hepatitis C, First Edition. Edited by Geoffrey W. McCaughan, John G. McHutchison and Jean-Michel Pawlotsky.
© 2012 Blackwell Publishing Ltd. Published 2012 by Blackwell Publishing Ltd.

Table 14.1 Rates of end of treatment (EOT) response and SVR in genotype 2 and genotype 3 patients treated with pegylated interferon and ribavirin [1,3,4,6–9].

Study	EOT	SVR
Hadziyannis et al. [1]		
ITT	431/492 (88)	398/492 (81)
Per protocol		
Shiffman et al. [6]		
ITT	1247/1469 (85)	965/1469 (65)
Per protocol	1247/1333 (94)	965/1319 (73)
Von Wagner et al. [7]		
ITT	135/153 (88)	119/153 (78)
Per protocol	135/144 (94)	119/135 (88)
Mangia et al. [4]		
ITT	235/283 (83)	217/283 (77)
Per protocol	235/274 (86)	217/274 (79)
Dalgard et al. [9]		
ITT	377/428 (88)	326/428 (76)
Per protocol	377/403 (94)	326/403 (81)
Lagging et al. [3]		
ITT	294/380 (77)	258/380 (68)
Per protocol	294/324 (91)	/324 (79)
Ferenci et al. [8]		
ITT	240/282 (85)	187/282 (66)
Per protocol	240/250 (96)	187/250 (75)

ITT, intention to treat.
Per protocol analyses did not include patients who were lost to follow-up.

ACCELERATE trial [6] the main variables associated with relapse after antiviral therapy were infection with genotype 3 (versus genotype 2), baseline viral load (>400 000 IU/ml), age > 45 years, weight > 80 kg, and bridging fibrosis or cirrhosis. Importantly, SVR was significantly lower among patients without a rapid virologic response (RVR, defined as undetectable HCV RNA at week 4 of therapy) (Figure 14.1). SVR in patients who achieved rapid virologic response (RVR) reached 85% in the 24-week treatment arm and 79% in the 16-week treatment arm. The same figures for patients who did not achieve RVR were respectively 45% and 26%. The significant differences in SVR reflect the higher relapse rate in the latter group (non-RVR). From this and other studies it is obvious that there is a subset of patients with G2/G3 chronic hepatitis C who have suboptimal response to standard of care treatment. What can we do to prevent treatment failure in these patients?

The first strategy to increase efficacy is treatment compliance, which should be encouraged in all individuals undergoing therapy. The second strategy might be to increase the dose of ribavirin or to extend treatment duration in those individuals with a high probability of not achieving SVR. Regretfully, there are very few evidence-based data regarding these two strategies in treatment-naïve patients.

As stated above, a fixed 800 mg dose of ribavirin is considered optimal in G2/G3-infected patients. However, most studies assessing the efficacy of abbreviated treatment regimens have used 1000–1200 mg/d of ribavirin, and one may speculate that the high rates of SVR in short treatment regimens might be explained by the high dose of ribavirin administered. Nevertheless, there are no data supporting this hypothesis. The Hadziyannis et al. study [1] was not designed to explore if weight-based ribavirin administration would be beneficial in slow virologic responders, but a retrospective analysis of the data from this trial partially addressed this question [10]. In this study, there were no significant differences in relapse rates among non-RVR who underwent treatment with 800 mg/d versus 1000–1200 mg/d of ribavirin (26% versus 24%). Moreover, Ferenci and collaborators [8] have recently shown that the dose of ribavirin can be further reduced without compromising efficacy. In this study 282 G2/G3 treatment-naïve patients were randomized to 24 weeks of treatment with ribavirin 800 mg/day or 400 mg/day plus peginterferon alfa-2a. The study did not find significant differences in the rate of SVR between both groups (69% versus 64%, respectively). Unfortunately, a separate subanalysis on the impact of the ribavirin dosing in individuals who did not achieve a RVR was not reported.

Regarding the possibility of extending the duration of therapy in patients with low chances to achieve SVR, the data are very limited. A retrospective analysis of data from the Hadziyannis et al. study compared the rates of SVR among non-rapid virologic responders who underwent 24 versus 48 weeks of treatment [10]. Relapse rates were significantly lower (8%) in patients who underwent 48 weeks of peglyated interferon alfa-2a plus ribavirin compared to those who were treated for 24 weeks (25%) (Figure 14.2). This would support that extending treatment duration to 48 weeks may be useful in patients who did not achieve an RVR. It is important to notice, however, that the number of patients included in this retrospective data analysis was relatively small. More recent data do not support the potential value of extended treatment duration, at least in G3-infected patients. In fact, Mangia and coworkers

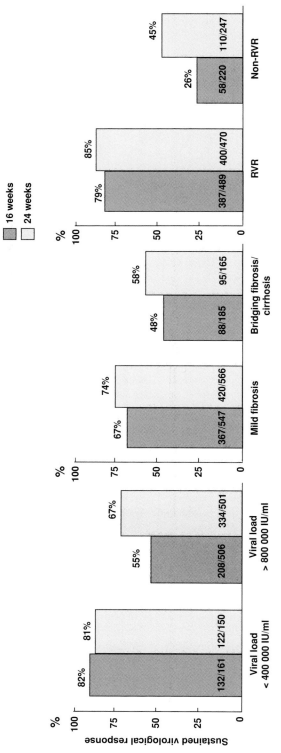

Figure 14.1 Rates of SVR in G2/G3 patients depending on baseline viral load, liver fibrosis, and rapid virologic response [6].

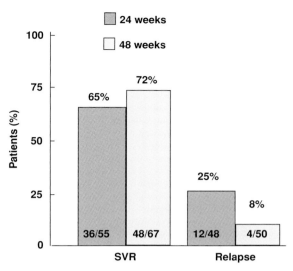

Figure 14.2 Rates of SVR and relapse in G2/G3 patients depending on the duration of therapy [10].

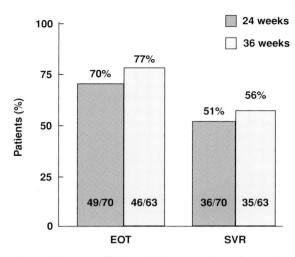

Figure 14.3 Rates of SVR in G2/G3 patients depending on the duration of therapy [11].

[11] analyzed whether extended duration of therapy with pegylated interferon alfa-2b and weight-based ribavirin was useful in G3 infected patients who did not achieve an RVR. In a multicenter Italian study 414 G3-infected patients were randomized to a standard 24-week regimen ($n = 207$) or to a variable treatment duration regimen ($n = 207$). In the latter group, patients who achieved an RVR underwent 12 weeks of treatment and those who did not achieve an RVR were treated for 36 weeks. In non-rapid virologic responders, the end of treatment and SVR were similar for patients treated for 24 or 36 weeks (Figure 14.3). Obviously, the data argue against longer treatment duration regimens in naïve G3-infected patients who do not achieve an RVR. However, a controlled clinical trial evaluating a 48-week duration is still lacking.

Studies evaluating the efficacy of short treatment regimens have recently shown that there are patients who may benefit from a short course (12–16 weeks) of treatment. However, the latter studies have also demonstrated that, similar to what is found with standard of care (24 weeks) treatment regimens, some variables predict treatment failure (mainly relapse) when short duration regimens are used: age >45 years, significant fibrosis or cirrhosis, body mass index above 30, high viral load (>400 000 IU/ml), and, most importantly, the lack of an RVR [12]. In order to reduce the rates of treatment failure, short treatment regimens should be avoided in individuals with any of these characteristics.

Management of Relapse or Non-response to Antiviral Therapy

Investigation of compliance in past treatment courses is probably the first issue that requires investigation in patients who experienced a treatment failure: taking the full dose of ribavirin and interferon, as well as completing the entire duration of the treatment, are important to prevent virologic relapse or non-response [12–14]. In individuals who were not compliant or in whom treatment was interrupted, the reasons for dose reduction or treatment discontinuation need to be carefully investigated. Adverse events such as anxiety, depression, neutropenia, or anemia could be properly managed in a second course of therapy, and thus the chances of completing a full treatment course (and thereby achieving an SVR) are increased. Intervention on some of the host factors that are associated with a poor response to therapy may also be helpful to increase the chances of viral clearance. Obesity, defined as a body mass index higher than 30, as well as insulin resistance and hepatic steatosis, have been shown to decrease the likelihood of viral clearance following antiviral therapy [14]. Dietary changes and exercise in order to decrease weight and treatment of insulin resistance may be helpful in some patients who did not respond to an initial course of therapy [15].

There are a number of studies that have assessed the efficacy of re-treatment in patients who failed a first course of therapy [16–31]. As expected, most of these studies included a large number of G1-infected patients and thus data on G2/G3-infected individuals are limited. As shown in Table 14.2, the efficacy of re-treatment varies greatly depending on the study: causes that explain the differences are various, such as different treatment regimens as initial therapy, baseline characteristics of patients, and the inclusion criteria. Probably, HALT-C and, particularly, EPIC are the two studies that have provided the more solid information on re-treatment of G2/G3 patients [25,28]. Both studies were focused on patients with advanced fibrosis and were designed to evaluate the efficacy of a second course of therapy (48 weeks) in previous non-responders; in the two studies patients who did not achieve a virologic response following 12–20 weeks of re-treatment were randomized to long-term peginterferon therapy versus no treatment. In this chapter we will not analyze the results of maintenance therapy.

The EPIC study [25] recruited relapsers and non-responders to a previous course of interferon (standard or pegylated) plus ribavirin. Only individuals with significant liver fibrosis were included (F2–F4). A total of 2293 patients (367 infected with G2/G3) were re-treated with peginterferon alfa-2b (1.5 μg/kg/wk) plus weight-based ribavirin (800–1400 mg/d) for 48 weeks. Overall 22% (497/2293) of individuals achieved SVR; among G2/G3 patients 55% (203/367) were sustained virologic responders. The variables that were independently related to SVR in a multivariate regression analysis were genotype (2/3 versus 1), baseline METAVIR score (F2 versus F4, F3 versus F4), baseline viral load (<600 000 IU/ml versus > 600 000 IU/ml), previous treatment (interferon/ribavirin versus peginterferon/ribavirin), and previous response (relapse versus non-response). The specific data for G2/G3 patients are shown in Figure 14.4. An important observation from this study was the predictive value of early virologic response: SVR occurred in 70% (196/281) of individuals with undetectable HCV RNA (<125 IU/ml) at week 12.

The results of the HALT-C trial [28] are similar to those discussed above. The study included non-responders to interferon or interferon plus ribavirin; non-response was defined as having detectable HCV RNA in serum for at least 12 weeks and within 4 weeks of completing therapy. All patients had advanced fibrosis (F3 or F4). Re-treatment consisted in peginterferon alfa-2a (180 μg/wk) and ribavirin (1000–1200 mg/d). A total of 604 patients (57 infected with G2/G3) had undetectable HCV RNA (<100 IU/ml) at week 20 and remained on therapy for 48 weeks. Overall, only 18% of patients achieved an SVR. The figure for G2/G3 patients was 60%. Variables inde-

pendently related to SVR were genotype 2 or 3, previous interferon monotherapy (as compared to combination treatment), absence of cirrhosis, and a viral load <1 500 000 IU/ml.

A recent meta-analysis [32] tried to analyze the factors that were associated with SVR in previous non-responders to interferon and ribavirin therapy. The meta-analysis included randomized controlled studies or prospective cohort studies; patients were non-responders to standard or pegylated IFN and ribavirin combination treatment. Importantly, non-response was defined as the presence of HCV RNA 3 or 6 months after treatment initiation. Re-treatment was performed with pegylated interferon and ribavirin. After review, a total of 14 full papers (including close to 4000 patients) fulfilled the inclusion criteria. Data on SVR rates according to genotype infection (1 versus non-1) were reported in only seven trials. SVR was significantly higher in non-1 genotype patients (34%) as compared to genotype 1 individuals (16%) ($p < 0.001$).

It seems clear from all these studies (Table 14.2) that re-treatment of G2/G3 patients can be successful in a significant proportion of individuals, particularly if they received interferon monotherapy, were relapsers to a previous course of treatment, have low viral load and mild fibrosis at baseline, and, more importantly, if they cleared HCV RNA by week 12. In most of these studies the duration of therapy was 48 weeks and the dose of ribavirin was weight based. Thus, the current recommendation might be to re-treat these patients for 48 weeks and with weight-dosed ribavirin; treatment should be interrupted in patients who do not clear HCV RNA by week 12.

Management of Relapse in Patients Who Underwent Short Treatment Regimens

In a recent study, Mangia and collaborators [5] assessed the efficacy of re-treatment in patients with chronic hepatitis C infected with G2/G3 who underwent a short treatment regimen and relapsed. An initial cohort of 718 G2/G3 infected patients underwent treatment with pegylated interferon alfa-2b and ribavirin (1000–1200 mg/d); 496 (69%) were rapid virologic responders and underwent a 12-week course of treatment. SVR was achieved in 409 (82%) whereas 67 (14%) were relapsers. Relapse was independently related to a low platelet count (probably reflecting advanced fibrosis) and high body mass index. Importantly, 43 relapsers agreed on a second course of treatment (24 weeks) and 30 (70%) achieved a SVR. Though the population included in this study is a "selected" cohort of

Table 14.2 Randomized trials of pegylated interferon plus ribavirin for the re-treatment of chronic hepatitis C: results in non-1 genotypes.

Study	n	Patient type and previous therapy	Re-treatment regimen	EOT (%)	SVR (%)		
					All	R	NR
Poynard et al. [25]	367[a]	Non-responders (137), relapsers (173), or treatment failures (57) to IFN/Peg-IFN plus RBV	Peginterferon alfa-2b plus RBV (WB) for 48 weeks	77[c]	55	61	46
Carr et al. [17]	197[b]	Previous IFN or IFN plus RBV treatment; non-response or relapse	IFN plus RBV or Peginterferon alfa-2b plus RBV (induction phase in some patients)	70	59	n.a.	n.a.
Jacobson et al. [20]	26[a]	Non-responders to IFN or IFN plus RBV, relapsers to combination therapy	Peginterferon alfa-2b plus RBV for 48 weeks	n.a.	31		
Shiffman et al. [28]	57[a]	Non-response to IFN or IFN plus RBV	Peginterferon alfa-2a plus ribavirin (WB) for 48 weeks	79	60	—	60
Mangia et al. [5]	43[a]	Relapsers to pegylated interferon and ribavirin (WB) for 12 weeks (rapid virologic responders)	Peginterferon alfa-2b plus ribavirin (WB) for 24 weeks	77	70		
Krawitt et al. [22]	24[a]	Non-responders (7) or relapsers (17) to IFN monotherapy or IFN plus RBV	Peginterferon alfa-2b plus RBV for 48 weeks	n.a.	58	59	57
Parise et al. [24]	37[a]	Non-responders (27) or relapsers (10) to IFN plus RBV	Peginterferon alfa-2a plus RBV for 48 weeks	n.a.	53	70	46
Sherman et al. [27]	59[a]	Non-responders (28) or relapsers (31) to IFN monotherapy or IFN plus RBV	Peginterferon alfa-2a plus RBV for 24-48 weeks (most of them 48 weeks)	n.a.	47	55	39
Taliani et al. [29]	20[a]	Non-responders to IFN plus RBV	Peginterferon alfa-2b plus RBV (WB) for 48 weeks	40	30	—	30
Basso et al. [16]	28[a]	Relapsers to IFN plus RBV	Peginterferon alfa-2b (1 μg/kg/w) plus RBV (WB) for 24 weeks	86	79	—	79
Ciancio et al. [18]	17[a]	Non-responders to IFN plus RBV	Peginterferon alfa-2a plus RBV (WB) ± amantadine for 48 weeks	76	76	—	76
Sagir et al. [26]	21[a]	Non-responders (13) or relapsers (8) to IFN or IFN plus RBV	IFN or Peg-IFN plus RBV (WB) for 24 weeks	52	38		
Jensen et al. [21]	31[b]	Non-response to Peginteferon alfa-2b plus RBV	Peginterferon alfa-2a plus RBV (WB) for 48–72 weeks	n.a.	~25[d]		~25
Moucari et al. [31]	34[b]	Relapsers or non-responders to standard IFN plus RBV	Peginterferon alfa-2b plus RBV (WB)	n.a.	43	60	29

[a]Genotypes 2 and 3, [b]Non-1 genotype, [c]Undetectable HCV RNA at week 12, [d]>50% genotype 4. IFN, interferon; RBV, ribavirin; WB, weight-based.

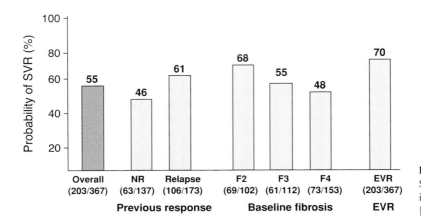

Figure 14.4 Variables associated with SVR in previous non-responders to interferon/peginterferon plus ribavirin [25].

relapsers (12-week treatment regimen), the data are relevant since treatment compliance was excellent: 96% of individuals received 80% of both ribavirin and interferon for 80% of the expected time. The study clearly suggests that short antiviral regimens are not appropriate in G2/G3 patients with advanced fibrosis and in those with obesity; however, the data also demonstrate that re-treatment with a longer regimen (24 weeks) is effective in most of them.

Future Therapies for Patients Who Experienced a Treatment Failure

Other types of interferon molecules (such as consensus interferon) have been used in non-responders to standard of care therapy, but most of the data were obtained in genotype 1 infected patients. A great effort has been made in the past few years to develop new drugs directly targeting HCV proteins. Two new protease inhibitors will be available to treat HCV-infected patients during 2011. Currently, almost all available data have been obtained in G1 infected patients. Telaprevir has been tested in a small cohort of G2-infected patients both in monotherapy and combined with pegylated interferon and ribavirin [33]. In both cases, significant reductions in viral load (3 to 5.3 $\log_{10}$) have been obtained. Regretfully, the efficacy in G3 infected patients appears to be very low. Recent data obtained with nucleoside and non-nucleoside polymerase inhibitors have shown that these drugs may be very effective in the treatment of G2/G3 infection.

Addendum: In the past few months there have been a number of studies evaluating the potential role of *IL28B*

genotypes in individuals infected with G2/G3 undergoing antiviral therapy. Although the results are still a matter of controversy, it appears that a favorable *IL28B* background might be associated with higher SVR rates in those individuals who do not achieve an RVR [34].

Acknowledgments

We are grateful to Kristian Bjøro and Neil Buss for providing some additional data.

References

1. Hadziyannis SJ, Sette H, Jr., Morgan TR, *et al.* Peginterferon-alpha2a and ribavirin combination therapy in chronic hepatitis C: a randomized study of treatment duration and ribavirin dose. *Ann Intern Med* 2004;140(5):346–55.
2. Dalgard O, Bjøro K, Hellum KB, *et al.* Treatment with pegylated interferon and ribavarin in HCV infection with genotype 2 or 3 for 14 weeks: a pilot study. *Hepatology* 2004; 40(6):1260–65.
3. Lagging M, Langeland N, Pedersen C, *et al.* Randomized comparison of 12 or 24 weeks of peginterferon alpha-2a and ribavirin in chronic hepatitis C virus genotype 2/3 infection. *Hepatology* 2008;47(6):1837–45.
4. Mangia A, Santoro R, Minerva N, *et al.* Peginterferon alfa-2b and ribavirin for 12 vs. 24 weeks in HCV genotype 2 or 3. *N Engl J Med* 2005;352(25):2609–17.
5. Mangia A, Minerva N, Bacca D, *et al.* Determinants of relapse after a short (12 weeks) course of antiviral therapy and re-treatment efficacy of a prolonged course in patients with chronic hepatitis C virus genotype 2 or 3 infection. *Hepatology* 2009;49(2):358–63.

6. Shiffman ML, Suter F, Bacon BR, *et al.* Peginterferon alfa-2a and ribavirin for 16 or 24 weeks in HCV genotype 2 or 3. *N Engl J Med* 2007;357(2):124–34.

7. von Wagner M, Huber M, Berg T, *et al.* Peginterferon-alpha-2a (40KD) and ribavirin for 16 or 24 weeks in patients with genotype 2 or 3 chronic hepatitis C. *Gastroenterology* 2005; 129(2):522–7.

8. Ferenci P, Brunner H, Laferl H, *et al.* A randomized, prospective trial of ribavirin 400 mg/day versus 800 mg/day in combination with peginterferon alfa-2a in hepatitis C virus genotypes 2 and 3. *Hepatology* 2008;47(6):1816–23.

9. Dalgard O, Bjøro K, Ring-Larsen H, *et al.* Pegylated interferon alfa and ribavirin for 14 versus 24 weeks in patients with hepatitis C virus genotype 2 or 3 and rapid virological response. *Hepatology* 2008;47(1):35–42.

10. Willems B, Hadziyannis S, Morgan TR, *et al.* Should treatment with peginterferon plus ribavirin be intensified in patients with HCV genotype 2/3 without a virological response? *J Hepatol* 2007;46:S6.

11. Mangia A, Bandiera F, Montalto G, *et al.* Individualized treatment with combination of peginterferon alpha 2b and ribavirin in patients infected with HCV genotype 3. *J Hepatol* 2010;53:1000–1005.

12. Zeuzem S, Rizzetto M, Ferenci P, Shiffman ML. Management of hepatitis C virus genotype 2 or 3 infection: treatment optimization on the basis of virological response. *Antivir Ther* 2009;14(2):143–54.

13. Tarantino G, Craxi A. Optimizing the treatment of chronic hepatitis due to hepatitis C virus genotypes 2 and 3: a review. *Liver Int* 2009;29(Suppl 1):31–8.

14. Heathcote J. Retreatment of chronic hepatitis C: who and how? *Liver Int* 2009;29(Suppl 1):49–56.

15. Romero-Gomez M, Diago M, Andrade RJ, *et al.* Treatment of insulin resistance with metformin in naïve genotype 1 chronic hepatitis C patients receiving peginterferon alfa-2a plus ribavirin. *Hepatology* 2009;50(6):1702–8.

16. Basso M, Torre F, Grasso A, *et al.* Pegylated interferon and ribavirin in re-treatment of responder-relapser HCV patients. *Digest Liver Dis* 2007;39(1):47–51.

17. Carr C, Hollinger FB, Yoffe B, *et al.* Efficacy of interferon alpha-2b induction therapy before retreatment for chronic hepatitis C. *Liver Int* 2007;27(8):1111–18.

18. Ciancio A, Picciotto A, Giordanino C, *et al.* A randomized trial of pegylated-interferon-alpha2a plus ribavirin with or without amantadine in the re-treatment of patients with chronic hepatitis C not responding to standard interferon and ribavirin. *Aliment Pharmacol Ther* 2006;24(7):1079–86.

19. Herrine SK, Brown RS, Jr., Bernstein DE, *et al.* Peginterferon alfa-2a combination therapies in chronic hepatitis C patients who relapsed after or had a viral breakthrough on therapy with standard interferon alpha-2b plus ribavirin: a

pilot study of efficacy and safety. *Digest Dis Sci* 2005;50(4):719–26.

20. Jacobson IM, Gonzalez SA, Ahmed F, *et al.* A randomized trial of pegylated interferon alpha-2b plus ribavirin in the retreatment of chronic hepatitis C. *Am J Gastroenterol* 2005;100(11):2453–62.

21. Jensen DM, Marcellin P, Freilich B, *et al.* Re-treatment of patients with chronic hepatitis C who do not respond to peginterferon-alpha2b: a randomized trial. *Ann Intern Med* 2009;150(8):528–40.

22. Krawitt EL, Ashikaga T, Gordon SR, *et al.* Peginterferon alfa-2b and ribavirin for treatment-refractory chronic hepatitis C. *J Hepatol* 2005;43(2):243–9.

23. Mathew A, Peiffer LP, Rhoades K, McGarrity T. Sustained viral response to pegylated interferon alpha-2b and ribavirin in chronic hepatitis C refractory to prior treatment. *Digest Dis Sci* 2006;51(11):1956–61.

24. Parise E, Cheinquer H, Crespo D, *et al.* Peginterferon alfa-2a (40KD) (PEGASYS) plus ribavirin (COPEGUS) in retreatment of chronic hepatitis C patients, nonresponders and relapsers to previous conventional interferon plus ribavirin therapy. *Braz J Infect Dis* 2006;10(1):11–16.

25. Poynard T, Colombo S, Bruix J, *et al.* Peginterferon alfa-2b and ribavirin: effective in patients with hepatitis C who failed interferon-alfa/ribavirin therapy. *Gastroenterology* 2009;136:1618–28.

26. Sagir A, Heintges T, Akyazi Z, *et al.* Relapse to prior therapy is the most important factor for the retreatment response in patients with chronic hepatitis C virus infection. *Liver Int* 2007;27(7):954–9.

27. Sherman M, Yoshida EM, Deschenes M, *et al.* Peginterferon alfa-2a (40KD) plus ribavirin in chronic hepatitis C patients who failed previous interferon therapy. *Gut* 2006;55(11):1631–8.

28. Shiffman ML, Di Bisceglie AM, Lindsay KL, *et al.* Peginterferon alfa-2a and ribavirin in patients with chronic hepatitis C who have failed prior treatment. *Gastroenterology* 2004;126(4):1015–23.

29. Taliani G, Gemignani G, Ferrari C, *et al.* Pegylated interferon alfa-2b plus ribavirin in the retreatment of interferon-ribavirin nonresponder patients. *Gastroenterology* 2006;130(4):1098–106.

30. Yoshida EM, Sherman M, Bain VG, *et al.* Re-treatment with peginterferon alfa-2a and ribavirin in patients with chronic hepatitis C who have relapsed or not responded to a first course of pegylated interferon-based therapy. *Can J Gastroenterol* 2009;23(3):180–84.

31. Moucari R, Ripault MP, Oules V, *et al.* High predictive value of early viral kinetics in retreatment with peginterferon and ribavirin of chronic hepatitis C patients non-responders to standard combination therapy. *J Hepatol* 2007;46(4):596–604.

32. Camma C, Cabibbo G, Bronte F, *et al.* Retreatment with pegylated interferon plus ribavirin of chronic hepatitis C

non-responders to interferon plus ribavirin: a meta-analysis. *J Hepatol* 2009;51(4):675–81.

33. Foster GR, Hezode C, Bronowicki JP. Activity of telaprevir alone or in combination with peginterferon alfa 2a and ribavirin in treatment naïve genotype 2 and 3 hepatitis C

patients: interim results of the study C209. *J Hepatol* 2009; 50:S22.

34. Afdhal NH, McHutchison JG, Zeuzem S, *et al.* Hepatitis C pharmacogenetics: state of the art in 2010. *Hepatology* 2011; 53:336–45.

15 Hepatitis C Genotype 4 Therapy: Progress and Challenges

Sanaa M. Kamal

Department of Gastroenterology and Liver Disease, Ain Shams Faculty of Medicine, Cairo, Egypt, and Department of Gastroenterology, Tufts School of Medicine, Boston, USA

HCV Genotype 4: Shifting Epidemiology

Hepatitis C genotype 4 (HCV-4) is the most frequent cause of chronic hepatitis C in the Middle East, North Africa and sub-Saharan Africa [1–3]. The global epidemiology of HCV-4 is difficult to establish given that most epidemiologic studies focused on the prevalence and distribution of HCV-4 in Egypt, the country with the highest worldwide incidence and prevalence of HCV, with rates reaching 14% [2], where HCV-4 is responsible for 90% of HCV infections [1,3–8]. The prevalence of HCV-4 is 50% in the Kingdom of Saudi Arabia (KSA) [9,10], 30% in Syria [11], 76% in the Gaza Strip [12], and 6% in Jordan [13]. A few epidemiologic studies showed prevalence of HCV-4 in several African countries such as Gabon, Nigeria, the Central African Republic, Cameroon, and Tanzania [3,14–18].

HCV-4 has recently spread to southern Europe through immigration and injecting drug use. The prevalence rates of HCV-4 have shown steady increases in France [19,20], Italy [21], Greece [22], and Spain [23]. In France, the prevalence of HCV-4 increased from 4% in 1990 to more than 11% in a decade [19,20]. In Europe, most HCV-4 cases are clustered among injecting drug users (IVDUs) and patients co-infected with human immunodeficiency virus (HIV) [19–26]. A recent study showed that HCV-4 was the second most frequently detected genotype, being detected in 23% of a large cohort of HIV-positive men who have sex with men (MSM) from England, the Netherlands, France, Germany, and Australia [26].

Treatment of Chronic HCV-4 Naïve Patients

HCV-4 comprises approximately 20% of the world's HCV-infected population [18]. However, these patients have been underrepresented in the large multicenter clinical trials [27,28] due to the limited prevalence of this genotype in Europe and the United States. As a result, data regarding the responsiveness of genotype 4 has been limited. The treatment of chronic hepatitis genotype 4 has evolved over the past decade. Initially, conventional interferon alfa monotherapy administered at a dose of 3–5 mIU three times a week resulted in disappointing sustained virologic response (SVR) rates ranging between 5% and 10% [29,30]. Addition of ribavirin improved SVR rates to almost 35% [31,32], which were similar to SVR in HCV genotype 1 patients but lower than HCV genotype 2 and 3 patients [27,28]. These SVR rates led to the concept that HCV-4 was a "difficult to treat" genotype.

A steady improvement in the overall response rates of chronic HCV-4 to anti-hepatitis C therapy was achieved with the introduction of pegylated interferon alfa-2, which resulted in dramatic improvement in SVR rates when compared with conventional IFN alfa [33–49] (Figure 15.1). A meta-analysis of studies conducted until 2003 that included genotype 4 patients showed significantly higher SVR rates among genotype 4 patients receiving Peg-IFN alfa plus ribavirin than in those receiving conventional IFN alfa plus ribavirin (55% versus 30%, $p = 0.0088$) [39]. Controlled randomized and

Advanced Therapy for Hepatitis C, First Edition. Edited by Geoffrey W. McCaughan, John G. McHutchison and Jean-Michel Pawlotsky.
© 2012 Blackwell Publishing Ltd. Published 2012 by Blackwell Publishing Ltd.

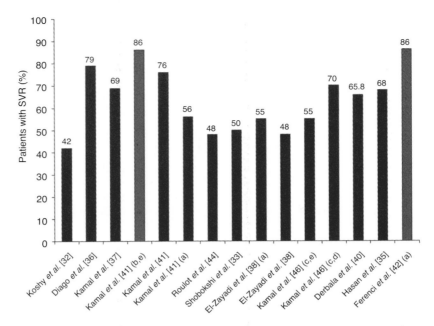

Figure 15.1 Sustained response rates to pegylated interferon and ribavirin therapy in patients with chronic hepatitis genotype 4 therapy. Patients were treated for 48 weeks with Peg-IFN and RBV, except for (a) shorter treatment duration: 24 weeks or 36 weeks; (b) shorter therapy: 24 weeks based on RVR; and (c) randomized trial comparing (d) Peg-IFN alfa-2a to (e) Peg-IFN alfa-2b. Adapted from Kamal and Nasser [18].

non-randomized clinical trials demonstrated high SVR rates ranging between 50% and 79% in chronic HCV-4 patients receiving Peg-IFN alfa-2b plus ribavirin [33–49] (Figure 15.2).

The overall SVR rates in patients with chronic HCV-4 treated with Peg-IFN alfa and ribavirin in the Middle East, specifically Egypt, the Kingdom of Saudi Arabia, and Qatar [37,38,41,46,47], were slightly higher

than SVR rates in patients with chronic HCV-4 from Europe or sub-Saharan Africa [44,47,48,49]. Retrospective analysis of SVR rates in French, Egyptian, and African patients with chronic HCV-4 showed an overall better response in Egyptian patients infected with the 4a subtype [44,47]. The overall SVR rates were highest in Egyptians (63%), followed by Europeans (51%) and sub-Saharan Africans (39%). In multivariate analysis, two factors were associated independently with SVR: the Egyptian origin of transmission and the absence of severe fibrosis [44,47]. Spanish [48] and Greek [49] studies evaluating the response of chronic HCV-4 treatment-naïve patients showed that treatment by pegylated interferon alfa-2b and ribavirin gives a more rapid decrease of HCV RNA level and a better SVR rate (62% versus 13%) in Egyptians than in non-Egyptians. To date, the reason for the difference in SVR rates is not clear. Possible explanations could be differences in patients' ethnic background, HCV-4 subtype, or the mode of transmission or duration of infection. Egyptian patients acquired the infection in most cases through anti-schistosomal therapy while most of the non-Egyptian patients acquired the infection through illicit drug use [44,47–49].

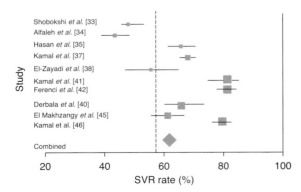

Figure 15.2 Meta-analysis of pegylated interferon and ribavirin therapy clinical trials in chronic hepatitis C.

Thus, the SVR rates in chronic HCV-4 patients are better than those achieved in genotype 1 patients. Table 15.1 summarizes the response rates of HCV-4 to pegylated interferon and ribavirin therapy. The next step in optimizing HCV-4 therapy is to adopt an individualized approach to therapy designed according to host and viral characteristics to determine the duration of therapy and the therapeutic options for special patient populations.

Duration of Chronic HCV-4 Therapy

The optimization of treatment duration is critical in ensuring that SVR rates are maximized without exposing the patient to an unnecessarily long treatment regimen that may have unfavorable implications in terms of cost and tolerability. The duration of therapy for chronic HCV-4 had been 48 weeks until emerging data from clinical trials on chronic HCV genotypes 1, 2, and 3 [50,51] demonstrated that shorter treatment durations based on pre-treatment and on-treatment criteria do not jeopardize patients' chances to maintain SVR.

The question of optimal treatment duration for genotype 4 chronic hepatitis C patients was addressed by a few prospective randomized studies and non-randomized studies. In one study [37], patients were randomized to receive Peg-IFN alfa-2b (1.5 mcg/kg/week) plus ribavirin (1000–1200 mg/day) for 24, 36, or 48 weeks. Overall, SVR rates were significantly higher in patients receiving treatment for 36 or 48 weeks than in those treated for 24 weeks (66% and 69% versus 29%; $p = 0.001$ for each comparison). Relapse during follow-up was highest among patients treated for 24 weeks (20 of 45, 44%) but relatively rare among the longer treatment arms, with no significant difference between the 36-week and 48-week treatment regimens. Baseline viral load and undetectable HCV RNA at week 12 were predictors of SVR [37].

A non-randomized study [38] allocated patients to 24 or 48 weeks of Peg-IFN alfa-2b and ribavirin or triple therapy of interferon alf-2b, ribavirin, and amantadine, according to financial affordability of the patients. The overall SVR rates were higher in patients treated with pegylated interferon and ribavirin combination therapy compared to those treated with triple therapy (64% versus 30%, respectively). Similar virologic outcomes were achieved in patients receiving Peg-IFN alfa plus ribavirin for 24 or 48 weeks (SVR, 48.6% versus 55.0%, $p = 0.517$).

Rapid virologic response (RVR), defined as an undetectable serum HCV RNA level at week 4 of therapy, emerged as an important factor for determining the duration of pegylated interferon-alfa and ribavirin therapy according to treatment-related viral kinetics [50–52]. To date, two studies have shown that 24 weeks of therapy is sufficient to induce SVR in patients with chronic HCV-4 achieving RVR. The first study [41] assessed the predictability of response in patients with chronic HCV-4 and determined the efficacy of a variable shorter duration Peg-IFN alfa-2b plus ribavirin treatment regimen based on viral load at weeks 4 and 12. Participants were randomly assigned to either standard fixed duration of 48 weeks (control group, $n = 50$) or shorter durations of 24 or 36 weeks based on patterns of viremia at therapy weeks 4 and 12. Patients with undetectable HCV RNA at weeks 4 and 12 treated with Peg-IFN alfa-2b and ribavirin for 24 weeks and 36 weeks, respectively, achieved high SVR rates with significantly fewer adverse events and better compliance. After controlling for predictors, low baseline histologic grade and stage were associated with SVR ($p < 0.029$) in all groups [41].

The second study [42] was conducted on 516 chronic HCV patients infected with genotype 1 ($n = 450$) or genotype 4 ($n = 66$) treated with Peg-IFN plus ribavirin. Patients with HCV-4 more frequently had an RVR than those with genotype 1 (45% versus 26%). Moreover, 86% of HCV-4 patients with RVR achieved SVR after 24 weeks of treatment compared to 78% of HCV-1 patients with RVR and the same duration of treatment.

Taken together, the results of the clinical trials [41,42] demonstrate that in chronic HCV-4, a 24-week regimen of peginterferon alfa-2a plus ribavirin 1000/1200 mg/day is appropriate to treat patients who achieve an RVR by week 4 of therapy. A 36-week regimen might be sufficient for patients with complete early virologic response (EVR) [43]. A proposed algorithm for duration of Peg-IFN alfa-2 and ribavirin is presented in Figure 15.3. However, larger randomized clinical trials are still needed to further optimize the duration of therapy.

The Efficacy of Different Pegylated Interferon Formulations in HCV-4 Infections

Most clinical trials assessing the treatment of chronic HCV-4 patients used either Peg-IFN alfa-2a or Peg-IFN alfa-2b in combination with ribavirin [35–49]. Recently, two Italian studies [53,54] demonstrated that Peg-IFN

Table 15.1 Overview of studies of Peg-IFN alfa and ribavirin in patients with chronic hepatitis C genotype 4.

Reference	Study design	Country (location)	Number of HCV-4 patients	Treatment	Therapy duration (weeks)	RVR (%)	EVR[a] (%)	EOTR[b] (%)	SVR[c] (%)
Randomized clinical trials									
Kamal et al. [37]	Prospective, double-blind, randomized study of Egyptian patients with HCV-4	Egypt	260	Peg-IFN alfa-2b 1.5 mcg/kg/wk + RBV 1000–1200 mg/d[d] for 24 weeks (n = 95)	24	n.a.	69	48	29
				Peg-IFN alfa-2b 1.5 mcg/kg/wk + RBV 1000–1200 mg/d[d] for 36 weeks (n = 96)	36		68	68[e]	66[f]
				Peg-IFN alfa-2b 1.5 mcg/kg/wk + RBV 1000–1200 mg/d[d] for 48 weeks (n = 69)	48		69	70[g]	69[f]
Ferenci et al. [42]	Prospective trial investigating response-guided therapy	Austria	66	Peg-IFN alfa-2a (180 μg/wk + RBV 1000 or 1200 mg/day according to virologic response at week 4	24 48 72	45	NR	NR	87
Kamal et al. [46]	Prospective randomized trial comparing the efficacy and safety of Peg-IFN alfa-2a and Pet-IFN alfa-2b	Egypt	217	Peg-IFN alfa-2a (180 μg/wk plus ribavirin 1000 or 1200 mg/day for 48 weeks (n = 109)	48	41.3	cEVR: 46.9 pEVR: 39.1	77	70[h]
				Peg-IFN alfa-2b 1.5 mcg/kg/wk plus ribavirin 1000–1200 mg/d[d] for 48 weeks (n = 108)	48	27.78	cEVR 26.9 pEVR: 30.8	70	55[h]
Kamal et al. [41]	Prospective, treatment duration based on virologic response at week 4 or 12 in Egyptian patients with chronic HCV-4	Egypt	308	Peg-IFN alfa-2b 1.5 mcg/kg/wk + RBV 1000–1200 mg/d[d] according to virologic response at week 4 or 12, respectively	24 36 48	22	cEVR: 79 pEVR: 160	90 86 70	86 (RVR) 76 (cEVR) 58 (pEVR)

Study	Design	Country	n	Regimen	Duration (weeks)				SVR
Rossignol et al. [64]	Phase II, randomized, double-blind, placebo-controlled	Egypt	97	Peg-IFN alfa-2a + RBV for 48 weeks ($n = 40$)	48	38	NR	NR	50
				Nitazoxanide monotherapy for 12 weeks followed by nitazoxanide + Peg-IFN alfa-2a for 36 weeks ($n = 28$)	48	64			64
				Nitazoxanide monotherapy for 12 weeks followed by nitazoxanide + Peg-IFN alfa-2a + RBV for 36 weeks ($n = 28$)	48				79
Alfaleh et al. [34]	Randomized, parallel-group study of Saudi patients with HCV	Kingdom of Saudi Arabia	59	Peg-IFN alfa-2b 100 mcg/wk + RBV 800 mg/d ($n = 28$)[i]	48		NR	67.9	42.9
				IFN alfa-2b 3 MU three times a week + RBV 800 mg/d ($n = 31$)[i]	48			54.8	32.3
Open label prospective trials									
El-Zayadi et al. [38]	Non-randomized prospective open label	Egypt	180	Peg-IFN alfa-2b 100 mcg/wk + RBV 1000–1200 mg/d[d] ($n = 40$)	48		72.5	65.0	55.0[j]
				Peg-IFN alfa-2b 100 mcg/wk + RBV 1000–1200 mg/d ($n = 70$)	24		72.9	65.7	48.6[k]
				IFN alfa-2b 3 MU[l] + RBV 1000–1200 mg/d + AMD 200 mg/d ($n = 70$)	24		54.3	47.1	28.6
Hasan et al. [35]	Open-label, prospective study of treatment-naïve HCV-4 patients in Kuwait	Kuwait	66	Peg-IFN alfa-2b 1.5 mcg/kg/wk + RBV 1000–1200 mg/d[d]	48		78	77	68
Derbala et al. [40]	Open label prospective	Qatar	73	Peg-IFN alfa-2a 180 mcg/wk + RBV 1200 mg/d for ($n = 38$)	48		NR	77[m]	68[n]
				IFN alfa-2b 3 MU three times a week + RBV 1200 mg/d ($n = 35$)	48			40.0	25.7

(Continued)

Table 15.1 (*Continued*)

Reference	Study design	Country (location)	Number of HCV-4 patients	Treatment	Therapy duration (weeks)	RVR (%)	EVR[a] (%)	EOTR[b] (%)	SVR[c] (%)
Shobokshi et al. [33]	Open-label study of Saudi and Egyptian patients with chronic HCV-4	Kingdom of Saudi Arabia		Peg-IFN alfa-2a 180 mcg/wk + RBV 800 mg/d	48		NR	NR	50
				Peg-IFN alfa-2a 180 mcg/wk	48				28
				IFN alfa-2a 4.5 MU three times a week plus RBV 800 mg/d	48				30
Trapero-Marugan et al. [48]	Open-label study of Spanish patients with chronic HCV G4	Spain	29	IFN alfa-2b 3 MU three times/week + RBV 800–1000 mg/d (n = 19)	48		NR	NR	55
				Peg-IFN alfa-2b (1.5 µg/kg/week) + RBV (1–1.2 g/day) (n = 10)					
El Makhzangy et al. [45]	Prospective open label trial	Egypt	95	Peg-IFN alfa-2a (180 µg/wk) + RBV 1000 or 1200 mg/day	48		NR	NR	61

Retrospective and post hoc analysis

Reference	Study design	Country (location)	Number of HCV-4 patients	Treatment	Therapy duration (weeks)	RVR (%)	EVR[a] (%)	EOTR[b] (%)	SVR[c] (%)
Roulot et al. [44]	A retrospective study	France	242	Peg-IFN alfa-2b 1.5 mcg/kg/wk + RBV 1000–1200 mg/d[d]	48		n.a.	n.a.	48: Egyptians 37: French 25: Africans
Elefsiniotis et al. [49]	A retrospective study	Greece	58	Peg-IFN alfa-2b 1.5 mcg/kg/wk + RBV 1000–1200 mg/d	48		63.8		53.4
Diago et al. [36]	Post hoc analysis of patients with HCV-4 from two large, double-blind clinical trials		98	Study 1: Peg-IFN alfa-2a 180 mcg/wk + RBV 1000–1200 mg/d[d] (n = 13)			NR	NR	79
				Study 2: Peg-IFN alfa-2a 180 mcg/wk + RBV 800–1200 mg/d[d] for 24 or 48 weeks	48				
				High-dose RBV (n = 24)	48				63
				Low-dose RBV (n = 8)	48				67
				High-dose RBV (n = 12)	24				0
				Low-dose RBV (n = 5)	24				

Therapy of HIV/HCV genotype 4 co-infected patients

Study	Description	Country	n	Treatment	Weeks			
Legrand-Abravanel et al. [57]	A case control study of patients with HCV-4 in France; 13 of 28 were HIV co-infected		28	Peg-IFN alfa-2b 1.5 mcg/kg/wk + RBV 1000–1200 mg/d[d]	48	50		32[o]
Soriano et al. [56]	A retrospective analysis of open-label clinical trials in G4 patients with HCV and HIV co-infection[p]		42	IFN alfa 3 MU three times a week (n = 9); IFN alfa 3 MU three times a week + RBV 800 mg/d (n = 11); Peg-IFN alfa-2b 1.5 mcg/wk + RBV 800 mg/d (n = 22)	48	NR		11.1, 9.1, 22.7
Martin-Carbonero et al. [58]	A retrospective analysis of open-label clinical trials in G4 patients with HCV and HIV co-infection in Italian and Spanish studies	Italy Spain	75	Peg-IFN alfa-2b and alfa-2a	48	42	60	55

Therapy of HCV-G4 non-responders

Study	Description	Country	n	Treatment	Weeks			
Hasan et al. [55]	Open-label, prospective controlled trial of Egyptian and Kuwaiti patients		63	Peg-IFN alfa-2b, 1.5 µg/kg concomitantly with RBV 1000–1200 mg per day	48	21	NR	5
				Peg-IFN alfa-2b, 1.5 µg/kg concomitantly with RBV 1000–1200 mg per day + amantadine 200 mg per day	48	42	NR	7

Therapy of chronic HCV-G4 in thalassemia major patients

Study	Description	Country	n	Treatment	Weeks			
Inati et al. [62]	Open-label, prospective controlled trial of Lebanese patients		20	Peg-IFN alfa-2a 180 mg/week monotherapy	48	NR	NR	30
				Peg-IFN alfa-2a 180 mg/week plus RBV		NR	NR	62.5
Kamal et al. [63]	Randomized trial of Egyptian patients		78	Peg-IFN alfa-2b, 1.5 µg/kg	48	19	21	18
				Peg-IFN alfa-2b, 1.5 µg/kg + RBV 800 mg/day		30	48	45

Table 15.1 (*Continued*)

Reference	Study design	Country (location)	Number of HCV-4 patients	Treatment	Therapy duration (weeks)	RVR (%)	EVR[a] (%)	EOTR[b] (%)	SVR[c] (%)
Therapy of acute HCV-4									
Kamal *et al.* [61]	Randomized controlled trial of Egyptian patients with acute HCV-4	Egypt	40	Peg-IFN alfa-2b monotherapy	24	NR	NR		80
				Peg-IFN alfa-2b + RBV	24				85
Kamal *et al.* [59]	Randomized controlled trial of Egyptian patients with acute HCV-4	Egypt	53	Peg-IFN alfa-2b monotherapy	12	NR	NR	88	84
Kamal *et al.* [60]	Randomized controlled trial of Egyptian patients with acute HCV-4	Egypt	40	Peg-IFN alfa-2b monotherapy	8	85	79	NR	67
					12	85	88	NR	82
					24	88	94	NR	91

Source: Adapted from Kamal and Nasser [18].

AMD, amantadine; EVR, early virologic response (cEVR, complete EVR; pEVR, partial EVR); HCV, hepatitis C virus; Peg-IFN, pegylated interferon; RBV, ribavirin; SVR, sustained virologic response.

[a]EVR was defined as undetectable HCV RNA or a $\geq 2 \log_{10}$ decrease at week 12.

[b]End-of-treatment response was defined as undetectable HCV RNA at the end of the scheduled treatment period.

[c]SVR was defined as undetectable HCV RNA at the end of a 24-week follow-up period.

[d]RBV was administered according to a weight-based administration schedule.

[e]$p = 0.04$.

[f]$p = 0.001$ versus 24-week treatment regimen.

[g]$p = 0.02$.

[h]$p = 0.017$ versus Peg-IFN alfa-2b.

[i]Data presented for genotype 4 patients only.

[j]$p = 0.006$.

[k]$p = 0.015$ versus induction dose regimen.

[l]Interferon was administered daily for the first four weeks of the study and then thrice weekly for the remaining 20 weeks.

[m]$p < 0.002$ versus conventional IFN.

[n]$p < 0.05$ versus conventional IFN.

[o]SVR occurred in 15% of HIV/HCV co-infected patients and in 50% of HCV mono-infected patients.

[p]Patients were allocated to treatment groups according to personal financial ability to afford treatment.

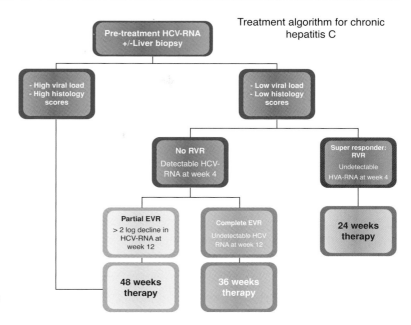

Treatment algorithm for chronic hepatitis C

Figure 15.3 A proposed algorithm for treatment of chronic hepatitis C genotype 4. Adapted from Kamal [76].

alfa-2a plus ribavirin produced significantly higher over-all SVR rates (68.8% and 66%, respectively) than Peg-IFN alfa-2b plus ribavirin (54.4% and 54%, respectively) in Italian patients infected with chronic HCV-4. Another randomized clinical trial [46] enrolling a large cohort of patients with chronic HCV-4 showed that SVR rates were significantly higher in Egyptian patients treated with Peg-IFN alfa-2a and ribavirin ($n = 109$) compared to those treated with Peg-IFN alfa-2b and ribavirin ($n = 108$) (70.6% versus 54.6%, respectively; $p = 0.017$). The relapse rates were 5.1% for Peg-IFN alfa-2a and 15.7% for Peg-IFN alfa-2b ($p = 0.0019$). Head-to-head clinical trials comparing the efficacy and safety of the two Peg-IFN alfa formulations in chronic HCV-4 patients are particularly important in countries with high prevalence of HCV-4 to maximize the SVR rates, prevent progression of liver disease, and increase the cost benefit of therapy.

HCV-4 Therapy in Special Populations

Treatment of Non-Responders

Treatment of non-responders is a challenge across all genotypes. Management of chronic HCV-4 patients who did not respond to interferon-based therapies has not been studied except in one small trial [55], which assessed the efficacy and safety of peginterferon plus ribavirin with or without amantidine in 63 non-responders to conven-

tional interferon therapy. Patients were randomized to receive either weekly peginterferon alfa-2b, 1.5 μg/kg, and ribavirin 1000–1200 mg, or peginterferon and ribavirin as in group A, plus amantadine. Only one patient (5%) treated with dual therapy and three patients (7%) treated with triple therapy achieved SVR. Further clinical trials are required to investigate management options for this population.

Treatment of Chronic HCV and HIV Co-Infections

Although in Europe, HCV-4 is frequent among HCV and HIV co-infected patients, few clinical trials have studied the efficacy of Peg-IFN and ribavirin therapy in patients with HIV and HCV-4 co-infection [56–58]. In a case series study, SVR rates of 16.7% were obtained in genotype 4 patients co-infected with HIV receiving various IFN-based antiviral therapies [56]. Overall, SVR was attained by 11.1% of patients receiving IFN alfa monotherapy, 9.1% of patients receiving IFN alfa plus ribavirin combination therapy, and 22.7% of patients receiving Peg-IFN alfa-2b (1.5 mcg/week) plus ribavirin (800 mg/day). In another study [57], end of treatment response and SVR rates were lower in HIV/HCV-4 co-infected patients than in HCV mono-infected patients (30% versus 66%, $p = 0.06$; 15% versus 50%, $p = 0.06$, respectively) receiving Peg-IFN alfa plus ribavirin (1000–1200 mg/day) for 48 weeks, although in neither case did the difference between cohorts achieve statistical significance. The SVR rates of <20% reported in co-infected patients are clearly lower than the SVR rates reported in HCV mono-infected genotype 4 patients receiving combination therapy with Peg-IFN alfa plus ribavirin (50–79%) [57]. An Italian-Spanish study [58] assessed the efficacy of Peg-IFN and ribavirin therapy in 75 HCV-4 patients co-infected with HIV. The overall SVR was 28% in Spanish patients and 34% in Italian HCV-4 patients. These studies suggest that co-infected HCV-4 patients are considered a difficult-to-treat population.

Treatment of Acute HCV Genotype 4

A few clinical trials have addressed the optimal treatment regimen in acute HCV-4 and demonstrated high SVR with IFN-based therapies compared with no treatment [59–61]. These studies showed that acute hepatitis patients infected with genotype 4 have higher rates of SVR compared to genotype 1 infections. In one study [60], SVR was achieved in 60% and 88% of genotype 1 patients and in 93% and 100% of genotype 4 patients after 12 and 24 weeks of treatment, respectively.

Treatment of Thalassemia Major Patients with Chronic HCV-4 Infection

Although many thalassemia patients are infected with HCV, treatment of these patients has not yet been established. A randomized study [62] evaluated the efficacy of peginterferon alfa with or without ribavirin therapy in 20 patients with thalassemia and HCV-4. SVR occurred in 4 of 12 and 5 of 8 patients in the monotherapy and combination groups (30% and 62.5%; $p = 0.19$), respectively. Transfusion requirements rose by 34% in the combination arm ($p = 0.08$). In another study [63], the overall SVR rates were 46% with peginterferon alfa-2b and 64% with peginterferon alfa-2b plus ribavirin combination therapy. However, the adverse events and withdrawals were more frequent with peginterferon alfa-2b plus ribavirin combination therapy than with peginterferon alfa-2b alone. Combination therapy was associated with a temporary increase in transfusion requirements.

Emerging New Regimen for Treatment of Chronic HCV-4

A phase II, randomized, double-blind, placebo-controlled study of nitazoxanide treatment for 24 weeks in 50 patients with chronic hepatitis C genotype 4 was conducted to evaluate safety with prolonged administration and to determine the antiviral efficacy of nitazoxanide monotherapy [64]. The study sequentially allocated 97 Egyptian patients with chronic HCV-4 into three treatment arms: peginterferon alfa-2a and ribavirin for 48 weeks ($n = 40$), nitazoxanide monotherapy for 12 weeks followed by nitazoxanide plus peginterferon alfa-2a for 36 weeks ($n = 28$), or nitazoxanide monotherapy for 12 weeks followed by nitazoxanide plus peginterferon alfa-2a and ribavirin for 36 weeks ($n = 28$).

The percentages of patients with RVR, defined as undetectable serum HCV RNA at week 4 of combination therapy, and SVR were significantly higher in patients given the triple therapy compared with the standard of care (64% versus 38%, $p = 0.048$, and 79% versus 50%, $p = 0.023$, respectively). Patients given nitazoxanide plus peginterferon alfa-2a had intermediate rates of RVR (54%) and SVR (61%). Adverse events were similar across treatment groups except for a higher rate of anemia in the groups receiving ribavirin. In the nitazoxanide group, virologic responses were maintained through the end of treatment with no virologic breakthroughs. Of note, the use of nitazoxanide was associated with reduced relapse rates (3/20 patients in the peginterferon plus nitazoxanide arm, and 1/23 patients in the triple arm with peginterferon, ribavirin, and nitazoxanide) versus 10/30 patients in the standard-of-care arm [64].

Recent studies have suggested that Peg-IFN and ribavirin are likely to be supplanted soon by the addition of specifically targeted antiviral therapy for HCV (STAT-C). Resistance to new antivirals such as HCV protease inhibitors and emergence of potentially resistant strains of HCV are likely to develop. It is important to investigate the response to STAT-C of patients with chronic HCV-4 in various geographic areas and ethnic groups, and the development of resistance or adverse events.

Personalizing Chronic HCV-4 Therapy

Personalizing Therapy According to On-Treatment Viral Kinetics

Some studies have addressed the predictors of SVR in HCV-4. RVR and EVR have been identified as independent predictors of SVR in genotype 4 infected chronic hepatitis C patients, regardless of their baseline parameters [41,42]. Among baseline criteria, a study showed that a low baseline histologic grade and stage ($p < 0.029$), low baseline body mass index ($p = 0.013$), and low baseline HCV RNA ($p < 0.001$) were significantly associated with SVR [43]. Similarly, another study found a significant association between SVR and severe fibrosis (Metavir score >F2) (OR = 0.4, 95% CI: 0.2–0.8), and presence of steatosis (OR = 0.5, 95% CI: 0.3–0.97) [48].

Personalizing Therapy According to Hepatic Steatosis and Fibrosis

Moderate to severe steatosis with or without sinusoidal fibrosis is present in about 70% of patients with chronic HCV-4 [18,41,47]. Advanced fibrosis and steatosis have been associated with lower SVR rates [41,47]. Treatment outcomes were improved in genotype 4 patients with mild liver disease compared to those patients with more advanced liver disease. In patients receiving Peg-IFN alfa-2b plus ribavirin (1000–1200 mg/day) for 48 weeks, SVR rates were significantly higher among those with no or mild fibrosis (F0 [no fibrosis]–F2 [portal fibrosis with rare septa]) than in those with severe fibrosis or cirrhosis (F3 [numerous septa without cirrhosis]–F4 [cirrhosis]) (84% versus 29%, $p < 0.0002$). SVR was independently associated with HOMA-IR < 2 ($p = 0.001$, OR = 5.314, 95% CI = 1.953–14.459), and non-severe fibrosis ($p < 0.001$, OR = 8.059, 95% CI = 2.512–25.855) [47].

Personalizing Therapy According to Host Genetics

Currently, it is not clear why patients with chronic hepatitis C respond differently to Peg-IFN alfa and ribavirin therapy despite comparable baseline host characteristics such as age, gender, and BMI or viral factors such as genotype and baseline viral load. African and Hispanic patients do not respond as well to IFN alfa-based therapies as Caucasians and Asians do [65–68]. Even among patients infected with HCV-4, Egyptians and French show an overall better response to Peg-IFN alfa and ribavirin regimen compared to patients of African ancestry [44,47]. The altered response of different populations and ethnic groups to therapy is intriguing and raises important questions on how ancestry and genetic variants influence HCV disease, individuals' response to therapy, and development of adverse events.

The link between *IL28B* and the outcome of HCV reported by several groups has revolutionized our understanding of host determinants of treatment response in order to personalize therapy and maximize response. Several studies have reported relevant *IL28B* polymorphisms on chromosome 19 associated with interferon therapy outcome. Patients with the CC genotype had greater likelihood of achieving SVR compared with patients who had the CT and TT genotypes. The CC genotype was associated with higher frequency in Europeans, African Amer-

icans, and Hispanics [69–74]. However, most genome-wide association studies (GWAS) focused on HCV genotypes 1, 2, and 3, the prevalent genotypes in Europe and the United States. One study that included a limited number of Egyptians living in Austria infected with HCV-4 identified *IL28B* genotype and RVR as important predictors of SVR [75]. Individualization of HCV therapy according to criteria such as *IL28B* genotype and RVR treatment could be a valuable tool for maximizing efficacy and cost-effectiveness of therapy in countries with high prevalence of HCV-4 infections, such as Egypt and other African countries, as well as European countries with evolving HCV-4 infections.

Conclusions and Future Prospects

Hepatitis C genotype 4 is responsible for about 20% of hepatitis C infections worldwide and is rapidly spreading to the West through immigration and injecting drug use. Personalized medicine offers the potential to tailor hepatitis C genotype 4 therapy according to patients' genetic profile, pre-treatment host and viral characteristics, and on-treatment viral kinetics to increase the effectiveness of existing and new therapies, minimize adverse events, and maximize cost benefit of therapy. Further research is needed to investigate the response of HCV-4 to emerging specifically targeted antiviral therapy for HCV (STAT-C).

References

1. World Health Organization. *Global Alert and Response, Hepatitis C.* Geneva, Switzerland: World Health Organization; 2002. Available at: www.who.int/csr/disease/hepatitis/whocdscsrlyo2003/en/index.html. Accessed June 8, 2011.
2. Lavanchy D. Evolving epidemiology of hepatitis C virus. *Clin Microbiol Infect* 2011;17:107–15.
3. Simmonds P. Genetic diversity and evolution of hepatitis C virus: 15 years on. *J Gen Virol* 2004;85(Pt 11):3173–88.
4. Egyptian Ministry of Health. Annual report, 2007. Available at www.mohp.gov.eg/Main.asp. Accessed May 25, 2011.
5. Abdel-Aziz F, Habib M, Mohamed MK, *et al.* Hepatitis C virus (HCV) infection in a community in the Nile Delta: population description and HCV prevalence. *Hepatology* 2000;32:111–15.
6. Ray SC, Arthur RR, Carella A, *et al.* Genetic epidemiology of hepatitis C virus throughout Egypt. *J Infect Dis* 2000;182:698–707.
7. Angelico M, Renganathan E, Gandin C, *et al.* Chronic liver disease in the Alexandria governorate, Egypt: contribution

of schistosomiasis and hepatitis virus infections. *J Hepatol* 1997;26(2):236–43.

8. Kamal S, Madwar M, Bianchi L, *et al.* Clinical, virological and histopathological features: long-term follow-up in patients with chronic hepatitis C co-infected with *S. mansoni*. *Liver* 2000;20:281–9.

9. Shobokshi OA, Serebour FE, Skakni L, *et al.* Hepatitis C genotypes and subtypes in Saudi Arabia. *J Med Virol* 1999;58(1):44–8.

10. Al-Knawy B, Okamoto H, El-Mekki A, *et al.* Distribution of hepatitis C genotype and co-infection rate with hepatitis G in Saudi Arabia. *Hepatol Res* 2002;24(2):95–8.

11. Abdulkarim AS, Zein NN, Germer JJ, *et al.* Hepatitis C virus genotypes and hepatitis G virus in hemodialysis patients from Syria: identification of two novel hepatitis C virus subtypes. *Am J Trop Med Hyg* 1998;59:571–6.

12. Shemer-Avni Y, el Astal Z, Kemper O, *et al.* Hepatitis C virus infection and genotypes in Southern Israel and the Gaza Strip. *J Med Virol* 1998;56:230–33.

13. Bdour S. Hepatitis C virus infection in Jordanian haemodialysis units: serological diagnosis and genotyping. *J Med Microbiol* 2002;51:700–704.

14. Xu, L-Z, Larzul D, Delaporte E, *et al.* Hepatitis C virus genotype 4 is highly prevalent in central Africa (Gabon). *J Gen Virol* 1994;75:2393–8.

15. Ndjomou J, Pybus OG, Matz B. Phylogenetic analysis of hepatitis C virus isolates indicates a unique pattern of endemic infection in Cameroon. *J Gen Virol* 2003;84:2333–41.

16. Njouom R, Frost E, Deslandes S, *et al.* Predominance of hepatitis C virus genotype 4 infection and rapid transmission between 1935 and 1965 in the Central African Republic. *J Gen Virol* 2009;90(Pt 10):2452–6.

17. Wansbrough-Jones MH, Frimpong E, Cant B, *et al.* Prevalence and genotype of hepatitis C virus infection in pregnant women and blood donors in Ghana. *Trans R Soc Trop Med H* 1998; 92, 496–499.

18. Kamal S, Nasser I. Hepatitis C genotype 4: what we know and what we don't yet know. *Hepatology* 2008;47(4):1371–83.

19. Payan C, Roudot-Thoraval F, Marcellin P, *et al.* Changing of hepatitis C virus genotype patterns in France at the beginning of the third millennium: the GEMHEP GenoCII Study. *J Viral Hepatisis* 2005;12:405–13.

20. Nicot F, Legrand-Abravanel F, Sandres-Saune K, *et al.* Heterogeneity of hepatitis C virus genotype 4 strains circulating in south-western France. *J Gen Virol* 2005;86:107–14.

21. Ansaldi F, Bruzzone B, Salamaso S, *et al.* Different seroprelavence and molecular epidemiology pattern of hepatitis C virus infection in Italy. *J Med Virol* 2005;76:327–32.

22. Katsoulidou A, Sypsa V, Tassopoulos NC, *et al.* Molecular epidemiology of hepatitis C virus (HCV) in Greece: temporal trends in HCV genotype-specific incidence and molecular characterization of genotype 4 isolates. *J Viral Hepat* 2006;13(1):19–27.

23. Fernandez-Arcas N, Lopez-Siles J, Trapero S, *et al.* High prevalence of hepatitis C virus subtypes 4c and 4d in Malaga (Spain): phylogenetic and epidemiological analyses. *J Med Virol* 2006;78(11):1429–35.

24. Franco S, Tural C, Clotet B, Martínez MA. Complete nucleotide sequence of genotype 4 hepatitis C viruses isolated from patients co-infected with human immunodeficiency virus type 1. *Virus Res* 2007;123(2):161–9.

25. de Bruijne J, Schinkel J, Prins M, *et al.* Emergence of hepatitis C virus genotype 4: phylogenetic analysis reveals three distinct epidemiological profiles. *J Clin Microbiol.* 2009;47(12):3832–8.

26. van de Laar T, Pybus O, Bruisten S, *et al.* Evidence of a large, international network of HCV transmission in HIV-positive men who have sex with men. *Gastroenterology* 2009;136(5):1609–17.

27. Fried MW, Shiffman ML, Reddy KR, *et al.* Peginterferon alfa-2a plus ribavirin for chronic hepatitis C virus infection. *N Engl J Med* 2002;347(13):975–82.

28. Manns MP, McHutchison JG, Gordon SC, *et al.* Peginterferon alfa-2b plus ribavirin compared with interferon alfa-2b plus ribavirin for initial treatment of chronic hepatitis C: a randomised trial. *Lancet* 2001;358(9286):958–65.

29. Zylberberg H, Chaix ML, Brechot C. Infection with hepatitis C virus genotype 4 is associated with a poor response to interferon-alpha. *Ann Intern Med* 2000;132:845–6.

30. Kamal SM, Madwar MA, Peters T, *et al.* Interferon therapy in patients with chronic hepatitis C and schistosomiasis. *J Hepatol* 2000;32:172–4.

31. Koshy A, Madda JP, Marcellin P, *et al.* Treatment of hepatitis C virus genotype 4-related cirrhosis: ribavirin and interferon combination compared with interferon alone. *J Clin Gastroenterol* 2002;35(1):82–5.

32. Koshy A, Marcellin P, Martinot M, Madda JP. Improved response to ribavirin interferon combination compared with interferon alone in patients with type 4 chronic hepatitis C without cirrhosis. *Liver* 2000;20:335–9.

33. Shobokshi A, Serebour PE, Skakni L, *et al.* Combination therapy of peginterferon alfa-2a (40KD) (PEGASYS®) and ribavirin (COPEGUS®) significantly enhance sustained virological and biochemical response rate in chronic hepatitis C genotype 4 patients in Saudi Arabia. *Hepatology* 2003;38(Suppl):636A (abstract).

34. Alfaleh FZ, Hadad Q, Khuroo MS, *et al.* Peginterferon a-2b plus ribavirin compared with interferon a-2b plus ribavirin for initial treatment of chronic hepatitis C in Saudi patients commonly infected with genotype 4. *Liver Int* 2004;24:568–74.

35. Hasan F, Asker H, Al-Khaldi J, *et al.* Peginterferon alfa-2b plus ribavirin for the treatment of chronic hepatitis C genotype 4. *Am J Gastroenterol* 2004;99:1733–7.

36. Diago M, Hassanein T, Rodes J, *et al.* Optimized virologic response in hepatitis C virus genotype 4 with peginterferon-alpha2a and ribavirin. *Ann Intern Med* 2004;140:72–3.

37. Kamal SM, El Tawil AA, Nakano T, *et al.* Peginterferon alpha-2b and ribavirin therapy in chronic hepatitis C genotype 4: impact of treatment duration and viral kinetics on sustained virological response. *Gut* 2005;54:858–66.

38. El-Zayadi A-R, Attia M, Barakat EMF, *et al.* Response of hepatitis C genotype-4 naive patients to 24 weeks of peg-interferon-a2b/ribavirin or induction-dose interferon-a2b/ribavirin/amantadine: a non-randomized controlled study. *Am J Gastroenterol* 2005;100:2447–52.

39. Khuroo MS, Khuroo MS, Dahab ST. Meta-analysis: a randomized trial of peginterferon plus ribavirin for the initial treatment of chronic hepatitis C genotype 4. *Aliment Pharmacol Ther* 2004;20(9):931–8.

40. Derbala MF, Al Kaabi SR, El Dweik NZ, *et al.* Treatment of hepatitis C virus genotype 4 with peginterferon alfa-2a: impact of bilharziasis and fibrosis stage. *World J Gastroenterol* 2006;12:5692–8.

41. Kamal S, Kamary S, Shardell M, *et al.* Pegylated interferon alpha-2b plus ribavirin in patients with genotype 4 chronic hepatitis C: the role of rapid and early virologic response. *Hepatology* 2007;46(6):1732–40.

42. Ferenci P, Laferl H, Scherzer TM, *et al.* Peginterferon alfa-2a and ribavirin for 24 weeks in hepatitis C type 1 and 4 patients with rapid virological response. *Gastroenterology* 2008;135(2):451–8.

43. Jessner W, Gschwantler M, Formann E, *et al.* Very early viral kinetics on interferon treatment in chronic hepatitis C virus genotype 4 infection. *Antivir Ther* 2008;13(4):581–9.

44. Roulot D, Bourcier V, Grando V, *et al.* Epidemiological characteristics and response to peginterferon plus ribavirin treatment of hepatitis C virus genotype 4 infection. *J Viral Hepatitis* 2007;14(7):460–7.

45. El Makhzangy H, Esmat G, Said M, *et al.* Response to pegylated interferon alfa-2a and ribavirin in chronic hepatitis C genotype 4. *J Med Virol* 2009;81(9):1576–83.

46. Kamal SM, Ahmed A, Mahmoud S, *et al.* Enhanced efficacy of pegylated interferon alpha-2a over pegylated interferon and ribavirin in chronic hepatitis C genotype 4: a randomized trial and quality of life analysis. *Liver Int* 2011;31(3):401–11.

47. Moucari R, Ripault MP, Martinot-Peignoux M, *et al.* Insulin resistance and geographical origin: major predictors of liver fibrosis and response to peginterferon and ribavirin in HCV-4. *Gut* 2009;58(12):1662–9.

48. Trapero-Marugan M, Moreno-Monteagudo JA, Garcia-Buey L, *et al.* Clinical and pathological characteristics and response to combination therapy of genotype 4 chronic hepatitis C patients: experience from a Spanish center. *J Chemother* 2007;19(4):423–7.

49. Elefsiniotis IS, Vezali E, Mihas C, Saroglou G. Predictive value of complete and partial early virological response on sustained virological response rates of genotype-4 chronic hepatitis C patients treated with PEG-interferon plus ribavirin. *Intervirology* 2009;52(5):247–51.

50. Zeuzem S, Pawlotsky JM, Lukasiewicz E, *et al.* International, multicenter, randomized, controlled study comparing dynamically individualized versus standard treatment in patients with chronic hepatitis C. *J Hepatol* 2005;43(2):250–57.

51. Mangia A, Minerva N, Bacca D, *et al.* Individualized treatment duration for hepatitis C genotype 1 patients: a randomized controlled trial. *Hepatology* 2008;47(1):43–50.

52. Poordad F, Reddy KR, Martin P. Rapid virologic response: a new milestone in the management of chronic hepatitis C. *Clin Infect Dis* 2008;46(1):78–84.

53. Ascione A, Luca MD, Tartaglione MT, *et al.* Peginterferon alfa-2a plus ribavirin is more effective than peginterferon alfa-2b plus ribavirin for treating chronic hepatitis C virus infection. *Gastroenterology* 2010;138(1):116–22.

54. Rumi M, Aghemo A, Prati GM, *et al.* Randomized study of peginterferon-alpha2a plus ribavirin vs peginterferon-alpha2b plus ribavirin in chronic hepatitis C. *Gastroenterology* 2010;138(1):108–15.

55. Hasan F, Al-Khaldi J, Asker H, *et al.* Peginterferon alpha-2b plus ribavirin with or without amantadine for the treatment of non-responders to standard interferon and ribavirin. *Antivir Ther* 2004;9(4):499–503.

56. Soriano V, Nunez M, Sanchez-Conde M, *et al.* Response to interferon-based therapies in HIV-infected patients with chronic hepatitis C due to genotype 4. *Antiviral Ther* 2005;10:167–70.

57. Legrand-Abravanel F, Nicot F, Boulestin A, *et al.* Pegylated interferon and ribavirin therapy for chronic hepatitis C virus genotype 4 infection. *J Med Virol* 2005;77:66–9.

58. Martín-Carbonero L, Puoti M, García-Samaniego J, *et al.* Response to pegylated interferon plus ribavirin in HIV-infected patients with chronic hepatitis C due to genotype 4. *J Viral Hepat* 2008;15(10):710–15.

59. Kamal SM, Fouly AE, Kamel RR, *et al.* Peginterferon alfa-2b therapy in acute hepatitis C: impact of onset of therapy on sustained virologic response. *Gastroenterology* 2006;130:632–8.

60. Kamal SM, Moustafa KN, Chen J, *et al.* Duration of peginterferon therapy in acute hepatitis C: a randomized trial. *Hepatology* 2006;43:923–31.

61. Kamal SM, Ismail A, Graham CS, *et al.* Pegylated interferon alpha therapy in acute hepatitis C: relation to hepatitis C virus-specific T cell response kinetics. *Hepatology* 2004;39(6):1721–31.

62. Inati A, Taher A, Ghorra S, *et al.* Efficacy and tolerability of peginterferon alpha-2a with or without ribavirin in thalassaemia major patients with chronic hepatitis C virus infection. *Br J Haematol* 2005;130(4):644–6.

63. Kamal S, Fouly A, Mohamed S, *et al.* Peginterferon alpha-2b therapy with and without ribavirin in patients with thalassemia: a randomized study. 2006;44(Suppl 2):S217.

64. Rossignol JF, Elfert A, El-Gohary Y, Keeffe EB. Improved virologic response in chronic hepatitis C genotype 4 treated with nitazoxanide, peginterferon, and ribavirin. *Gastroenterology* 2009;136(3):856–62.

65. Satapathy SK, Lingisetty CS, Proper S, *et al.* Equally poor outcomes to pegylated interferon-based therapy in African Americans and Hispanics with chronic hepatitis C infection. *J Clin Gastroenterol* 2007;44(2):140–45.

66. Muir AJ, Bornstein JD, Killenberg PG. Peginterferon alfa-2b and ribavirin for the treatment of chronic hepatitis C in blacks and nonhispanic whites. *N Engl J Med* 2004;350:2265–71.

67. Jeffers L, Cassidy W, Howell CD, *et al.* Peginterferon alfa-2a (40kd) and ribavirin for black American patients with chronic hepatitis C virus genotype 1. *Hepatology* 2004;39:1702–8.

68. Conjeevaram HS, Fried MW, Jeffers LJ, *et al.* Peginterferon and ribavirin treatment in African American and Caucasian American patients with chronic hepatitis C genotype 1. *Gastroenterology* 2006;31:470–77.

69. Ge D, Fellay J, Thompson A, *et al.* Genetic variation in IL28B predicts hepatitis C treatment-induced viral clearance. *Nature* 2009;461:399–401.

70. Tanaka Y, Nishida N, Sugiyama M, *et al.* Genome-wide association of IL28B with response to pegylated interferon-alpha and ribavirin therapy for chronic hepatitis C. *Nature Genet* 2009;41:1105–10.

71. Suppiah V, Moldovan M, Ahlenstiel G, *et al.* IL28B is associated with response to chronic hepatitis C interferon-alpha and ribavirin therapy. *Nature Genet* 2009;41:1100–104.

72. Montes-Cano MA, Garcia-Lozano JR, Abad-Molina C, *et al.* Interleukin-28B genetic variants and hepatitis virus infection by different viral genotypes. *Hepatology* 2010;52:33–7.

73. Tillmann HL, Thompson AJ, Patel K, *et al.* A polymorphism near IL28B is associated with spontaneous clearance of acute hepatitis C virus and jaundice. *Gastroenterology* 2010;139(5):1586–92.

74. Thompson AJ, Muir AJ, Sulkowski MS, *et al.* Interleukin-28B polymorphism improves viral kinetics and is the strongest pretreatment predictor of sustained virologic response in genotype 1 hepatitis C virus. *Gastroenterology* 2010;139(1):120–29.

75. Stättermayer AF, Stauber R, Hofer H, *et al.* Impact of IL28B genotype on the early and sustained virologic response in treatment naïve patients with chronic hepatitis C. *Clin Gastroenterol Hepatol* 2011;9(4):344–50.

76. Kamal SM. Hepatitis C genotype 4 therapy: increasing options and improving outcomes. *Liver Int* 2009; 29 (Suppl 1):39–48.

16 Antivirals in Acute Hepatitis C

Heiner Wedemeyer

Department of Gastroenterology, Hepatology and Endocrinology, Medizinische Hochschule Hannover, Hannover, Germany

Diagnosis of Acute Hepatitis C

The diagnosis of acute hepatitis C is based on the detection of HCV RNA, while initially anti-HCV antibodies may be undetectable for several weeks after suspected infection [1]. In some cases of HIV-positive patients the time to anti-HCV seroconversion was more than 1 year [2]. If seroconversion could not be documented and patients were already anti-HCV-positive, acute hepatitis C had been defined in several trials as sudden onset of acute hepatitis with at least 10-fold elevated alanine amino-transferase (ALT) levels in the absence of any other liver disease and documented normal liver enzymes or negative anti-HCV tests in the preceding 1–2 years [3,4].

Diagnostic tests in patients with suspected acute hepatitis C should include determination of viral load and HCV genotype. Early viral kinetics may be useful to predict spontaneous viral clearance [5], while controversial data exist to what extent different HCV genotypes may be associated with spontaneous viral clearance [6]. Biochemical and hematologic parameters can determine disease activity. Both high bilirubin and ALT levels are associated with HCV clearance [7,8]. Single nucleotide polymorphisms (SNPs) in the region of IL28B (lambda-3 interferon) are also associated with likelihood of HCV clearance after acute infection [9]. IL28B variants may predict spontaneous recovery from HCV infection, in particular in asymptomatic non-icteric acute HCV infection [10]. Other causes of acute hepatitis must be excluded (see Figure 16.1). All patients with acute hepatitis C should also be tested for HIV co-infection.

Prevention of HCV Transmission

There are currently no vaccines available to prevent HCV infection [11]. Thus, HCV transmission can only be avoided by education and strict adherence to hygienic standards. The incidence of acute hepatitis C has declined in most Western countries during the past two decades – mainly due to the introduction of screening of blood products for HCV antibodies and more recently also for HCV RNA. Nevertheless, acute HCV infections continue to occur in risk populations such as intravenous drug addicts [12]. *Drug users* should therefore be educated about modes of HCV transmission and should be tested regularly for anti-HCV [13]. In addition, minor community exposures such as dental treatment or other *medical treatments* still contribute substantially to HCV transmission even in developed countries. The Spanish Acute HCV study group identified hospital admission as a significant risk factor for acquiring HCV infection, with about two thirds of all cases being associated with nosocomial acquisition of HCV [14]. In the German Hep Net Acute HCV study cohort, hospital admission was the only identifiable risk factor in 38 out of 254 (15%) patients with acute hepatitis C [15].

HCV transmission by needle stick injury occurred in less than 1% of cases in European studies [16]. Factors associated with a higher likelihood of HCV transmission after occupational exposure are a high HCV viral load in the index patient, the amount of transmitted fluid, and the duration between contamination of the respective needle and injury [17]. The management of occupational exposures should consider that HCV is rather stable in fluids for several days or even weeks [18]. Persons who experience an injury with an HCV-contaminated needle should be tested for HCV RNA within 2–4 weeks. Anti-HCV and ALT testing may be performed after 12 and 24 weeks [1].

The risk to *acquire HCV sexually* is extremely low in individuals with stable partnerships and avoiding any injuries. Cohort studies including >500 HCV infected patients followed over periods of more than 4 years could

Advanced Therapy for Hepatitis C, First Edition. Edited by Geoffrey W. McCaughan, John G. McHutchison and Jean-Michel Pawlotsky.
© 2012 Blackwell Publishing Ltd. Published 2012 by Blackwell Publishing Ltd.

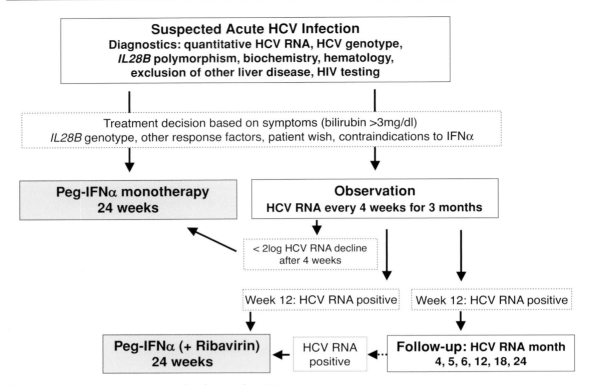

Figure 16.1 Suggested treatment algorithm for acute hepatitis C.

not identify cases of confirmed HCV transmission. Thus, several guidelines do not recommend the general use of condoms in monogamous relationships. However, this statement does not hold true for HIV-positive homosexual men. Recently, several outbreaks of acute hepatitis C have been described in populations of men who have sex with men (MSM) [19].

Caesarean sections are not recommended for *HCV-infected pregnant women* to prevent HCV transmission as the vertical transmission rate is low (at 1–6%). Transmission might be higher for girls than for boys and in HIV-positive mothers [20]. Children of HCV-infected mothers should be tested for HCV RNA as maternal anti-HCV antibodies can be detected for several months after birth. Mothers with chronic hepatitis C are allowed to breastfeed their children as long as they are negative for HIV and do not use intravenous drugs.

Treatment of Acute Hepatitis C

Successful treatment of acute hepatitis C virus (HCV) infection by interferon alfa-based therapies has been shown to be possible in the majority of patients. Treatment of acute hepatitis C should be considered not only because chronic HCV infection can lead to further serious clinical sequelae like liver cirrhosis or hepatocellular carcinoma, but also because HCV viremia may be associated with a risk for transmission of HCV to other persons. In addition, HCV infection can have significant social, legal, and economic consequences, especially for health care workers. While treatment of acute hepatitis C with type I interferons is well established, there has been some debate about timing, dose and duration therapy is optimal considering efficacy, side effects, and costs [21].

Early treatment of acute hepatitis C with recombinant interferon alpha was highly effective, with sustained virologic response (SVR) rates of up to 98% [4]. Importantly, no combination with ribavirin was necessary to achieve these high response rates when acute hepatitis C was treated early. Follow-up studies confirmed that virologic response rates are durable after the end of therapy and thus successful treatment can be considered as cure from HCV infection [22]. Subsequent studies investigating pegylated interferons to treat acute hepatitis C showed similarly high response rates [3]. Factors associated with response to treatment were the dose of peginterferon alfa [23] and, most importantly, adherence to therapy. One of the largest prospective trials was performed by the German Hep Net [24]. This study reflected to a large extent the "real-life" setting as patients were included not only by 18 university hospitals but also by 26 municipal hospitals and even by 9 gastroenterologists in private practice. The intent-to-treat and the adherent-to-therapy analyses showed SVR rates of 71% and 89%, respectively. Only 70 patients were adherent to therapy and a rather high number of patients (15%) were lost to follow-up. Additionally, 8 individuals had to stop treatment due to side effects and only 4 of those achieved an SVR. Thus, selection of patients, guidance and motivation, as well as management of side effects are key determinants of successful treatment in particular in acute hepatitis C. This experience was confirmed by studies from Switzerland [25], Italy [26], and Australia [27].

Timing of Therapy

Data on optimal timing of treatment of acute hepatitis C is limited since the heterogeneous studies and case series are rather difficult to compare. Several investigators delayed treatment for 12 weeks after the acquisition of HCV or after the clinical onset of hepatitis. Nomura *et al.* compared early "immediate" treatment with a very delayed treatment, starting treatment only after 1 year showing a superiority of the early approach for Japanese patients [28]. We would suggest that treatment can be delayed for up to 3 months after the onset of hepatitis in individuals with symptomatic acute hepatitis C, while immediate treatment should be considered if the patients are infected with genotype 1. If frequent monitoring of HCV RNA levels is possible, HCV RNA kinetics may also be considered for timing of therapy as repeated measurement of HCV RNA may predict spontaneous clearance of acute hepatitis C [5]. *IL28B* genotyping may also be used to decide whether treatment should be initiated early [29]. It could be reasonable to delay treatment particularly in individuals with favorable *IL28B* genotypes as these patients have a much higher chance of spontaneous HCV clearance. Finally, the patient's wishes need to be taken into account.

Duration of Therapy

Most trials using pegylated interferon alfa-2b have treated patients for 24 weeks. However, shorter therapies are very

likely to be possible [23,30], in particular in individuals with baseline parameters associated with a high likelihood of achieving an SVR.

Is Ribavirin Needed to Treat Acute Hepatitis C?

The use of ribavirin is very well established in the treatment of chronic hepatitis C. However, and maybe also surprisingly, there is currently no need to use ribavirin in patients with acute hepatitis C since 9 out of 10 patients can be treated successfully with interferon alfa alone. Ribavirin can be associated with significant side effects and costs and thus combination therapy of acute hepatitis is not needed in most patients [31]. The mode of action of ribavirin against hepatitis C is still largely undefined [32]. Clinically, the main effect of ribavirin is that the antiviral efficacy of interferon alfa is enhanced with improved early kinetics and fewer relapses after the end of treatment. In acute hepatitis C, however, interferon is still fully active against HCV. In this setting there are also no differences in responses against different HCV genotypes. Thus, the potential benefits of ribavirin are very minor. Still, if there is a high likelihood that interferon is not sufficient, ribavirin could be added, for example, patients with delayed HCV RNA kinetics during treatment, genotype 1 infection, and low or normal baseline ALT values may be considered as candidates of combination treatment of Peg-IFNa and ribavirin. As adherence to therapy is the main determinant of successful treatment of acute hepatitis, the unnecessary addition of ribavirin may reduce patient compliance due to the additional side effect profile.

In the Australian Trial of Acute Hepatitis C (ATAHC) acute HCV mono-infection was treated with peginterferon alone while acute HCV in HIV-infected patients was treated with combination therapy [33]. The authors reported similar rates of RVR but greater HCV RNA reductions at weeks 8 and 12 in the co-infected patients, suggesting an effect of RBV on third-phase viral kinetics. However, a number of patients were treated relatively late in the course of their acute HCV infection and may not necessarily be considered as "acute" HCV infection.

Conclusions

Interferon alfa therapy of acute hepatitis C is well established. Response rates are high and pegylated interferon can be recommended with an anticipated high rate of SVR as monotherapy. While ribavirin administration is usually not required to attain SVR, the absence of markers to identify the small number of patients who may benefit from the addition of ribavirin, and its marked effect in chronic hepatitis C, may lead some physicians to use it especially if begun relatively late in the course of acute infection. Asymptomatic patients with genotype 1 infection should be treated as early as possible while treatment may be delayed in individuals presenting with significant symptoms, at high ALT levels, in patients with genotype 2 or 3 infections, and those with favorable *IL28B* genotypes. Currently, we still would recommend a 24-week course of treatment although shorter treatment regimens are likely to be effective in a significant proportion of patients.

References

1. Craxi A. EASL clinical practice guidelines: management of hepatitis C virus infection. *J Hepatol* 2011;Feb 28 [Epub ahead of print].

2. Vogel M, Boesecke C, Rockstroh JK. Acute hepatitis C infection in HIV-positive patients. *Curr Opin Infect Dis* 2011;24(1):1–6.

3. Wiegand J, Deterding K, Cornberg M, Wedemeyer H. Treatment of acute hepatitis C: the success of monotherapy with (pegylated) interferon alpha. *J Antimicrob Chemother* 2008;62(5):860–65.

4. Santantonio T, Wiegand J, Tilman GJ. Acute hepatitis C: current status and remaining challenges. *J Hepatol* 2008;49(4):625–33.

5. Hofer H, Watkins-Riedel T, Janata O, *et al*. Spontaneous viral clearance in patients with acute hepatitis C can be predicted by repeated measurements of serum viral load. *Hepatology* 2003;37(1):60–64.

6. Lehmann M, Meyer MF, Monazahian M, *et al*. High rate of spontaneous clearance of acute hepatitis C virus genotype 3 infection. *J Med Virol* 2004;73(3):387–91.

7. Gerlach JT, Diepolder HM, Zachoval R, *et al*. Acute hepatitis C: high rate of both spontaneous and treatment-induced viral clearance. *Gastroenterology* 2003;125(1):80–88.

8. Mosley JW, Operskalski EA, Tobler LH, *et al*. Viral and host factors in early hepatitis C virus infection. *Hepatology* 2005;42(1):86–92.

9. Thomas DL, Thio CL, Martin MP, *et al*. Genetic variation in IL28B and spontaneous clearance of hepatitis C virus. *Nature* 2009;461(7265):798–801.

10. Tillmann HL, Thompson AJ, Patel K, *et al*. A polymorphism near IL28B is associated with spontaneous clearance of acute hepatitis C virus and jaundice. *Gastroenterology* 2010;139(5):1586–92.

11. Torresi J, Johnson D, Wedemeyer H. Progress in the development of preventive and therapeutic vaccines for hepatitis C virus. *J Hepatol* 2011;Jan 12 [Epub ahead of print].

12. Aitken CK, Lewis J, Tracy SL, *et al*. High incidence of hepatitis C virus reinfection in a cohort of injecting drug users. *Hepatology* 2008;48(6):1746–52.

13. Backmund M, Reimer J, Meyer K, *et al*. Hepatitis C virus infection and injection drug users: prevention, risk factors, and treatment. *Clin Infect Dis* 2005;40(Suppl 5):S330–35.

14. Marti Nez-Bauer E, Forns X, Armelles M, *et al*. Hospital admission is a relevant source of hepatitis C virus acquisition in Spain. *J Hepatol* 2007;48(1):20–27.

15. Deterding K, Wiegand J, Gruner N, Wedemeyer H. Medical procedures as a risk factor for HCV infection in developed countries: do we neglect a significant problem in medical care? *J Hepatol* 2008;48(6):1019–20.

16. Kubitschke A, Bader C, Tillmann HL, *et al*. [Injuries from needles contaminated with hepatitis C virus: how high is the risk of seroconversion for medical personnel really?]. *Internist (Berl)* 2007;48(10):1165–72.

17. Yazdanpanah Y, De CG, Migueres B, Lot F, Campins M, Colombo C, *et al*. Risk factors for hepatitis C virus transmission to health care workers after occupational exposure: a European case-control study. *Clin Infect Dis* 2005 Nov 15;41(10):1423–1430.

18. Ciesek S, Friesland M, Steinmann J, Becker B, Wedemeyer H, Manns MP, *et al*. How stable is the hepatitis C virus (HCV)? Environmental stability of HCV and its susceptibility to chemical biocides. *J Infect Dis* 2010 Jun 15;201(12):1859–1866.

19. van de Laar TJ, Matthews GV, Prins M, Danta M. Acute hepatitis C in HIV-infected men who have sex with men: an emerging sexually transmitted infection. *AIDS* 2010;24(12):1799–1812.

20. European Paediatric Hepatitis C Virus Network. Effects of mode of delivery and infant feeding on the risk of mother-to-child transmission of hepatitis C virus. European Paediatric Hepatitis C Virus Network. *BJOG-Int J Obstet Gy* 2001;108(4):371–7.

21. Wedemeyer H, Jackel E, Wiegand J, *et al*. Whom? When? How? Another piece of evidence for early treatment of acute hepatitis C. *Hepatology* 2004;39(5):1201–03.

22. Wiegand J, Jackel E, Cornberg M, *et al*. Long-term follow-up after successful interferon therapy of acute hepatitis C. *Hepatology* 2004;40(1):98–107.

23. De Rosa FG, Bargiacchi O, Audagnotto S, *et al*. Dose-dependent and genotype-independent sustained virological response of a 12 week pegylated interferon alpha-2b treatment for acute hepatitis C. *J Antimicrob Chemother* 2006;57(2):360–63.

24. Wiegand J, Buggisch P, Boecher W, *et al*. Early monotherapy with pegylated interferon alpha-2b for acute hepatitis C infection: the HEP-NET acute-HCV-II study. *Hepatology* 2006;43(2):250–56.

25. Broers B, Helbling B, Francois A, *et al.* Barriers to interferon-alpha therapy are higher in intravenous drug users than in other patients with acute hepatitis C. *J Hepatol* 2005;42(3):323–8.

26. De Rosa FG, Bargiacchi O, Audagnotto S, *et al.* Twelve-week treatment of acute hepatitis C virus with pegylated interferon-alpha-2b in injection drug users. *Clin Infect Dis* 2007;45(5):583–8.

27. Dore GJ, Hellard M, Matthews GV, *et al.* Effective treatment of injecting drug users with recently acquired hepatitis C virus infection. *Gastroenterology* 2010;138(1): 123–35.

28. Nomura H, Sou S, Tanimoto H, *et al.* Short-term interferon-alfa therapy for acute hepatitis C: a randomized controlled trial. *Hepatology* 2004;39(5):1213–19.

29. Grebely J, Petoumenos K, Hellard M, *et al.* Potential role for interleukin-28B genotype in treatment decision-making in recent hepatitis C virus infection. *Hepatology* 2010;52(4):1216–24.

30. Delwaide J, Bourgeois N, Gerard C, *et al.* Treatment of acute hepatitis C with interferon alpha-2b: early initiation of treatment is the most effective predictive factor of sustained viral response. *Aliment Pharmacol Ther* 2004;20(1):15–22.

31. Kamal SM, Ismail A, Graham CS, *et al.* Pegylated interferon alpha therapy in acute hepatitis C: relation to hepatitis C virus-specific T cell response kinetics. *Hepatology* 2004;39(6):1721–31.

32. Hofmann WP, Herrmann E, Sarrazin C, Zeuzem S. Ribavirin mode of action in chronic hepatitis C: from clinical use back to molecular mechanisms. *Liver Int* 2008;28(10):1332–43.

33. Matthews GV, Grebely J, Hellard M, *et al.* Differences in early virological decline in individuals treated within the Australian Trial in Acute HCV suggest a potential benefit for the use of ribavirin. *J Hepatol* 2010;52(Suppl. 1):28.

17 Antivirals in Cirrhosis and Portal Hypertension

Diarmuid S. Manning and Nezam H. Afdhal

Beth Israel Deaconess Medical Center, Harvard Medical School, Boston, MA, USA

Introduction

Chronic hepatitis C results in cirrhosis in up to 40% of infected patients [1] and represents one of the critical stages in the natural history of hepatitis C virus (HCV). It is estimated that 2–3% of chronically infected patients will develop cirrhosis each year. The complications of hepatitis C are predominantly seen in those patients who have progressed to cirrhosis, and include hepatic decompensation, portal hypertension with bleeding, and the development of hepatocellular carcinoma (HCC) [2]. In the cirrhotic patient, the risk of developing HCC is between 1% and 3% per year [3,4] and decompensation is approximately 4% per year [3].

Approximately 30% of patients with cirrhosis will develop portal hypertension. Variceal hemorrhage occurs in between 25% and 40% of patient with varices and is more common in patients with elevated hepatic venous pressure gradient above 12 mmHg and those with large varices [5]. Despite improvements in pharmacological, endoscopic, and interventional radiologic treatments, the mortality from an episode of variceal hemorrhage is still between 20% and 30%. On the basis of these figures, prevention of variceal hemorrhage remains extremely important.

The aims of treatment of patients with cirrhosis due to chronic hepatitis C include:

1 Prevention of progression of disease and hepatic decompensation.

2 Reduction of risk of development of HCC.

3 Possible regression of cirrhosis.

4 Elimination of hepatitis C prior to liver transplantation to prevent recurrence of HCV post-transplant and improve outcome of transplantation.

There is a growing body of evidence that all of the aims can be achieved to some degree but only effectively in those patients who have sustained virologic response (SVR) with eradication of HCV.

The best data exist for the beneficial effect of SVR on the natural history, where we have long-term follow-up data for over 10 years, which suggests a dual effect by resolution of both portal hypertension and reduced inflammation with improvement in liver function [6]. A recent study by Mallet and colleagues retrospectively examined 96 patients who had been treated with an interferon-based regimen and had at least one post-treatment liver biopsy [6]. Overall 18 of 96 patients had regression of cirrhosis, including 8 whose post-treatment liver biopsies showed F0–F1 fibrosis. They measured a number of endpoints: ascites, hepatic encephalopathy, variceal bleeding, spontaneous bacterial peritonitis, HCC, and liver transplantation. The incidence of the combined endpoint was 0 per 100 patient years in the group who showed regression of cirrhosis and 4 in those who did not show regression of cirrhosis [6]. Similar results have been seen in a large retrospective study of 920 patients with compensated cirrhosis by Bruno et al. [7] where there was significant relative risk reduction in the 124 patients who achieved SVR in the endpoints of liver-related death, hepatic decompensation, and HCC (Figure 17.1). In several recent retrospective series that followed cirrhotic patients post-SVR, the beneficial effects of SVR were clearly seen for reduction in development of liver decompensation but HCC still occurred, although at a markedly reduced rate [8–10]. We would recommend that even after an SVR, patients with established cirrhosis should still have HCC screening. Overall we can state that treatment of HCV and achievement of SVR can improve natural history in

Advanced Therapy for Hepatitis C, First Edition. Edited by Geoffrey W. McCaughan, John G. McHutchison and Jean-Michel Pawlotsky.
© 2012 Blackwell Publishing Ltd. Published 2012 by Blackwell Publishing Ltd.

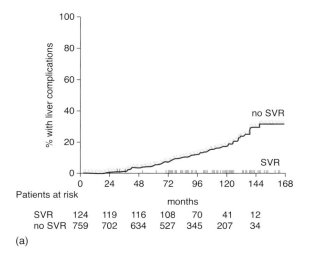

(a)

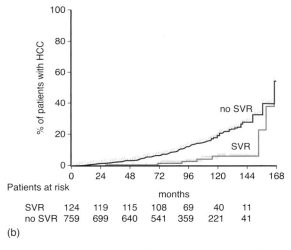

(b)

Figure 17.1 Impact of SVR on disease progression in cirrhosis. 920 patients in total with 142 cirrhotic patients achieving SVR, p < 0.001 Adapted from Bruno *et al.* [7].

compensated cirrhosis and strongly recommend that these patients be considered for treatment.

In decompensated cirrhosis the data on benefits of therapy are a little less robust due to both the relatively low numbers of patients treated and the low rate of SVR seen in this population. We would caution that in some patients the reverse can occur and treatment can induce worsening of liver function and induce decompensation. The real benefit of SVR in decompensated patients is the potential for prevention of recurrence of HCV post-transplant.

In summary, the beneficial effects of SVR in cirrhotic patients have been confirmed and they represent an important population for HCV therapy. However, treat-

ment in this group is challenging and requires significant expertise in side effect management both to optimize efficacy and to ensure safe treatment.

Compensated Cirrhosis

The current standard of care for the treatment of chronic hepatitis C is the combination of pegylated interferon alpha (Peg-IFN) and ribavirin (RBV) [11,12]. This combination leads to an SVR of 56% overall, compared to 44% in patients treated with standard interferon alfa-2a and RBV [11,12]. There is data on treatment of compensated cirrhosis for both Peg-IFN monotherapy [13] and combination with RBV, and overall there is a reduced SVR compared to patients without cirrhosis. SVR rates for Peg-IFN alfa-2a 90 mcg versus 180 mcg once a week were 5% and 12% for genotype 1 and 29% and 51% for genotypes 2 and 3 [13]. In many clinical trials, fibrosis stage 3 (bridging fibrosis) is combined in the analysis with cirrhosis, which can confound the results. In a large US study, WIN-R, 499 patients with cirrhosis were compared to 3724 non-cirrhotic patients in a sub-analysis of the effect of cirrhosis on SVR [14]. SVR rates were significantly higher in patients with F0–F3 fibrosis (43%) than those with cirrhosis (32%), and this effect was more pronounced in genotype 1 patients, where only 25% of patients with cirrhosis who received an optimal weight-based dose of RBV had an SVR.

There are two currently available pegylated interferon alfa preparations: pegylated interferon alfa-2a and -2b. The IDEAL study compared these two preparations in patients with hepatitis C, genotype 1 infection [15]. There does not appear to be any significant difference in SVR between these two preparations, at least in patients infected with hepatitis C, genotype 1. Again, in this study, there was a lower SVR in patients with advanced fibrosis (F3 or F4) when compared to those patients with earlier stages of fibrosis. Interestingly, the SVR seen in genotypes 2 and 3 patients appears to be independent of the degree of fibrosis, and cirrhosis has less of a predictive effect in these interferon-sensitive genotypes, where SVR can be as high as 70% [11,12]. More recently, pharmacogenomic studies from the IDEAL trial have discovered a series of polymorphisms in the vicinity of the *IL28B* gene, which predict interferon sensitivity in genotype 1 HCV patients [16]. Regression analysis shows that this *IL28B* polymorphism is more important than the stage of fibrosis in predicting response, and this may represent a useful baseline predictor in aiding therapeutic decisions for cirrhotic patients.

The majority of clinical trials in HCV have excluded patients with thrombocytopenia and since platelet count is a good surrogate for portal hypertension and hypersplenism, so by extrapolation these studies have really predominantly included well-compensated cirrhotics. DiMarco and colleagues performed a trial of Peg-IFN alfa-2b 1 μg/kg with RBV at a fixed dose of 800 mg for 52 weeks in 51 patients with presumed cirrhosis and portal hypertension [17]. Portal hypertension was diagnosed by the presence of varices, platelet count less than 100 000 per dl, or splenomegaly. The SVR rate by intention to treat was 22% and the major predictors were low baseline viral load and HCV RNA negativity at 12 weeks with no patients who were positive at 12 weeks achieving HCV RNA negativity by week 24. Interestingly, SVR in genotypes 2 and 3 was over 80%, establishing the value of treating these patients with favorable genotype. Unfortunately, severe side effects occurred in 37% of the study population, who had to discontinue treatment prematurely.

Decompensated Cirrhosis

Treatment of decompensated cirrhosis (Child-Turcotte-Pugh [CTP] class B) is controversial, associated with increased risk of significant adverse outcomes, less effective in terms of SVR, and should only be undertaken in experienced centers affiliated with liver transplant programs. Crippin and colleagues first treated 15 cirrhotic patients awaiting liver transplant in 2002 using conventional IFN alfa-2b monotherapy at a low dose of 1 mU daily [18]. There were 20 severe adverse events, including hematologic, worsening of liver failure, and infections. No patients achieved an SVR. The patients in this trial had a mean CTP score of 11.9 ± 1.2 and were probably too advanced for IFN-based treatment. Thomas and colleagues subsequently treated a small group of 20 patients with mean CTP score of 10 with 5 mU IFN daily and used granulocyte colony stimulating factor (GCSF) for support of neutropenia [19]. Twelve of twenty patients were virus-free prior to transplant and 20% achieved an SVR. Forns and colleagues added low-dose RBV 800 mg to IFN alfa-2b 3 mU in 30 patients awaiting liver transplant who had an estimated 4 months to wait before transplant [20]. Nine patients were HCV RNA negative prior to transplant and six remained HCV-free post-transplant. The largest study was performed by Everson and colleagues, who used a low-dose accelerating regimen (LADR) with

standard IFN and RBV, in 124 patients including CTP A, B, and C classes [21]. The overall SVR was 24%, 11% in genotype 1, and 50% in genotypes 2 and 3. Interestingly, 10 patients with an SVR underwent liver transplant and in none of these patients did HCV recur post-transplant.

Iacobellis and colleagues evaluated Peg-IFN alfa-2b 1 mcg/kg weekly with RBV 800–1000 mg for 24 weeks in patients with CTP classes B and C cirrhosis [22]. Only 41% of patients were able to tolerate treatment, with an SVR of 7% in genotypes 1 and 4 and 30% in genotypes 2 and 3 but none seen in patients with CTP class C. Infections were a serious side effect and by multivariate analysis related to a neutrophil count of <900 cells/μl on treatment and CTP class C, and the authors concluded that treatment should be avoided for CTP class C. Multiple other small studies have also evaluated Peg-IFN and RBV up to the full dose and durations used for standard of care in non-cirrhotics. The overall trend in these trials is similar to that seen in compensated patients, with the best results seen in patients with favorable genotypes 2 and 3 (up to 50%), low baseline viral load, and early viral clearance at week 4 and 12. The majority of these trials confirm the beneficial effects of SVR on liver function and CTP score but controversy still exists whether SVR can prevent the complications of portal hypertension and HCC development.

Maintenance Interferon

Patients with significant fibrosis/compensated cirrhosis (Metavir stage 3/4 or Ishak 4–6) who failed standard antiviral therapies are felt to be the optimal candidates for maintenance therapies. Interferon has a wide variety of antiviral and immune modulating functions, making it an obvious candidate for maintenance therapy. Originally, a small pilot study was conducted in 1999 in HCV nonresponders to determine if histologic progression could be halted [23]. This randomized controlled trial was conducted in 53 patients who received 6 months of interferon alfa-2b therapy, in whom HCV RNA remained positive but a histological response was seen; 27 patients were assigned to continue standard interferon (3 MU three times a week) for 24 months and 26 patients discontinued treatment and were observed, with the two groups well matched demographically. In patients receiving maintenance interferon there was a significant improvement in serum ALT level, log HCV RNA titer, and hepatic inflammation. In fact, after 30 months of treatment, there was a mean reduction in fibrosis score (from 2.5 to 1.7) with

80% of patients showing histologic improvement. Further evidence of benefit with maintenance interferon was seen in patients in whom therapy was withdrawn, where discontinuation of interferon was associated with an increase in fibrosis score and histological progression (30%).

These findings led to three major clinical trials investigating the use of maintenance Peg-IFN to prevent the progression in chronic hepatitis C infection [24–26] (see Table 17.1):

1 *HALT-C: Hepatitis C Antiviral Long Term Treatment Against Cirrhosis.* This study was a National Institutes of Health (NIH) sponsored study that recruited 1145 patients from 10 different sites into a lead-in phase. The patients (interferon non-responders) with chronic HCV and advanced fibrosis (Ishak stage 3–6) were randomized to a combination of pegylated interferon (Pegasys®) 180 μg/week and ribavirin (1000–1200 mg/day) for 24 weeks. There were 662 non-responders, and 151 relapsers from the lead-in phase put forward into the maintenance study. In addition, an external express cohort with the same inclusion/exclusion criteria and persistent HCV infection were inserted to make a total of 1050 patients (428 cirrhotic, 622 non-cirrhotic) for the maintenance study, of whom 517 were randomized to pegylated interferon (Pegasys®) 90 μg/week and 533 to untreated control. The majority of the patients in the study were genotype 1 (>90%), with high viral load (>log 6), and were stratified equally for baseline characteristics. The patients were followed with clinical, serum, radiologic assessment (at 3–6 month intervals), and liver biopsy at 1.5 and 3.5 years for histologic assessment. The primary outcomes were clinical (evidence of hepatic decompensation as shown by (i) increase in CPT score to 7 or higher; (ii) variceal hemorrhage; (iii) ascites; (iv) spontaneous bacterial peritonitis; (v) hepatic encephalopathy; (vi) HCC development; and (vii) death) and histological parameters (development of cirrhosis on liver biopsy with progression of Ishak fibrosis score by 2 points or more). Secondary outcomes include quality of life, serious adverse events, events requiring dose reductions, and development of presumed hepatocellular carcinoma. The trial lasted 4 years including the 6-month lead-in phase [24].

In this study maintenance therapy with Peg-IFN did not result in a reduction in clinical events or histological fibrosis improvement. However, there was an improvement in viral load, serum ALT, and necroinflammatory scores in the group treated with Peg-IFN alfa-2a.

2 *COPILOT (Colchicine versus PEGINTRON Long-Term Trial).* This study recruited 555 patients with chronic hepatitis C from 40 sites in the United States (supported by Schering-Plough Corp.). It compared weight-based low-dose peginterferon alfa-2b (subcutaneous injection of 0.5 mcg/kg/wk, one-third the dose used in standard HCV combination therapy) versus colchicine (0.6 mg orally, twice daily), an antifibrotic medication, in 555 chronic hepatitis C patients with advanced liver fibrosis (Ishak 3–6) who previously failed interferon-based therapies. It was a four-year study with similar baseline characteristics in the two study arms. Over the four years of the randomized study, investigators monitored the patients to determine how many reached a primary endpoint, defined as death, liver transplant, hepatocellular carcinoma, variceal bleeding, or liver failure (increase in CTP by 2 points with ascites, jaundice, or encephalopathy). They analyzed their findings for all 555 patients, who received at least one dose of their assigned drug, in two ways: (i) based on all events that occurred during the entire four years of the study, regardless of whether a patient was still taking their assigned drug or not (the "intent-to-treat" or ITT analysis), and (ii) based on only the events that occurred while patients were taking their assigned drug (the "on-drug" analysis). The investigators presented the data at the European Association for the Study of Liver Diseases (EASL) meeting in Milan, Italy 2008 [25]. A primary endpoint was reached by 17.8% (51/286) of patients in the peginterferon alfa-2b group versus 20.4% (55/269) in the colchicine group in the ITT analysis, and by 12.2% (35/286) and 16.0% (43/269) patients, respectively, in the on-drug analysis (treatment differences were not statistically significant). Among patients who had portal hypertension (42.3% and 48.0% of patients in the peginterferon alfa-2b and colchicine groups, respectively), peginterferon alfa-2b therapy resulted in significantly improved event-free survival in both the ITT and on-drug analyses (Wilcoxon $p = 0.041$ and 0.028, respectively). Further, variceal bleeding, a complication of portal hypertension, was almost abolished with peginterferon alfa-2b in both the ITT (10 versus 1 patients) and the on-drug (10 versus 0 patients) analyses. In the ITT analysis, hepatocellular carcinoma occurred in 7.7% and 5.9% of patients in the peginterferon alfa-2b and colchicine groups, respectively, a non-significant difference. A total of 49% of patients discontinued their medication before the end of the four-year study, with 36% due to failure to comply and 13% due to side effects.

This study indicates that maintenance Peg-IFN alfa-2b is effective in HCV cirrhotic patients with portal hypertension as it improves the event-free survival in this subgroup of patients; however final publication of the study results are awaited.

Table 17.1 Maintenance therapy trials

	HALT-C	COPILOT	EPIC 3
Patient selection	Ishak 4–6	Ishak 3–6	Metavir 2–4
Liver disease	CTP ≤6	CTP ≤ 7	CTP ≤ 6
Total number	1400	555	1700
Maintenance number	1050	555	616
Maintenance therapy	Peg-IFN alfa-2a	Peg-IFN alfa-2b	Peg-IFN alfa-2b
Dose	90 mcg	0.5 mcg/kg	0.5 mcg/kg
Arms	Placebo	Colchicine	Placebo
Run-in period	Yes (24 weeks)	No	Yes (12 weeks)
Duration (years)	3.5	4	3–5
Clinical outcomes			
Peg/control (%)	21 versus 24%	17 versus 24%	
Histology			
Fibrosis	No difference	n.a.	No difference
Inflammation	Improved	n.a.	Improved
Portal hypertension	No difference	Improved ($p < 0.02$)	Improved ($p < 0.02$)

Source: Adapted from Di Bisceglie *et al.* [24], Afdhal *et al.* [25], and Bruix *et al.* [26].

3 *EPIC (Efficacy of Peg-IFN in Chronic Hepatitis C).* This was the largest study to date to evaluate the re-treatment of patients with chronic hepatitis C infection, with advanced fibrosis, who had failed at least 12 weeks of interferon-based therapy previously [26]. Initially, this prospective, multicenter, open-label study evaluated the efficacy and safety of peginterferon alfa-2b (1.5 μg/kg/wk) plus weight-based ribavirin (800–1400 mg/day) in 2333 chronic HCV-infected patients with significant fibrosis/cirrhosis. A total of 497 patients (22%) achieved an SVR, with response rates better in patients previously treated with standard interferon/ribavirin compared to Peg-IFN/ribavirin (25% versus 17%) and also in relapsers compared to non-responders (38% to 14%).

Patients who did not respond to re-treatment by week 12 were offered entry into the maintenance interferon study arm, which assessed the histologic benefits of low-dose (0.5 mcg/kg) and long-term (3–5 years) peginterferon alfa-2b treatment in patients with F2/F3 metavir fibrosis score. The majority of patients had genotype 1 (92%) and high viral loads (70% viral load >600 000 IU/l) and were stratified equally for baseline characteristics.

The investigators presented the maintenance data (up to 3 years) at the EASL meeting in Vienna, Austria, in 2008. In the primary analysis, the maintenance Peg-IFN alfa-2b group ($n = 270$) showed no difference with the control observation group ($n = 270$) in fibrosis response. However, in sub-group analysis in patients treated for >2.5 years there was a trend toward improvement (21% versus 14%). A large group of patients (35%, 192/540) had no post-maintenance biopsy (Peg-IFN alfa-2b, $n = 88$; observation, $n = 104$) and were hence classed as no change, making the interpretation of these results difficult.

There was a significant difference in inflammatory score (≥1 point improvement in Metavir activity score) between the two groups, with the maintenance Peg-IFN alfa-2b group having a significant improvement in inflammatory activity compared to the control group (20% versus 9%).

The mean duration of treatment was 2.3 years among patients receiving Peg-IFN alfa-2b and 2.4 years among the control group. In the 348 patients with pre-re-treatment and end-of-treatment liver biopsies, the mean duration between the biopsies was 3.6 years in the Peg-IFN alfa-2b group and 3.9 years in the control group. There were major adverse events in 20% (53/270) of patients in the Peg-IFN alfa-2b group and 11% (31/270) of patients in the control observed group.

This study suggests that maintenance Peg-IFN alfa-2b improves inflammatory activity but does not improve fibrosis or prevent progression. However, as there were large numbers of patients who did not get a post-maintenance liver biopsy, which likely affected the analysis, the results from the 5-year analysis will provide more definitive information on improvement in fibrosis.

In conclusion, when we evaluate the three large trials we are finally left with some controversy based on the study designs and endpoints. We can certainly conclude that maintenance had no effect overall on histology for fibrosis progression or regression but there was a clear improvement in necroinflammation. Whether with a longer duration this would affect fibrosis is unclear but we can conclude that this did not occur with 4 years of treatment. The overall results on clinical outcome were also not favorable but both Peg-IFN alfa-2b studies with 0.5 μg/kg showed a distinct benefit in the subgroup with portal hypertension. Since IFN has been shown to reduce portal pressure, there is both a mechanism for this effect and a potential rationale to use this relatively well-tolerated treatment in patients with cirrhosis and portal hypertension.

Side Effects

The treatment of cirrhosis with IFN and RBV is challenging due to the side effect profile seen in these patients. In the cirrhosis studies, both compensated and decompensated, the discontinuation rates can reach above 40%. All the expected side effects of therapy are seen in cirrhotic patients but in particular the hematological side effects can be much more severe in this population [27,28].

Management of Thrombocytopenia

Thrombocytopenia has been reported in up to 70% of patients with cirrhosis [29]. In addition, thrombocytopenia is a common side effect of interferon alfa treatment and can lead to difficulty with starting antiviral therapy and maintenance of full-dose interferon [30]. Thrombocytopenia in cirrhosis is due to a combination of hypersplenism and underproduction of thrombopoeitin. Thrombopoeitin is a growth factor produced in the liver and involved in proliferation of megakaryocytes and platelet production. Thrombocytopenia can prevent patients from starting IFN therapy, and most trials exclude patients with platelet counts <80 000/ml and so the SVR rates in these patients is unknown. In addition, discontinuation and dose reduction for thrombocytopenia is common in HCV cirrhosis trials.

There are a number of therapeutic approaches under development for the management of thrombocytopenia including eltrombopag, a thrombopoeitin receptor agonist, recombinant human IL-11, and various thrombopoeitin mimetics. Eltrombopag is currently being tested in phase III studies in over 1000 patients with cirrhosis (ENABLE trials) to examine whether it will allow initiation and maintenance of treatment with interferon alfa in patients with cirrhosis and HCV. A recent randomized phase II study of eltrombopag in patients with HCV showed that 4 weeks of therapy led to platelet counts of >100 000/μl in up to 95% of patients versus 0% in the placebo group ($p < 0.001$) [31]. In addition, continuing eltrombopag for 12 weeks allowed significantly more patients to complete 12 weeks of antiviral treatment (up to 65%, compared to 6% in the placebo group).

Management of Neutropenia

Cirrhotic patients often have low total white cell counts secondary to hypersplenism and are very susceptible to Peg-IFN induced neutropenia. Antonini et al. reported 73 infections in 23% of 319 subjects treated with Peg-IFN [32]. Infection was independent of type of IFN and neutrophil count but was associated with age >60 years. However, cirrhotic patients already have increased risk of infections and in one trial in patients awaiting liver transplant there was an association of severe infections including spontaneous bacterial peritonitis (SBP) and bacteremia associated with poor liver function, low white cell count, and use of Peg-IFN. We currently recommend the use of filigrastin in patients with cirrhosis on IFN when the neutrophil count falls below 750 cells/ml.

Conclusions

One of the most challenging groups of patients with hepatitis C to treat are those with cirrhosis. Treatment has clearly been shown to improve long-term outcomes and survival in patients who have SVR and treatment should be offered to patients with cirrhosis and a CTP score <8 (CTP class B). Side effects, including thrombocytopenia, neutropenia, infections, and progression of liver disease, are more common in patients with cirrhosis and these patients should be treated in experienced liver centers. Active management of side effects is important to increase the efficacy of treatment but overall SVR rates are reduced in cirrhotic patients compared to non-cirrhotics. New therapies with direct acting antiviral agents need to be evaluated in both compensated and decompensated cirrhotic patients with the goal of safely improving SVR. Maintenance therapy should be reserved for patients with portal hypertension and esophageal varices who have failed to obtain an SVR with standard therapy.

References

1. Rustgi VK. The epidemiology of hepatitis C infection in the United States. *J Gastroenterol* 2007;42(7):513–21.
2. Niederau C, Lange S, Heintges T, *et al.* Prognosis of chronic hepatitis C: results of a large, prospective cohort study. *Hepatology* 1998;28(6):1687–95.
3. Fattovich G, Giustina G, Degos F, *et al.* Morbidity and mortality in compensated cirrhosis type C: a retrospective follow-up study of 384 patients. *Gastroenterology* 1997;112(2):463–72.
4. Hu KQ, Tong MJ. The long-term outcomes of patients with compensated hepatitis C virus-related cirrhosis and history of parenteral exposure in the United States. *Hepatology* 1999;29(4):1311–16.
5. Grace ND. Prevention of initial variceal hemorrhage. *Gastroenterol Clin N Am* 1992;21(1):149–61.
6. Mallet V, Gilgenkrantz H, Serpaggi J, *et al.* Brief communication: The relationship of regression of cirrhosis to outcome in chronic hepatitis C. *Ann Intern Med* 2008;149(6):399–403.
7. Bruno S, Stroffolini T, Colombo M, *et al.* Sustained virological response to interferon alfa is associated with improved outcome in HCV related cirrhosis: a retrospective study. *Hepatology* 2007;45:579–87.
8. Veldt BJ, Heathcote EJ, Wedemeyer H, *et al.* Sustained virologic response and clinical outcomes in patients with chronic hepatitis C and advanced fibrosis. *Ann Intern Med* 2007;147(10):677–84.
9. Morgan TR, Ghany MG, Kim HY, *et al.* Outcome of sustained virological responders with histologically advanced chronic hepatitis C. *Hepatology* 2010;52(3):833–44.
10. George SL, Bacon BR, Brunt EM, *et al.* Clinical, virologic, histologic, and biochemical outcomes after successful HCV therapy: a 5-year follow-up of 150 patients. *Hepatology.* 2009;49(3):729–38.
11. Fried MW, Shiffman ML, Reddy KR, *et al.* Peginterferon alfa-2a plus ribavirin for chronic hepatitis C virus infection. *N Engl J Med* 2002;347(13):975–82.
12. Manns MP, McHutchison JG, Gordon SC, *et al.* Peginterferon alfa-2b plus ribavirin compared with interferon alfa-2b plus ribavirin for initial treatment of chronic hepatitis C: a randomised trial. *Lancet* 2001;358(9286):958–65.
13. Heathcote EJ, Shiffman ML, Cooksley WG, *et al.* Peginterferon alfa-2a in patients with chronic hepatitis C and cirrhosis. *N Engl J Med* 2000;343(23):1673–80.
14. Jacobson IM, Brown RS, Jr., Freilich B, *et al.* Peginterferon alfa-2b and weight-based or flat-dose ribavirin in chronic hepatitis C patients: a randomized trial. *Hepatology* 2007;46(4):971–81.
15. McHutchison JG, Lawitz EJ, Shiffman ML, *et al.* Peginterferon alfa-2b or alfa-2a with ribavirin for treatment of hepatitis C infection. *N Engl J Med* 2009;361(6):580–93.
16. Thompson AJ, Muir AJ, Sulkowski MS, *et al.* IL28B polymorphism improves viral kinetics and is the strongest pretreatment predictor of SVR in HCV-1 patients. *Gastroenterology* 2010;139(1):120–29.
17. Di Marco V, Almasio PL, Ferraro D, *et al.* Peg-interferon alone or combined with ribavirin in HCV cirrhosis with portal hypertension: a randomized controlled trial. *J Hepatol* 2007;47:484–91.
18. Crippin JS, McCashland T, Terrault N, *et al.* A pilot study of the tolerability and efficacy of antiviral therapy in hepatitis C virus infected individuals awaiting liver transplant. *Liver Transpl* 2002;8:350–55.
19. Thomas RM, Brems JJ, Guzman-Hartmann G, *et al.* Infection with chronic hepatitis C virus and liver transplantation: a role for interferon therpay before transplantation. *Liver Transpl* 2003;9:905–15.
20. Forns X, Garcia-Retortillo M, Serrano T, *et al.* Antiviral therapy of patients with decompensated cirrhosis to prevent recurrence of hepatitis C after liver transplantation. *J Hepatol* 2003;39:389–96.
21. Everson JT, Forman L, Kugelmas M, *et al.* Treatment of advanced hepatitis C with a low accelerating dosage regimen of antiviral therapy. *Hepatology* 2005;42:255–62.
22. Iacobellis A, Siciliano M, Perri F, *et al.* Peginterferon alfa-2b and ribavirin in patients with hepatitis C virus and decompensated cirrhosis: a controlled study. *J Hepatol* 2007;46:206–12.
23. Shiffman ML, Hofmann CM, Contos MJ, *et al.* A randomized, controlled trial of maintenance interferon therapy for patients with chronic hepatitis C virus and persistent viremia. *Gastroenterology* 1999;117(5):1164–72.
24. Di Bisceglie AM, Shiffman ML, Everson GT, *et al.* Prolonged therapy of advanced chronic hepatitis C with low-dose peginterferon. *N Engl J Med* 2008;359(23):2429–41.
25. Afdhal NH, Levine R, Brown R, *et al.* Colchicine versus Peginterferon alfa 2b long term therapy: results of the 4 year COPILOT trial. *J Hepatol* 2008;48(Suppl 2):S4.
26. Bruix J, Poynard T, Colombo M, *et al.* Final Results of the EPIC3 cirrhosis maintenance trial: pegintron maintenance therapy in cirrhotic (METAVIR F4) HCV patients, who failed to respond to interferon/ribavirn (IR) therapy. *Gastroenterology* 2009;136(5 Suppl 1):A-798.
27. Bashour FN, Teran JC, Mullen KD. Prevalence of peripheral blood cytopenias (hypersplenism) in patients with nonalcoholic chronic liver disease. *Am J Gastroenterol* 2000;95(10):2936–9.
28. Dienstag JL, McHutchison JG. American Gastroenterological Association technical review on the management of hepatitis C. *Gastroenterology* 2006;130(1):231–64; quiz 214–7.

29. Afdhal NH, Esteban R. Introduction: thrombocytopenia in chronic liver disease – treatment implications and novel approaches. *Aliment Pharmacol Ther* 2007;26(Suppl 1):1–4.

30. Afdhal NH, McHutchison JG. Review article: pharmacological approaches for the treatment of thrombocytopenia in patients with chronic liver disease and hepatitis C infection. *Aliment Pharmacol Ther* 2007;26(Suppl 1):29–39.

31. McHutchison JG, Dusheiko G, Shiffman ML, *et al.* Eltrombopag for thrombocytopenia in patients with cirrhosis associated with hepatitis C. *N Engl J Med* 2007;357(22):2227–36.

32. Antonini MG, Babudieri S, Maida I, *et al.* Incidence of neutropenia and infections during combination treatment of chronic hepatitis C with pegylated alfa interferon 2a or alfa 2b plus ribavirin. *Infection* 2008;36:250–55.

18 Treatment of Recurrent Hepatitis C Following Liver Transplantation

Ed Gane

New Zealand Liver Transplant Unit, Auckland City Hospital, Grafton, New Zealand

Introduction

Liver failure and liver cancer from chronic hepatitis C are the most common indications for elective adult liver transplantation, accounting for almost 50% of cases. It is estimated that the demand for liver transplantation for chronic hepatitis C will treble over the next 20 years [1–4]. Recurrence of hepatitis C infection is universal and immediate following liver transplantation and associated with more rapid progression to cirrhosis and reduced graft and patient survival. Recurrence hepatitis C is now the greatest challenge facing the adult liver transplant program worldwide.

Management of recurrent hepatitis C has therefore become a major issue facing all adult liver transplant programs. The primary goal will be prevention of graft loss through delay in fibrosis progression. Although disease-modifying approaches (agents that inhibit fibrogenesis, apoptosis, and inflammation) are being pursued, the current approach is the use of antiviral therapy to eradicate or suppress established infection. Successful HCV eradication is the only factor associated with improved graft and patient survival following transplantation for hepatitis C [5].

The past decade has seen huge advances in antiviral therapy for chronic hepatitis C, with improvement in sustained virologic response (SVR) rates from <10% with standard interferon monotherapy to >60% with combination pegylated interferon plus ribavirin (the current standard-of-care).

However, liver transplant recipients with recurrent HCV infection represent a "born-to-lose" population, which possesses multiple baseline negative predictors for both early virologic response (EVR) and SVR to interferon:

1 High prevalence of HCV genotype 1 infection: this genotype accounts for almost 80% of patients transplanted for end-stage hepatitis C in the USA and more than 90% in Europe. HCV genotype 1 is also associated with more rapid fibrosis progression in the allograft and increased graft loss. Genotype 1 is the strongest baseline negative predictor of response to interferon-based therapies.

2 High prevalence of previous non-response to interferon-based therapy, which is a negative predictor for response.

3 High pre-treatment viremia level: levels increase 10- to 100-fold following liver transplantation, usually exceeding 10^6 units/ml [6–8]. More than 80% of liver transplant recipients with recurrent hepatitis C have a viral load greater than 400 000 IU/ml, associated with low response to interferon-based therapies.

4 Direct effects of immunosuppression on interferon efficacy. The initial antiviral effect (first-phase decline) is blunted in liver transplant recipients [9]. Both innate immune responses and HCV-specific T-cell immune responses are blunted in liver transplant recipients [10–12].

5 Poor adherence to antiviral therapy. More than 80% of patients must dose reduce and almost 30% must cease therapy because of adverse effects.

When determining the best approach for the treatment of recurrent hepatitis C, several issues need to be addressed: when should treatment be considered, who should be treated, and which agent(s) should be used.

Advanced Therapy for Hepatitis C, First Edition. Edited by Geoffrey W. McCaughan, John G. McHutchison and Jean-Michel Pawlotsky.
© 2012 Blackwell Publishing Ltd. Published 2012 by Blackwell Publishing Ltd.

Timing of Antiviral Therapy

The optimal timing of antiviral therapy in patients undergoing liver transplantation is not known. Antiviral strategies to prevent progressive graft injury from recurrent hepatitis C include: (i) pre-transplant treatment on the waiting list; (ii) peri-transplant prophylaxis; (iii) preemptive treatment; and (iv) treatment of established disease.

Pre-Transplant Treatment on the Wwaiting List

The rationale for treating transplant candidates while on the waiting list is to eradicate the virus prior to transplant. Unfortunately, combination pegylated interferon plus ribavirin is poorly tolerated in listed patients because of increased risks of neutropenia and thrombocytopenia, sepsis, and bleeding in patients with hypersplenism. In addition, Interferon-induced flares may precipitate acute decompensation and death in patients with advanced liver disease [13]. In a pilot study of 32 patients listed with Child-Turcotte-Pugh (CTB) class B or C cirrhosis (mean CPS $= 12 \pm 1$), less than half were suitable for interferon treatment. Of the 15 who were treated, only 33% had end-of-treatment virologic response (ETR) and none achieved SVR, 87% withdrew because of serious adverse events, namely sepsis, encephalopathy, or bleeding [14]. In a second study of patients listed for transplant but with less advanced disease (mean CPS $= 7 \pm 2$), a low accelerating dose regimen (initially interferon 1.5 mu three times a week and ribavirin 600 mg/day), was better tolerated, with serious adverse events in 19% and no deaths [15]. Thirty patients achieved SVR (24%), of whom half were delisted for improvement. Twelve patients were transplanted after successful SVR, none of whom have subsequently relapsed. These studies would support a cautious approach to antiviral therapy prior to liver transplantation. The most recent Asia and Pacific Association of the Study of the Liver consensus statement suggests that patients with decompensated hepatitis C should only be considered for treatment in an experienced liver unit, preferably a transplant center [16]. A low ascending dose regimen should be adopted, and supportive therapies to prevent variceal bleeding and infections and to correct cytopenias are recommended. One of the major issues in treating such patients is the catabolic effect of interferon-based therapies. This may exacerbate hypoalbminemia and precipitate the onset of clinical ascites and its complications of spontaneous bacterial peritonitis and hep-

atorenal syndrome. Thus treatment should be limited to those with CTP score ≤ 7, Mayo End-stage Liver Disease (MELD) score ≤ 18, without clinical ascites, and with baseline platelet count $>60\,000$, that is, only those transplant candidates with well-compensated disease, either listed for hepatocellular carcinoma or awaiting live-donor liver transplantation [17].

Peritransplant Prophylaxis

Because initial infection occurs immediately following reperfusion, prevention of allograft infection requires intra-operative neutralization of any virions circulating following removal of the native liver. In the analogous situation of transplantation for chronic hepatitis B, re-infection is prevented by very high-dose intravenous hepatitis B immunoglobulin (HBIG). Of note, HBIG prepared prior to the elimination of anti-HCV+ blood donors appeared to protect French patients transplanted for HBV/HCV co-infection from recurrent HCV infection [18]. It was postulated that these immunoglobulin preparations contained large amounts of polyclonal HCV anti-envelope antibodies, capable of neutralizing residual circulating hepatitis C virus, thereby preventing HCV infection of the graft. Chimpanzee studies conducted at the Centers for Disease Control (CDC) have demonstrated that a single dose of post-exposure hepatitis C immunoglobulin (HCIG) (prepared from HCV RNA+ donors) markedly prolonged the incubation period of acute HCV, while repeated doses reduced viremia levels in chronic infection [19]. However, the trials to date of high-dose IV hepatitis C immunoglobulin (both monoclonal and polyclonal) have failed to decrease either the incidence, time of onset, or severity of recurrent hepatitis C [20–22]. It is unlikely that passive immunoprophylaxis will be effective in chronic hepatitis C infection, which is associated with rapid evolution of new HCV quasispecies facilitating rapid immune escape. Recently, multiple different direct acting antiviral agents against HCV (inhibitors of HCV NS3/4A, 5A, and 5B) have entered clinical trials and combinations of different oral agents without cross-resistance are planned. Such combinations may provide safe and effective peri-operative prophylaxis to prevent recurrent hepatitis C infection of the allograft.

Pre-Emptive Treatment

The rationale for antiviral therapy in the very early post-transplant period is to treat early in the course of recurrent hepatitis C when quasispecies diversity [23] and viremia levels [24] are still low – both important predictors of SVR in non-transplant HCV infection. Although infection of the graft has already occurred at reperfusion, antiviral prophylaxis from early post-transplant should delay the onset of acute lobular hepatitis C in the graft and subsequent fibrosis progression [7,25]. The potential advantage of early therapy is that fibrosis will be minimal, an important predictor for SVR. Unfortunately, current antiviral therapies are poorly tolerated within the 3 months of transplant, due to renal dysfunction and cytopenias, which result from concomitant medications, viral infections, and persistent hypersplenism. In an early study with conventional interferon, 24 patients were randomized to receive 6 months interferon commencing at day 14 or no treatment. Although the onset of acute hepatitis was delayed in the prophylaxis group (408 versus 193 days), the severity of chronic hepatitis C was similar in both groups after 2 years [26]. In a second study, 86 patients were randomized to receive either conventional interferon or no treatment for 48 weeks starting within 2 weeks of transplantation [27]. Although interferon prophylaxis reduced the incidence of recurrent biochemical hepatitis at 1 year (27% versus 54%), there was no subsequent difference in patient and graft survival rates.

In the largest pre-emptive study with pegylated interferon plus ribavirin, 124 liver transplant recipients at the University of California, San Francisco were screened between 2 and 6 weeks post-transplant. More than 60% were excluded because of persistent cytopenias (usually anemia), renal dysfunction, rejection, or sepsis [28]. Of those actually treated, 85% required dose reduction and 40% were discontinued after a median of only 9 weeks. Despite adopting a low ascending dose regimen, less than 10% ever achieved full-dose ribavirin. The most frequent reasons for discontinuation were rejection and cytopenias. The use of growth factors had no impact on rate of dose reduction/discontinuation. Only 9% achieved SVR and almost 30% developed a serious adverse event during treatment. The disappointing results from this study have curbed enthusiasm for pre-emptive therapy with combination pegylated interferon plus ribavirin in the early months post-transplant. One other study has suggested that this approach should be used in patients with HCV genotypes 2 and 3, where high SVR rates have been reported.

On the basis that most problems were with ribavirin dosing, another study evaluated the safety and efficacy of 48 weeks pegylated interferon monotherapy administered from week 3 [29]. Although only 2/26 patients who received pegylated interferon achieved SVR (compared to 0/28 in the control group), pre-emptive therapy was associated with lower HCV RNA during treatment and less fibrosis post-treatment.

In a recent large, randomized, controlled, multicenter study of safety and efficacy of early pre-emptive therapy for the prevention of recurrent hepatitis C after liver transplantation (PHOENIX study), 115 patients were randomized to receive either pegylated interferon-alfa 2a (135 μg/week for 4 weeks followed by 180 μg/week for 44 weeks) plus ribavirin (400 mg p.o. daily escalating to 1200 mg p.o. daily for 48 weeks) or no treatment. No differences were observed in rate of SVR between those randomized to pre-emptive therapy (12/54) and those who switched to treatment (3/14). Rates of significant histologic recurrence, and patient and graft survival were similar in the two study arms [30].

Treatment of Established Disease

Most reports of antiviral therapy for recurrent hepatitis C have included patients with established chronic hepatitis in the allograft, who are at least 6 months post-transplant. There are a few reports of the safety and efficacy of antiviral therapy administered early post-transplant at the time of acute hepatitis C in the allograft. Most patients develop acute graft dysfunction from acute hepatitis C between 2 and 6 months post-transplant. Severe acute hepatitis C (early and persistent elevation of both serum HCV RNA levels and serum aminotransferases) has been associated with increased graft loss both from the rapidly progressive fibrosing cholestatic hepatitis syndrome and from late recurrent cirrhosis [31–33]. It has been postulated that starting antiviral therapy at the time of acute hepatitis C may prevent severe graft injury. In a recent study, such an approach (commencing therapy a mean 3.8 months post-transplant) achieved SVR in 35% of patients [34]. However, no long-term benefit was observed in non-responders, of whom 50% developed cirrhosis during follow-up.

As mentioned, the most popular antiviral strategy is targeting those recipients with established chronic liver disease and at highest risk for recurrent cirrhosis and graft loss. The best predictor of rapid fibrosis progression is the grade of necroinflammation and stage of fibrosis in the one-year protocol allograft biopsy [35–38].

Tolerability of Current Antiviral Therapy

When evaluating different antiviral regimens for the treatment of recurrent hepatitis C, it is important to consider not only their efficacy but also their safety and tolerability in liver transplant recipients.

Ribavirin

The most frequent adverse effect of ribavirin is dose-related hemolysis. Because red blood cells (RBCs) lack phosphorylase enzymes, ribavirin triphosphate (RTP) accumulates rapidly within RBC membranes. By directly competing with ATP, RTP may induce membrane oxidative damage, resulting in reduced red cell survival [39]. In the non-transplant registration studies for interferon and ribavirin, hemolysis necessitated dose reduction in 7% and dose withdrawal in less than 1% [40]. Unfortunately, hemolysis is more severe in liver [41–50] and kidney transplant recipients [51,52]. This reflects rapid accumulation of ribavirin following liver transplantation because of reduced renal clearance secondary to calcineurin-inhibitor nephrotoxicity and HCV-related glomerulonephritis [53]. In addition, calcineurin inhibitors may have a direct deleterious effect on RBC membrane fragility while azathioprine, another purine nucleoside analog, may competitively inhibit ribavirin metabolism. In a study of 72 liver transplant recipients receiving ribavirin, the mean creatinine clearance was only 45 ± 4 ml/min. More than 70% of transplant recipients developed significant hemolysis (defined as at least 15% reduction in hemoglobin) compared to less than 25% of subjects with normal renal function [54]. In studies of combination ribavirin plus either standard or pegylated interferon, ribavirin dose was reduced in 40–66% and stopped in 10–33%. Tolerability of ribavirin was particularly poor if commenced in the immediate post-transplant period. Strategies to improve ribavirin adherence include supportive transfusions and erythropoietin, although the latter is expensive and has not been associated with improved response rates in non-transplant patients [55]. Adjusting ribavirin dose according to a renal function algorithm is problematic. Regular monitoring of plasma ribavirin levels and adjusting daily dose to maintain trough plasma ribavirin levels at 10–15 mmol/l may improve adherence [56]. However, this assay (HPLC) is not yet widely available.

Interferon

The usual adverse effects of interferon alfa, including flu-like symptoms, anorexia, weight loss, and alopecia. occur with similar frequency after liver transplantation. Dose-related cytopenias are more common. Between 10% and 20% of liver transplant recipients receiving interferon cease treatment because of severe neutropenia and thrombocytopenia [42–47,49]. Transplant recipients are more susceptible because of co-existing hypersplenism, viral infections (CMV, HHV6), and myelosuppressive drugs (ganciclovir, cotrimoxazole, MMF). Interferon-induced depression may also be more common after liver transplantation [57]. Even in the absence of interferon, both liver transplantation and recurrent HCV infection may be additional risk factors for depression. Quality of life surveys report high depression scores in patients with recurrent HCV infection, which is attributed to direct effects of HCV and immunosuppressive agents and indirect effects of liver transplantation [26,58,59]. Almost 10% of liver transplant recipients stop interferon because of depression. Pre-emptive use of selective serotonin-reuptake inhibitors (SSRI) is often administered to prevent depression and facilitate interferon adherence [60].

Interferon treatment of chronic hepatitis C in renal transplant recipients has been associated with an increased risk of acute allograft dysfunction and loss secondary to severe rejection [61–63]. This has been attributed to IFN-induced up-regulation of HLA class I antigen expression [64]. Interferon alfa has also been associated with increased rates of both acute and chronic allograft rejection in renal transplant recipients. Although an early report of conventional interferon in liver transplant recipients reported an increased risk of chronic rejection (36%) [65], subsequent studies in liver transplant recipients have not confirmed any increased risk of acute allograft rejection during either standard or pegylated interferon with or without ribavirin [26,66–70]. However, there is recent concern that the incidence of chronic rejection may be increased in patients receiving pegylated interferon [71]. Reported cases have followed successful HCV RNA clearance, which improves graft function and accelerates calcineurin inhibitor clearance. The decreased calcineurin inhibitor levels may then precipitate a rejection episode. It is therefore essential that CNI levels are monitored frequently during antiviral therapy and maintenance doses adjusted in order to maintain adequate protection against rejection.

It would also seem reasonable, however, to avoid interferon alfa-based therapy in any patient with a history of chronic rejection or recurrent acute rejection [72].

Efficacy of Current Antiviral Therapy for Established Chronic Hepatitis

One issue when considering antiviral therapy for recurrent hepatitis C is which regimen to use and when to start.

However, current standard-of-care (pegylated interferon plus ribavirin) has poor efficacy and tolerability in transplant recipients. Favorable baseline predictors include viral load, genotype, and fibrosis stage. Early on-treatment responses are also useful – rapid virologic response (RVR) has excellent positive predictive value, while EVR has excellent negative predictive value and should be adopted as an early stopping rule [73,74].

There is an urgent need to develop more effective and better tolerated antiviral regimens for this area of unmet need. The introduction of direct-acting antivirals (polymerase and protease inhibitors) may provide new opportunities in the treatment of established recurrence and as pre- or peri-transplant prophylaxis to prevent recurrent infection.

Conventional Interferon Monotherapy

The earliest reports of treatment for recurrent hepatitis C with 6–12 months standard interferon alfa monotherapy were disappointing [65–67]. Although between 20% and 50% of patients achieved ETR, most relapsed and SVR was attained in <5%, and was limited to HCV non-1 genotype infections [75].

Ribavirin Monotherapy

Ribavirin is a non-interferon-inducing nucleoside analog, with multiple mechanisms of action against HCV. The direct inhibition of IMPDH will deplete intracellular GTP, thereby interrupting viral mRNA synthesis and viral RNA polymerase. Ribavirin may also trigger lethal mutagenesis, whereby increased HCV genomic mutations result in "error catastrophe" and HCV inhibition [76]. However, ribavirin therapy has minimal effect of HCV RNA levels or antigen expression [77–80].

Despite lack of any demonstrable antiviral effect, ribavirin monotherapy leads to normalization of serum aminotransferase levels and reduction in lobular inflammation in 50–70% of liver and kidney transplant recipients [41,80,81]. This is thought to reflect an indirect enhancement of HCV-specific T-cell immunity with switching from a predominantly TH2 to TH1 phenotype [82–84]. However, ribavirin monotherapy does not prevent progression of fibrosis [79,80].

When combined with interferon, ribavirin augments *in vitro* HCV-specific T-cell responses [85] and prevents post-treatment relapse, thereby increasing the SVR rate [40]. A recent study in liver transplant recipients with recurrent hepatitis C reported that long-term maintenance ribavirin monotherapy following combination pegylated interferon plus ribavirin improved histology, including fibrosis stage, but did not prevent virologic relapse rates [86].

Combined Conventional Interferon and Ribavirin

Since 1997, several centers have reported the safety and efficacy of 12 months combination conventional interferon plus ribavirin in liver transplant recipients with established chronic hepatitis C. Reported intention-to-treat SVR rates are between 17% and 27% (Figure 18.1) [42–49,87].

Unfortunately, adherence to both interferon and ribavirin has been poor, with 20–50% [47] of patients stopping treatment because of drug-related serious adverse events. Some centers have adopted initial low dose therapy (interferon 1 mU three times a week; ribavirin 200 mg b.i.d.) in order to reduce treatment withdrawal but the lower drug exposure may reduce subsequent SVR rates.

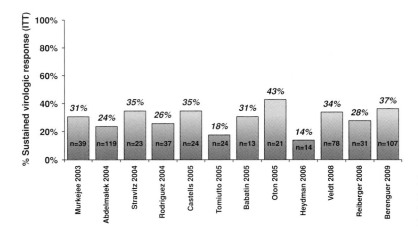

Figure 18.1 Efficacy of 48 weeks pegylated interferon plus ribavirin in liver transplant recipients with established recurrent hepatitis C.

Combination Pegylated Interferon and Ribavirin

Since combination pegylated interferon and ribavirin became the accepted standard-of-care (SOC) in non-transplant chronic hepatitis C infection, there have been many small uncontrolled pilot studies of the efficacy and safety of this SOC regimen in transplant recipients with recurrent hepatitis C [5,88–92]. Overall SVR rates are between 20% and 35%, significantly lower than those reported from studies with SOC in non-transplant hepatitis C.

Because of concerns that ribavirin toxicity was the major barrier to antiviral therapy post-liver transplantation, a recent randomized controlled study compared the safety and tolerability of pegylated interferon versus pegylated interferon monotherapy in recipients with established recurrent hepatitis C. Despite a marked increase in the incidence of serious adverse effects, dose reduction, and cessation, the addition of ribavirin was associated with a significant increase in SVR rate [71].

The PROTECT study, a large single-arm, multicenter, open-label study of 48 weeks combination pegylated interferon alfa-2b and ribavirin, was conducted in 125 liver transplant recipients with established recurrent hepatitis C at 25 US transplant centers. The reported sustained response rate was 24% in patients infected with HCV genotype 1 and 55% in those infected with HCV genotype 2/3. More than 50% of patients required dose reductions, while 30% discontinued therapy [93].

Predictors of Response to Antiviral Therapy for Recurrent Hepatitis C

Baseline Predictors for SVR

These include HCV genotype and fibrosis stage. SOC achieves SVR in 40–85% of transplant recipients with recurrent HCV genotype 2/3 infection compared to only 15–34% those with genotype 1 [5,86,94]. Severe fibrosis ($\geq$F3) is associated with SVR in <20%. This is problematic in that most consensus guidelines recommend delaying therapy until significant allograft injury has developed [16].

On-treatment Predictors for SVR

In non-transplant chronic hepatitis C infection, the most accurate predictors of SVR following SOC treatment of established recurrent hepatitis C are the early, on-treatment virologic responses: (i) the EVR, defined as HCV RNA after 12 weeks therapy decreased $\geq$2 log reduction from baseline; (ii) the complete early virologic response (cEVR), defined as undetectable HCV RNA after 12 weeks; and (iii) the RVR, defined as undetectable HCV RNA after 4 weeks [71,73,74,95,96]. In multiple studies of treatment of recurrent HCV infection, the strongest positive predictor for SVR was RVR (PPV 90–100%), while PPV for cEVR was 69–100% and for EVR only 49–65% [71]. In contrast, the strongest negative predictor for SVR (i.e., absence was associated with subsequent failure to achieve SVR) was EVR (NPV 89–100%) while the NPV of RVR was only 53–82%. These studies would support the adoption of a 12-week stopping rule for patients who fail to achieve EVR. There is no data yet to support reduced duration of therapy for those patients who achieve RVR.

A recent report of worsening outcomes with combination pegylated interferon plus ribavirin in patients with recurrent hepatitis C over the past decade is alarming [97]. In this large single-center experience, the SVR rate has almost halved during the past decade (from 47% to 24%). In a multivariate analysis, the authors identified increasing donor age and increasing stage of liver disease as the two independent variables associated with this reduced efficacy.

The role of immunosuppression on response to antiviral therapy is controversial. Cyclosporine and tacrolimus have opposing effects on HCV *in vitro*. While cyclosporine directly suppresses HCV replication *in vitro* through binding to cyclophilin B and inhibiting HCV RNA polymerase, tacrolimus indirectly enhances HCV replication *in vitro* through inhibition of phosphorylation and nuclear translocation of STAT-1, thereby blocking interferon signaling pathways [98,99].

Some studies have reported better SVR rates with SOC in patients receiving cyclosporine [95,97,100,101]. However, others have not, and a large multicenter, randomized study is needed to address this issue.

There is an urgent need to develop more effective and better-tolerated antiviral regimens for this area of unmet need. The introduction of direct-acting antivirals (polymerase and protease inhibitors) may provide new opportunities in the treatment of established recurrence and as pre- or peri-transplant prophylaxis to prevent recurrent infection.

Future Antiviral Strategies

The poor tolerability of ribavirin has encouraged the development of alternative, less toxic ribavirin analogues, of which viramidine (tarabivirin) is the most promising. This liver-targeting ribavirin prodrug is converted to active drug in the liver, thereby reducing RBC accumulation and subsequent haemolysis [102].

The poor efficacy and tolerability of current standard-of-care have driven the development of alternative therapeutic approaches in patients infected with HCV genotype 1. The development of the *in vitro* replicon and transgenic models for HCV replication have facilitated rapid development of direct-acting antiviral agents that directly inhibit HCV NS3 helicase, NS5A and NS5B RNA-dependent RNA polymerase. In clinical trials in non-transplant HCV, the addition of protease inhibitor improves the efficacy of current standard-of-care (pegylated interferon plus ribavirin) [103]. Combining two or more agents without cross-resistance may provide a safe and effective oral, interferon-free antiviral regimen for chronic hepatitis C infection. Such an approach may provide pre- and post-transplant suppression of recurrent hepatitis C, analogous to lamivudine plus adefovir in patients undergoing liver transplantation for HBV cirrhosis. This should be suitable for patients with advanced liver disease, enabling rescue from the waiting list, while perioperative administration may achieve the ultimate aim of universal prophylaxis against recurrent infection of the allograft.

Summary

Recurrent hepatitis C is now an important cause of graft loss following liver transplantation. Successful HCV eradication is the only factor associated with improved graft and patient survival following transplantation for hepatitis C [5].

However, current standard-of-care (pegylate interferon plus ribavirin) has poor efficacy and tolerability in transplant recipients. More than 80% of patients must dose reduce and almost 30% must cease therapy because of adverse effects. The biggest problem is severe hemolysis because of reduced renal clearance of ribavirin. Overall SVR rates are 20–30%, significantly lower than in non-transplant hepatitis C. Favourable baseline predictors include viral load, genotype, and fibrosis stage. Early on-treatment responses are also useful – RVR has excellent positive predictive value, while EVR has excellent negative predictive value and should be adopted as an early stopping rule.

Previously, only patients with severe recurrence were targeted for antiviral therapy, with disappointing results. The emphasis is now on earlier treatment of those patients most likely to develop severe graft injury.

The treatment and prevention of recurrent hepatitis C remains a priority area of "unmet need." The introduction of direct-acting antivirals (polymerase and protease inhibitors) may provide new opportunities in the treatment of established recurrence and as pre- or peri-transplant prophylaxis to prevent recurrent infection.

References

1. Armstrong G, Wasley A, Simard E, *et al.* Prevalence of HCV infection in the United States. *Ann Intern Med* 2006;144:705–14.
2. Wise M, Bialek S, Bell B, *et al.* Changing trends in HCV-related mortality in USA. *Hepatology* 2008;47:1128–35.
3. Davila J, Morgan R, Shaib Y, *et al.* HCV and increasing incidence of hepatocellular carcinoma: a population-based study. *Gastroenterology* 2004;127:1372–80.
4. Davis G, Albright J, Cook S. Projecting future complications of chronic hepatitis C in the United States. *Liver Transpl* 2003;9:331-8.
5. Berenguer M, Palau A, Aguilera V, *et al.* Clinical benefits of antiviral therapy in patients in recurrent HCV. *Am J Transpl* 2008;8:679–87.
6. Chazouilleres O, Kim M, Coombs C, *et al.* Quantitation of HCV RNA in liver transplant recipients. *Gastroenterology* 1994;106:994–9.
7. Gane E, Naoumov N, Qian K, *et al.* A longitudinal analysis of hepatitis C virus replication following liver transplantation, *Gastroenterology* 1996;110:167–77.
8. Everhart J, Wei Y, Eng H, *et al.* Recurrent and new HCV infection after liver transplantation. *Hepatology* 1999;29:1220–26.
9. Reiberger T, Rasoul-Rockenschaub S, Rieger A, *et al.* Efficacy of interferon in immunocompromised HCV patients after liver transplantation or with HIV co-infection. *Eur J Clin Invest* 2008;38:421–9.
10. Rosen H, Hinrichs D, Gretch D, *et al.* Association of multispecific CD4+ response to HCV and severity of recurrence after liver transplantation. *Gastroenterology* 1999;117:926–32.
11. Gruener N, Jung M, Ulsenheimer A, *et al.* Analysis of a successful HCV-specific CD8+ T cell response in patients with recurrent HCV-infection after orthotopic liver transplantation. *Liver Transpl* 2004;10:1487–96.
12. Schirren C, Zachoval R, Gerlach J, *et al.* Antiviral treatment of recurrent hepatitis C virus (HCV) infection after liver transplantation: association of a strong, multispecific, and long-lasting CD4 +T cell response with HCV-elimination. *J Hepatol* 2003;39:397–404.
13. Lock G, Reng C, Schölmerich J, *et al.* Interferon-induced hepatic failure in a patient with hepatitis C. *Am J Gastroenterol* 1999;94:2570–71.

14. Crippin J, McCashand T, Terrault N, *et al.* A pilot study of the tolerability and efficacy of antiviral therapy in hepatitis C-infected patients awaiting liver transplantation. *Liver Transpl* 2002;4:350–55.

15. Everson G, Trotter J, Forman L, *et al.* Treatment of advanced hepatitis C with a low accelerating dosage regimen of antiviral therapy. *Hepatology* 2005;42:255–62.

16. McCaughan G, Omato M, Dore G, Gane E, *et al.* APASL consensus statements on the diagnosis, management and treatment of hepatitis C Infection. *J Gastroen Hepatol* 2007;22:615–33.

17. Halprin A, Trotter J, Everson G, *et al.* Posttransplant eradication by pretransplant treatment in living donor liver transplant recipients. *Hepatology* 2001;34:244A.

18. Feray C, Gigou M, Samuel D, *et al.* Incidence of hepatitis C in patients receiving immunoglobulins after liver transplantation. *Ann Intern Med* 1998;128:810–16.

19. Krawczynski K, Alter M, Tankersley D, *et al.* Effect of immune globulin on prevention of experimental HCV infection. *J Infect Disease* 1996;173:822–8.

20. Willems B, Ede M, Marotta P, *et al.* HCV human immunoglobulins for the prevention of graft infection in HCV–related liver transplantation. *J Hepatol* 2002;36 (S1):32.

21. Davis G, Nelson D, Terrault N, *et al.* A randomised open-label study to evaluate the safety and pharmacokinetics of human hepatitis C immunoglobulin in liver transplant recipients. *Liver Transpl* 2005;11:941–9.

22. Schiano T, Charlton M, Younossi Z, *et al.* Monoclonal HCV-AbXTL68 in patients undergoing liver transplantation for HCV. *Liver Transpl* 2006;12:1381–9.

23. Moribe T, Hayashi N, Kanazawa Y, *et al.* Hepatitis C viral complexity detected by single strand conformation polymorphism and response to interferon therapy. *Gastroenterology* 1995;108(3):789–95.

24. Garcia-Retortillo M, Forns X, Feliu A, *et al.* Hepatitis C kinetics during and immediately after transplantation. *Hepatology* 2002;35:680–87.

25. Ballardini G, De Raffele E, Groff P, *et al.* Timing of reinfection and mechanisms of hepatocellular damage in transplanted HCV-infected liver. *Liver Transpl* 2002;8:10–20.

26. Singh N, Gayowski T, Wannstedt C, *et al.* Interferon-α for prophylaxis of recurrent viral hepatitis C in liver transplant recipients. *Transplantation* 1998;65:82–6.

27. Sheiner P, Boros P, Klion F, *et al.* The efficacy of prophylactic interferon alfa-2b in preventing recurrent hepatitis C after liver transplantation. *Hepatology* 1998;28:831–8.

28. Shergill A, Khalili M, Straley S, *et al.* Applicability, tolerability and efficacy of pre-emptive antiviral therapy in HCV-infected patients undergoing liver transplantation. *Am J Transplant* 2005;5:118–24.

29. Chalasani N, Manzarbeitia C, Ferenci P, *et al.* Peginterferon alfa-2a for hepatitis C after liver transplantation: two randomized, controlled trials. *Hepatology* 2005;41:289–98.

30. Bzowej N, Nelson D, Terrault D, *et al.* PHOENIX: a randomized controlled trial of peginterferon alfa-2a plus ribavirin as a prophylactic treatment after liver transplantation for hepatitis C virus. *Liver Transpl* 2011;17:528–38.

31. Sreekumar R, Gonzalez-Koch A, Maor-Kendler Y, *et al.* Early identification of recipients with progressive histologic recurrence of HCV after liver transplantation. *Hepatology* 2000;32:1125–30.

32. Shackel N, Jamias J, Rahman W, *et al.* Early high peak HCV load levels independently predict HCV-related liver failure post-transplantation. *Liver Transpl* 2009;15:709–18.

33. Pelletier S, Iezzoni J, Crabtree T, *et al.* Prediction of liver allograft fibrosis after transplantation for hepatitis C virus. *Liver Transpl* 2000;6:44–53.

34. Castells L, Vargas V, Allende H, *et al.* Combined treatment with pegylated interferon and ribavirin in the acute phase of HCV recurrence after liver transplantation. *J Hepatol* 2005;43:53–9.

35. Gane E, Portmann B, Naoumov N, *et al.* Long-term outcome of hepatitis C infection after liver transplantation. *N Engl J Med* 1996;334:821–7.

36. Prieto M, Bereguer M, Rayon J, *et al.* High incidence of allograft cirrhosis in HCV genotype 1b following transplantation. *Hepatology* 1999;29:250–56.

37. Firpi R, Abdelmalek M, Soldevila-Pico C, *et al.* One-year protocol liver biopsy can stratify fibrosis progression in liver transplant recipients with recurrent hepatitis C infection. *Liver Transpl* 2004;10:1240–47.

38. Neumann U, Berg T, Bahra M, *et al.* Fibrosis progression after liver transplantation in patients with recurrent hepatitis C. *J Hepatol* 2004;41:830–36.

39. De Franceschi L, Fattovich G, Turrini F, *et al.* Haemolytic anaemia induced by ribavirin therapy in patients with chronic HCV infection: role of membrane oxidative damage. *Hepatology* 2000;31:997–1004.

40. McHutchinson J, Gordon S, Schiff E, *et al.* Interferon 2b alone or in combination with ribavirin as initial treatment of chronic hepatitis C. *N Engl J Med* 1998;339:1485–92.

41. Cattral MS, Krajden M, Wanless IR, *et al.* A pilot study of ribavirin therapy for recurrent hepatitis C virus infection after liver transplantation. *Transplantation* 1996;61:1483–8.

42. Zamboni F, Franchello A, Lavezzo B, *et al.* Treatment of recurrent hepatitis C after liver transplantation with interferon alfa 2b and ribavirin. *J Hepatol* 2000;32:S265.

43. Bellati G, Alberti A, Belli L, *et al.* Therapy of chronic hepatitis C after liver transplantation: multicentre Italian experience. *J Hepatol* 1999;30(Suppl 1):51.

44. Ahmad J, Dodson S, Demetris A, *et al.* Recurrent hepatitis C after liver transplantation: a nonrandomised trial of interferon alfa alone versus interferon alfa plus ribavirin. *Liver Transpl* 2001;7:863–9.

45. Gopal D, Rabkin J, Corless C, *et al.* Treatment of progressive hepatitis C recurrence after liver transplantation

with combination interferon plus ribavirin. *Liver Transpl* 2001;7:181–90.

46. Alberti A, Belli L, Airoldi A, *et al.* Combined therapy with interferon and low dose ribavirin in posttransplantation recurrent hepatitis C: a pragmatic study. *Liver Transpl* 2001;7:870–76.

47. De Vera M, Smallwood G, Rosado K, *et al.* Interferon-alpha and ribavirin for the treatment of recurrent hepatitis C after liver transplantation. *Transplantation* 2001;71:678–86.

48. Menon K, Poterucha J, El-Amin O, *et al.* Treatment of posttransplantation recurrence of hepatitis C with interferon and ribavirin: lessons in tolerability and efficacy. *Liver Transpl* 2002;8:623–9.

49. Samuel D, Bizillon T, Feray C, *et al.* Combination interferon-alpha and ribavirin for recurrent HCV infection after liver transplantation: a randomised controlled study. *Hepatology* 2000;32:A542.

50. Reddy R, Fried M, Dickson R, *et al.* Interferon alfa-2b and ribavirin vs. placebo as early treatment in patients transplanted for hepatitis c end-stage liver disease: results of multicenter, randomized trial. *Gastroenterology* 2002;122:A199.

51. Garnier JL, Chevallier P, Dubernard JM, *et al.* Treatment of hepatitis C virus infection with ribavirin in kidney transplant patients. *Transplant Proc* 1997;29:783.

52. Daoud S, Garnier JL, Chossegros P, *et al.* Hepatitis C virus infection in renal transplantation. *Transplant Proc* 1995;27(2):1735.

53. Dumortier J, Ducos E, Scoazec J-Y, *et al.* Plasma ribavirin concentrations during treatment of recurrent hepatitis C with peginterferon alpha-2b and ribavirin combination after liver transplantation. *J Viral Hepatitis* 2006;13:538–43.

54. Jain AB, Eghtesad B, Venkataramanan R, *et al.* Ribavirin dose modification based on renal function is necessary to reduce hemolysis in liver transplant patients with hepatitis C virus infection. *Liver Transpl* 2002;8:1007–13.

55. Shiffman M, Salvatore J, Hubbard S, *et al.* Treatment of chronic hepatitis C genotype 1 with peginterferon, ribavirin and epoetin alpha. *Hepatology* 2007;46:371–9.

56. Rendina M, Schena A, Castellaneta N, *et al.* The treatment of chronic hepatitis C with peginterferon alfa-2a (40 kDa) plus ribavirin in haemodialysed patients awaiting renal transplant *J Hepatol* 2007;46:768–74.

57. Zdilar D, Franco-Bronson K, Buchler N, *et al.* Hepatitis C, interferon alfa and depression. *Hepatology* 2000;31:1207–11.

58. De Bona M, Ponton P, Ermani M, *et al.* The impact of liver disease and medical complications on quality of life and psychological distress before and after liver transplantation. *J Hepatol* 2000;33:609–15.

59. Forton D, Allsop J, Main J, *et al.* Evidence for a cerebral effect of HCV. *Lancet* 2001;358:38–39.

60. Musselman D, Lawson D, Gumnick J, *et al.* Paroxetine for the prevention of depression induced by high-dose interferon. *N Engl J Med* 2001;34:961–6.

61. Rostaing L, Modesto A, Baron E, *et al.* Acute renal failure in kidney transplant patients treated with interferon alpha 2b for chronic hepatitis C. *Nephron* 1996;74:512–16.

62. Kramer P, ten Kate FW, Bijnen AB, *et al.* Recombinant leucocyte interferon induces steroid-resistant acute vascular rejection episodes in renal transplant recipients. *Lancet* 1984;1:989–90.

63. Magnone M, Holley J, Shapiro R, *et al.* Interferon-alpha-induced acute renal allograft rejection. *Transplantation* 1995;59:1068–70.

64. Slater A, Klein J, Sonnerfield G, *et al.* The effects of interferon in a model of rat heart transplantation. *J Heart Lung Transpl* 1992;11:975–8.

65. Féray C, Samuel D, Gigou M, *et al.* An open trial of interferon alfa recombinant for hepatitis C after liver transplantation. *Hepatology* 1995;22:1084–9.

66. Wright T, Combs C, Kim M, *et al.* Interferon-alfa therapy for hepatitis C virus infection after liver transplantation. *Hepatology* 1994;20:773–9.

67. Gane E, Lo SK, Portmann BC, *et al.* A randomised study comparing ribavirin and interferon-alpha monotherapy for hepatitis C recurrence after liver transplantation. *Hepatology* 1998;27:1403–7.

68. Jain A, Demetris A, Manez R, *et al.* Incidence and severity of acute allograft rejection in liver transplant recipients treated with alfa interferon. *Liver Transpl Surg* 1998;4:197–203.

69. Ferenci P, Peck-Radosavljevic M, Vogel W, *et al.* 40 kDa Peginterferon alfa-2a (Pegasys) in post-liver transplant recipients with established recurrent hepatitis C: preliminary results of a randomized multicenter trial. *Hepatology* 2001; 34: 406A.

70. Stravitz R, Shiffman M, Sanyal A, *et al.* Effects of interferon on liver histology and allograft rejection in patients with recurrent hepatitis C following liver transplantation. *Liver Transpl* 2004;10:850–88.

71. Gane E, Strasser S, Crawford D, *et al.* A multicenter, randomized trial of combination pegylated interferon-alpha 2a plus ribavirin vs. pegylated interferon-alpha 2a monotherapy in liver transplant recipients with recurrent hepatitis C. *Hepatology* 2009;50(4 Suppl):393A.

72. Walter T, Dumortier J, Guillard O, *et al.* Rejection under alpha interferon therapy in liver transplant recipients. *Am J Transplant* 2007;7:177–84.

73. Hanouneh I, Miller C, Aucejo F, *et al.* Recurrent HCV after liver transplant: on treatment prediction of response to Peg/RBV. *Liver Transpl* 2008;14:53–8.

74. Oton E, Barcena R, Moreno-Planas J, *et al.* Hepatitis C recurrence after liver transplantation: viral and histologic response to full-dose PEG-interferon and ribavirin. *Am J Transpl* 2006;6:2345–55.

75. Cotler S, Ganger D, Kaur S, *et al.* Daily interferon for HCV infection in liver transplant recipients. *Transplantation* 2001;71:261–6.

76. Hong Z, Cameron CE. Pleiotropic mechanisms of ribavirin antiviral activities. *Prog Drug Res* 2002;59:41–69.

77. Dusheiko G, Main J, Thomas H, *et al*. Ribavirin treatment for patients with chronic hepatitis C: results of a placebo-controlled study. *J Hepatol* 1996;25:591–8.

78. Bodenheimer HC, Lindsay KKL, Davis GL, *et al*. Tolerance and efficacy of oral ribavirin treatment of chronic hepatitis C: a multicentre trial. *Hepatology* 1997;26:473–7.

79. Di Bisceglie AM, Conjeevaram HA, Fried MW, *et al*. Ribavirin as therapy for chronic hepatitis C. *Ann Intern Med* 1995;123:897–903.

80. Quadri R, Giostra E, Roskams T, *et al*. Immunological and virological effects of ribavirin in hepatitis C after liver transplantation. *Transplantation* 2002;73:373–8.

81. Gane E, Tibbs C, Ramage J, Portmann B, Williams R. Ribavirin therapy for hepatitis C infection following liver transplantation. *Transpl Int* 1995;8:61–4.

82. Ilyin G, Longouet S, Rissel M, *et al*. Ribavirin inhibits protein synthesis and cell proliferation induced by mitogenic factors in primary human and rate hepatocytes. *Hepatology* 1998;27:1687–94.

83. Ning Q, Brown D, Parado J, *et al*. Ribavirin inhibits viral-induced macrophage production of TNF-a, IL-1, fg12 prothrombinase and preserves TH1 cytokine production but inhibits TH2 cytokine response. *J Immunol* 1998;160:3487–93.

84. Hultgren C, Milich D, Weiland O, *et al*. The antiviral compound ribavirin modulates the T helper (Th) 1/Th2 subset balance in hepatitis B and C virus-specific immune responses. *J Gen Virol* 1998;79:2381–91.

85. Cramp M, Rossol S, Chokshi S, *et al*. Hepatitis C virus-specific T-cell reactivity during interferon and ribavirin treatment in chronic hepatitis C. *Gastroenterology* 2000;118:346–55.

86. Calmus Y, Duvoux C, Pageaux G, *et al*. Multicentre randomised trial in HCV-infected patients treated with pegylated IFN and ribavirin followed by ribavirin alone after liver transplantation. *Am J Transpl* 2008;8:A1617.

87. Bizollon T, Palazzo U, Ducerf C, *et al*. Pilot study of combination of Interferon alpha and ribavirin as therapy of recurrent hepatitis C after liver transplantation. *Hepatology* 1997;26:500–504.

88. Mukherjee S, Lyden E. Impact of Peg-IFN plus ribavirin on hepatic fibrosis in liver transplant patients with recurrent hepatitis C. *Liver Int* 2006;26:529–35.

89. Rodriguez-Luna H, Khatib A, Sharma P, *et al*. Treatment of recurrent HCV infection after liver transplantation with combination Peg-IFN alpha 2b and ribavirin. *Transplant* 2004;77:190–94.

90. Toniutto P, Fabris C, Fumo E, *et al*. Pegylated vs standard IFN in antiviral regimens for post-transplant recurrent hepatitis C. *J Gastroenterol Hepatol* 2005;20: 577–82.

91. Babatin M, Schindel L, Burak K, *et al*. Peg-IFN alpha 2b and ribavirin for recurrent hepatitis C after liver transplantation. *Can J Gastroenterol* 2005;19:359–65.

92. Heydtmann M, Freshwater D, Dudley T, *et al*. Peg-IFN alpha 2b for patients with HCV recurrence and graft fibrosis following liver transplantation. *Am J Transpl* 2006;6:825–33.

93. Gordon F, Brown R, Kwo P, *et al*. Peginteferon alfa-2b and ribavirin for hepatitis C recurrence post orthotopic liver transplantation: final results from the PROTECT study. *J Hepatol* 2010;52:S10–S11

94. Roche B, Sebagh M, Canfora M, *et al*. HCV therapy in liver transplant recipients: response predictors effect on fibrosis progression and importance of initial stage of fibrosis. *Liver Transpl* 2008;14:1766–77.

95. Carrion J, Marreo J, Fontana R, *et al*. Efficacy of antiviral therapy on HCV recurrence after liver transplantation. *Gastroenterology* 2007;132:1746–56.

96. Sharma P, Marrero J, Fontana R, *et al*. Sustained virologic response to therapy of recurrent hepatitis C after liver transplantation is related to early virologic response and dose adherence. *Liver Transpl* 2007;13:1100–108.

97. Berenguer M, Aguilera V, Prieto M, *et al*. Worse recent efficacy of antiviral therapy in liver transplant recipients with recurrent hepatitis C. *Liver Transpl* 2009;15: 738–46.

98. Henry SD, Metselaar HJ, Lonsdale RC, et al.Mycophenolic acid inhibits hepatitis C virus replication and acts in synergy with cyclosporin A and interferon-alpha. *Gastroenterology* 2006;131:1452–62.

99. Hirano K, Ichikawa T, Nakao K, *et al*. Differential effects of calcineurin inhibitors, tacrolimus and cyclosporin a, on interferon-induced antiviral protein in human hepatocyte cells. *Liver Transpl* 2008;14:292–8.

100. Bizollon T, Pradat P, Mabrut J, *et al*. Histologic benefit of retreatment by peg-IFN plus ribavirin in patients with recurrent hepatitis C. *Am J Transpl* 2007;7:448–53.

101. Cescon M, Grazi G, Cucchetti A, *et al*. Predictors of SVR after antiviral therapy for HCV recurrence following liver transplantation. *Liver Transpl* 2009;15:782–9.

102. Benhamou Y, Afdhal N, Nelson D, *et al*. A phase III study of the safety and efficacy of viramidine versus ribavirin in treatment-naïve patients with chronic hepatitis C: ViSER1 results. *Hepatology* 2009;50:717–26.

103. Jacobson I, McHutchison J, Dusheiko G, *et al*. Telaprevir for previously untreated chronic hepatitis C virus infection. *N Engl J Med* 2011;364:2405–16.

19 Antiviral Treatment in Chronic Hepatitis C Virus Infection with Extrahepatic Manifestations

Benjamin Terrier and Patrice Cacoub
Department of Internal Medicine, Hôpital Pitié-Salpêtrière; Université Pierre et Marie Curie, Paris, France

Introduction

Hepatitis C virus (HCV) infection is a worldwide disease that affects about 170 million persons. Following acute infection, development of chronic hepatitis in up to 80% of cases may lead to cirrhosis and hepatocarcinoma. With the discovery of HCV, it has been appreciated that HCV is not uniquely associated with chronic hepatic inflammation but also with many extrahepatic complications. Among these extrahepatic manifestations, mixed cryoglobulinemia (MC) and its clinical features hold the strongest association.

In this chapter, we will describe the most frequent reported extrahepatic manifestations, and discuss their treatment, in particular the role of antiviral therapy.

HCV-Associated Mixed Cryoglobulinemia Vasculitis

Pathophysiology of HCV-Associated MC

HCV exerts a chronic stimulus on the immune system, which may lead to the proliferation of B cell clones producing pathogenic immunoglobulin M (IgM) with rheumatoid factor (RF) activity. The basis for the strong association between this B cell response to HCV and the detection of an RF in MC vasculitis may lie in the structural and antigenic homologies between the N-terminal region of the HCV E2 envelope protein and the human immunoglobulin variable domains [1]. A possible contributory factor may be the ability of E2 envelope glycoprotein to bind CD81 B cell surface protein. CD81 on B cell surface may

provide a strong stimulatory signal if activated as part of a complex (CD19/CD21/CD81 complex) together with B-cell receptor (BCR) activation [2]. These findings strongly support the use of antiviral agents and B-cell depletion therapy in the management of HCV-associated MC vasculitis.

On the other hand, both CD4+ and CD8+ T cells accumulate in vasculitic nerve lesions with an increased expression of interferon (IFN)-γ and tumor necrosis factor (TNF)-α, associated with the absence of typical type 2 cytokines, pointing to a strong polarized type 1 immune response. These findings support the use of non-specific immunosuppressive agents in severe and refractory forms of MC vasculitis.

The mechanisms involved in HCV MC vasculitis are summarized in Figure 19.1.

Clinical and Laboratory Features of HCV-Associated MC

Circulating mixed cryoglobulins are frequently detected in HCV-infected patients (40–60%) whereas overt cryoglobulinemia vasculitis develops in only 5–10% of cases [3]. The most frequently targeted organs are skin, joints, nerves, and kidney. The disease expression is variable, ranging from mild clinical symptoms (purpura, arthralgia) to fulminant life-threatening complications (glomerulonephritis, widespread vasculitis). The most common clinical and immunologic manifestations of HCV-associated MC are shown in Table 19.1.

Skin is the most frequently involved target organ and is the direct consequence of the small-size vessel vasculitis. The main sign is a palpable purpura, which is

---

Advanced Therapy for Hepatitis C, First Edition. Edited by Geoffrey W. McCaughan, John G. McHutchison and Jean-Michel Pawlotsky.
© 2012 Blackwell Publishing Ltd. Published 2012 by Blackwell Publishing Ltd.

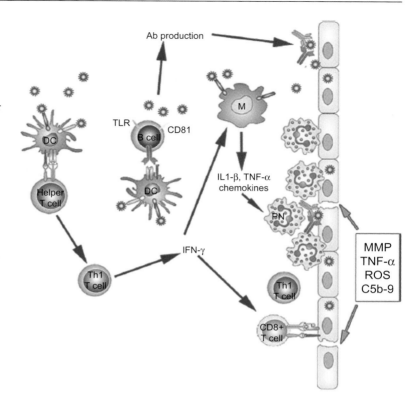

Figure 19.1 Mechanisms responsible for HCV MC vasculitis lesions. HCV may infect B cells by CD81 and induce a chronic stimulation. B cells produce antibodies against HCV that cross-link with IgM with RF activity and may form immune complex (i.e., cryoglobulin). Cryo vasculitis is characterized by immune complex mediated with tissue injury link to deposit of immune complexes and subsequent neutrophil recruitment and complement activation. Also, there is a presence of macrophages and T cells in vasculitic tissues and a predominant Th1 type cytokine differentiation. The last step of vasculitis lesions involves matrix metalloprotease (MMP), oxydative stress molecules (ROS), and proinflammatory cytokines like TNF-α. DC, dendritic cells; M, macrophages; PN, polymorphonuclear neutrophil.

reported in 70–90% of patients [4,5]. It always begins at the lower limbs and may extend to the abdominal area, less frequently to the trunk and upper limbs. Skin biopsy

Table 19.1 Clinical and immunologic findings in HCV-associated mixed cryoglobulinemia.

Findings	Percentage
Clinical	
Purpura	70–90
Weakness	60–80
Arthralgia	40–80
Peripheral neuropathy	8–55
Sicca syndrome	20–40
Renal involvement	20–35
Leg ulcers	10–20
Raynaud's phenomenon	3–15
Biological	
Rheumatoid factor	70–80
Type II cryoglobulin	70–80
Low C4 complement level	60–80

shows a non-specific leukocytoclastic vasculitis involving small-size vessels with inflammatory infiltrates and, in some cases, fibrinoid necrosis of the arteriolar walls and endovascular thrombi. Raynaud's phenomenon and acrocyanosis, which may evolve to digital ulcerations, can also occur.

Arthralgia is reported in 40–80% of HCV-infected patients with MC [6,7]. They are bilateral and symmetric, non-deforming and involving mainly knees and hands, more seldom elbows and ankles. Frank arthritis is rarely reported, being present in less than 10% of patients [6,7]. Rheumatoid factor activity is found in 70–80% of MC patients but is not correlated with the presence of joint disease as patients chronically infected with HCV in the absence of HCV MC or RF may have prominent joint symptoms. There is no evidence of joint destruction, and antibodies to cyclic citrullinated peptide, which are highly specific of rheumatoid arthritis, are absent [8].

MC-associated peripheral neuropathies are found in up to 70% of HCV-infected patients with MC [4,9,10]. Bilateral, more often asymmetric, polyneuropathies represent 45–70% of MC polyneuropathies and multiple mononeuropathies 30–55% [11–14]. Patients always present with sensory symptoms of the lower limbs, such as hypoesthesia and paresthesia, frequently painful. Second, they may develop a motor involvement. The clinical examination found a thermoalgic sensory deficiency of lower limbs, more seldom of upper limbs. More rarely, a motor deficiency involves the lower limbs. Electromyographic tests show an axonal involvement with alteration of the sensory potentials and the motor conduction velocities. When neuromuscular biopsy is performed, anatomopathological analysis often highlights moderate to severe axonal damage associated with a small-size vessel vasculitis (arterioles, venules, capillaries) and an inflammatory infiltrate only composed of monocytes and lymphocytes, without necrotizing angiitis. The differential diagnosis with a periarteritis nodosa (PAN)-like vasculitis may be difficult. It is noteworthy that when PAN-like lesions are present, they involve small and medium vessels with necrotizing vasculitis, and a mixed inflammatory infiltrate of monocytes, lymphocytes, and polymorphonuclear neutrophils is always evidenced [15]. The direct implication of the HCV is still debated but the evidence of a local replication of the HCV has never been proven, real-time polymerase chain reaction (RT-PCR) failing to demonstrate the presence of genomic negative-strand HCV RNA in neuromuscular biopsies [14,16]. The central nervous system can be rarely involved. Main manifestations are encephalopathy, convulsions, cerebral vasculitis with strokes, and cranial neuropathies [15,17,18].

HCV MC-associated renal manifestations are reported in 2–50% of patients [4,9,19]. The most frequent clinical and histologic picture is an acute or chronic type-I membranoproliferative glomerulonephritis (MPGN) with sub-endothelial deposits. It represents 70–80% of cryoglobulinemic renal diseases and it is strongly associated with the type II IgMκ MC [20–22]. The most frequent presentation is proteinuria with microscopic hematuria and a variable degree of renal insufficiency [23]. Acute nephrotic syndrome or acute nephritic syndrome can also reveal cryoglobulinemic renal involvement. New-onset arterial hypertension is seen in 80% of cases. Morphological features are characterized by an important monocyte infiltrate with double contours of the basement membrane, large, eosinophilic, and amorphous intra-luminal thrombi. Immunofluorescence study shows intra-glomerular sub-endothelial deposits of IgG, IgM (identical to those of the cryoprecipitates) and complement components. In addition, vasculitis of small renal arteries is present in one third of patients. Extra-capillary crescents are rarely observed [21].

Other organs may be more rarely involved by HCV MC vasculitis. Abdominal pains are reported and digestive bleeding may reveal a mesenteric vasculitis. Lungs can be involved without clinical symptoms but some patients may present moderate exercise dyspnea, dry cough, interstitial lung fibrosis, pleural effusions, or hemoptysis, which can be consequent of alveolar hemorrhages. A cardiac involvement may be revealed by mitral valvular damage, coronary vasculitis that may complicate myocardial infraction, pericarditis, or congestive cardiac failure. Finally, chronic fever may be associated with other clinical manifestations.

Biologically, cryoglobulins are defined by the presence of circulating immunoglobulins that precipitate as serum is cooled below core body temperature and resolubilize when re-warmed. Cryoglobulins are readily detectable in 40–60% of HCV-infected patients in most case series [3]. Cryoglobulins are immunochemically categorized into three types by the method of Brouet *et al.* [24]. Type I cryoglobulins are single monoclonal immunoglobulins usually found in lymphoproliferative disorders. Type II consists of polyclonal IgG with monoclonal rheumatoid factor activity. Type III are comprised of polyclonal IgG and polyclonal rheumatoid factor. During chronic HCV infection, cryoglobulins are type II and III, often referred to as MC [24]. Beside the detection of serum cryoglobulin itself, other laboratory abnormalities may provide surrogate evidence of the presence of cryoglobulinemia, such as low C4 serum level, depressed total hemolytic complement levels, monoclonal proteinemia, or rheumatoid factor activity. Hypocomplementemia is a sensitive and important finding in cryoglobulinemia vasculitis, being found in 70–90% of MC patients. Other immunologic abnormalities in HCV-infected patients, whether MC positive or negative, include antinuclear (17–41%), anti-cardiolipin (20–27%), anti-smooth muscle cell (9–40%), and anti-thyroglobulin (8–13%) antibodies [9,25].

Therapeutic Management of HCV-Associated MC

The discovery of HCV and the analysis of pathophysiologic mechanisms provided the opportunity to control HCV MC with: (i) antiviral therapy based on the belief that the underlying infection was driving immune complex formation and resultant vasculitis; (ii) B-cell depletion therapy targeting B cells that produce cryoglobulinemia; and (iii) non-specific immunosuppressive therapy targeting inflammatory cells present in vasculitic lesions. Moreover, potential adverse effects of immunosuppressive therapy with glucocorticoids and cytotoxic drugs on an underlying chronic viral infection were a matter of concern.

Antiviral Agents

The treatment of HCV infection (i.e., in the absence of HCV MC) has progressed dramatically over the past 20 years, with the standard of pegylated interferon alfa and ribavirin therapy now leading to sustained virologic clearance in nearly half of patients. The early attempts to control HCV MC with standard thrice weekly IFN-α was not surprisingly associated with a relatively poor response and a high relapse rate, especially in severe cases [26]. IFN-α monotherapy was effective in 50–100% of patients with purpuric skin lesions, but did not demonstrate efficacy on neurologic or renal involvement. Clinical improvement of HCV-related vasculitis correlated with virologic response. However, when follow-up was sufficient, most of the responders developed virologic and clinical relapses following IFN-α withdrawal [26–28]. Combination therapy with standard IFN-α plus ribavirin has provided much better short- and long-term results in patients with HCV-related vasculitis than historically reported with IFN-α. In three uncontrolled studies [29–31], combination therapy with standard IFN-α and ribavirin demonstrated enhanced efficacy on main HCV-related vasculitic manifestations (cutaneous, 100%; renal, 50%; and neurological, 25–75%). Two studies reported a loss of proteinuria and hematuria in sustained viral responders treated by IFN-α plus ribavirin [22,32]. No significant changes in renal function were noted in MC patients following anti-HCV therapy, regardless of the virologic response to treatment [22,32]. We recently reported in 72 consecutive HCV MC patients [33] that Peg-IFN-α plus ribavirin achieved a higher rate of complete clinical response (67.5% versus 56.2%) and virologic response (62.5% versus 53.1%) as compared with standard IFN-α plus ribavirin, regardless of HCV genotype and viral load. In multivariate analysis, an early virologic response at month 3 (OR 3.53, 95% CI 1.18 to 10.59) was independently associated with a complete clinical response of MC. A glomerular filtration rate lower than 70 ml/min (OR 0.18; 95% CI 0.05 to 0.67) was negatively associated with a complete clinical response of MC.

Although up to 70% of HCV MC patients exhibit sustained virologic response with Peg-IFN-α plus ribavirin combination for 13–14 months, 30% of patients remain refractory to this antiviral therapy. In such patients, specifically targeted antiviral therapy for HCV (STAT-C) could represent promising drugs to increase the viro-logic response rate and thus, the clinical and immunologic response [34,35].

B-Cell Depletion Therapy

Several Italian groups have initially reported on the efficacy of anti-CD20 monoclonal antibody, rituximab (RTX), in patients with HCV MC vasculitis resistant or intolerant to IFN-α monotherapy [36,37]. A complete clinical response was reported in 60–70% of cases, with cryoglobulin clearance in one third of patients. However, the absence of efficacy on HCV viral clearance and the high relapse rates supported the need for combined antiviral therapy to block the HCV infection trigger and obviate long-term liver complications of such a chronic infection. A recent clinical trial showed a superiority of a combination of RTX plus Peg-IFN alfa-2b plus ribavirin compared to Peg-IFN alfa-2b plus ribavirin in severe HCV-associated MC vasculitis. Triple therapy showed a more rapid improvement and a higher rate of kidney complete response, with a good safety profile [38]. The efficacy and tolerance of RTX with and without combined antiviral therapy in a large cohort of HCV vasculitis patients with a long-term follow-up was also recently reported [39]. RTX and Peg-IFN alfa-2b plus ribavirin induced a clinical complete (CR) and partial (PR) response in 80% and 15% of cases, respectively; an immunologic CR and PR in 67% and 33%, respectively; and a sustained virologic response in 55%. RTX alone induced a clinical CR and PR in 58% and 9% of patients, and immunologic CR and PR in 46% and 36%, respectively. Moreover, patients treated with RTX without antiviral therapy showed stable levels of HCV RNA and a slight increase of ALT levels (1.5, the upper limit of normal value at baseline, to 1.7 at the end of follow-up). These findings are reassuring regarding the use of RTX in HCV-infected patients, even in the absence of antiviral therapy.

However, in rare cases, RTX may form a complex with RF-positive IgMκ, leading to accelerated cryoprecipitation and to severe systemic reactions. Then, RTX should be administered with the use of 375 mg/m^2/week protocol (4 consecutive weeks) and plasma exchanges prior to RTX infusion in patients with high baseline values of MC [40].

Non-Specific Immunosuppressive Agents

Immunosuppressive agents are typically reserved for patients with severe disease manifestations such as membranoproliferative glomerulonephritis, severe neuropathy, and life-threatening complications. Traditionally, a combination of corticosteroids and immunosuppressants such as cyclophosphamide and azathioprine has been used for the control of severe vasculitis lesions while awaiting the generally slow response to antiviral treatments. In a large retrospective study of 105 patients with renal disease associated with cryoglobulinemia vasculitis, 80% were administered corticosteroids and/or cytotoxic agents, while 67% underwent plasmapheresis [23]. Despite this aggressive approach, long-lasting remission of the renal disease was achieved in only 14% of cases, and the 10-year survival rate was only 49%.

Corticosteroids, used alone or in addition to IFN-α, did not favorably affect the response of HCV-related vasculitic manifestations in two controlled studies [26,27]. In one randomized trial, methylprednisolone alone given for one year was associated with clinical response in 22% of patients, compared with 66% and 71% in patients receiving IFN-α or IFN-α plus methyprednisolone, respectively [28]. Low-dose corticosteroids may help to control minor intermittent inflammatory signs such as arthralgia, but do not succeed in cases of major organ involvement (i.e., neurologic, renal), or in the long-term control of vasculitis.

Plasmapheresis offers the theoretical advantage of removing the pathogenic cryoglobulins from the circulation of patients with HCV MC vasculitis. Immunosuppressive therapy is usually needed associated with plasma exchange in order to avoid the rebound increase in cryoglobulinemia that is commonly seen after discontinuation of apheresis. When used in combination with anti-HCV treatment, plasmapheresis did not modify the virologic response if IFN-α was given after each plasma exchange session [41].

Therapeutic Guidelines

It appears logical that aggressive antiviral therapy with Peg-IFN and weight-based ribavirin be considered as induction therapy for HCV MC with mild to moderate disease severity and activity (i.e., without rapidly progressive nephritis, motor neuropathy, or other life-threatening complications). The duration of therapy has not yet been rigorously determined but treatment courses longer than those merely based on genotype alone appear more likely to be effective, that is, at least 13 months [31].

In patients presenting with severe disease (i.e., progressive renal disease, progressive motor neuropathy, extensive skin disease, including ulcers and distal necrosis), an induction phase with RTX and/or plasmapheresis may be useful, before starting HCV treatment.

The therapeutic management of HCV-related MC vasculitis according to the clinico-biological presentation is summarized in Figure 19.2.

HCV-Associated B-Cell Non-Hodgkin Lymphoma

Pathophysiology of HCV-Associated B-Cell Non-Hodgkin Lymphoma

HCV exerts a chronic stimulus on the immune system, which may lead to the selection of abnormal clones, in

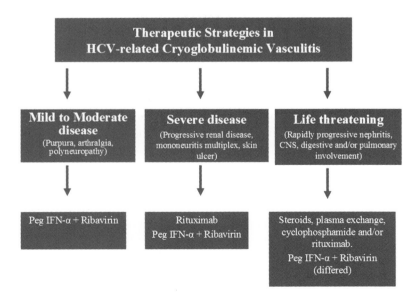

Figure 19.2 Treatment of HCV-related mixed cryoglobulinemia vasculitis according to the clinico-biological presentation. Reproduced from Saadoun et al. [32], with permission.

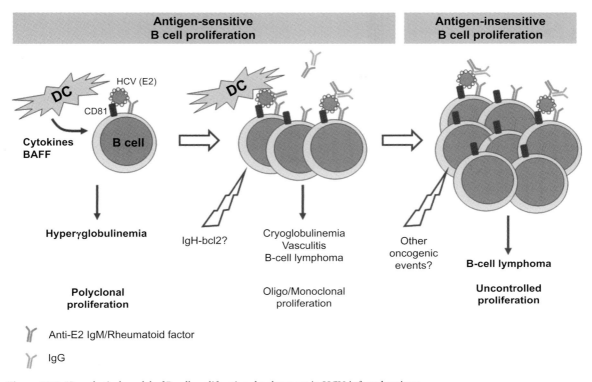

Figure 19.3 Hypothetical model of B-cell proliferation development in HCV-infected patients.

a scenario reminiscent of the role of *Helicobacter pylori* in gastric mucosal-associated lymphoid tissue (MALT) lymphoma. Previous findings seem to delineate a process that begins with HCV antigens stimulating B-cells, and evolves into an under-regulated polyclonal and subsequently monoclonal expansion, leading in some instances to frank malignancy (Figure 19.3).

Chronic antigenic stimulation may underlie the transformation process, as engagement of BCR on mature B cells can induce proliferation. Another regulatory element implicated is the B lymphocyte stimulator (BLyS), produced by marginal zone dendritic cells, which is an important survival signal that may also serve as a co-stimulatory proliferation signal. Genetic events could also support B-cell survival in HCV-related clonal expansion [2].

Characteristics of HCV-Associated B-Cell Non-Hodgkin Lymphoma

Monoclonal B cells producing pathogenic IgM with rheumatoid factor activity can be detected in patients with HCV-associated MC. A significant proportion of

monoclonal MC type II can evolve into overt B-cell non-Hodgkin lymphoma (B-NHL). In a multicenter Italian study, the estimated risk for lymphoproliferative disease was found to be 35-fold in patients with HCV-related MC compared with the general population [42]. In a meta-analysis, the prevalence of HCV infection in patients with B-NHL was found to be approximately 15% [43]. Epidemiologic studies have demonstrated the association between HCV infection and B-NHL [43–48]. Most common histologic subtypes of HCV-associated lymphomas are low-grade marginal zone lymphomas, such as splenic lymphoma with villous lymphocytes (SLVL) and MALT lymphomas, and more rarely with lymphoplasmacytic lymphomas and large B-cell lymphomas. MC is constantly present in HCV-associated SLVL [49]. The great argument for a clear association between HCV infection and SLVL was brought by a multicenter French study [50]. Among nine HCV-infected patients with SLVL, under combination course of IFN-α plus ribavirin without any immunosuppressive drug, seven patients experienced a complete hematologic response while remaining negative for HCV

RNA after a median follow-up of 27 months, one had a partial response, and another relapsed of SLVL concomitantly to virologic relapse (detectable levels of HCV RNA). A second treatment combining IFN-α and ribavirin resulted in a second virologic response with a persistent complete hematological response. Inversely, none of the six non-HCV infected patients with SLVL (control group) who received a 6-month course of IFN-α presented hematological response.

Overall, these data indicate a strong correlation between serum viral load and tumor burden in HCV-associated SLVL, and support the existence of a causal relationship between HCV chronic antigenic stimulation and the marginal zone lymphomatous process.

Other HCV-Associated Extrahepatic Manifestations

Fatigue

Fatigue is one of the most frequent HCV-associated extrahepatic manifestations with frequencies ranging from 35% to 67% according to studied cohorts and predefined criteria of fatigue. Severe fatigue, which causes degradation of daily social or professional activities, is found in 17–20% of patients [51,52]. A fibromyalgic syndrome, including fatigue, arthralgia, and myalgia, was present in 16–19% of patients [52,53].

The factors that may influence the occurrence of fatigue were also highlighted: female gender, cirrhosis, age over 50 years, depression, purpura, and presence of arthralgia or myalgia. There was no correlation with alcohol consumption, viral genotype or load, abnormal thyroid function, and type and level of cryoglobulinemia [51,52]. Under antiviral treatment, only virologic sustained responders obtained significant improvement on fatigue, which decreased by 50–70%, whereas prevalences of fatigue did not change among non-responders or relapsers. Nevertheless, fatigue may persist in one third of sustained responder patients and the factors that were associated with this included presence of other extrahepatic manifestation (OR = 7), depression (OR = 3), female gender (OR = 2.5), and cirrhosis (OR = 2) [51].

Sicca Syndrome

Several data have initially suggested association between HCV and Gougerot-Sjögren syndrome, considering the high frequency of MC in both diseases, and HCV salivary gland tropism (found in 50% of patients). However, although ocular and/or mouth Sicca syndrome is frequently found in HCV-infected patients, a definite Gougerot-Sjögren syndrome is rarer. There is no frank improvement of such Sicca syndrome under anti-HCV antiviral course, even after sustained virologic response [51].

Autoimmune Thrombocytopenia

The presence of thrombocytopenia in HCV-infected patients may result from several causes: peripheral destruction by hypersplenism, autoimmune thrombocytopenia with anti-platelet antibodies, central involvement by proliferative disease, thrombopoietin defect. In immunologic thrombocytopenic purpura, anti-HCV antibodies are found in 10–19% of patients [54,55]. Inversely, a thrombocytopenia was found in 41% of HCV infected patients versus 19% in HBV-infected patients. The efficacy of antiviral course of IFN and ribavirin in a certain number of autoimmune thrombocytopenia resistant to conventional treatments (steroids, disulone, immunosuppressive drugs, intravenous immunoglobulins) seems to enforce the hypothesis of a non-fortuity association between HCV infection and autoimmune thrombocytopenia [56,57].

Type 2 Diabetes Mellitus

Type 2 diabetes mellitus is more and more thought to be associated with HCV infection. In the majority of studies, which are mostly controlled, the prevalence of type 2 diabetes mellitus is significantly higher among HCV-infected patients (20–33%) than among HBV-infected (6.6–12%) and healthy control groups (5.6–11%) [58–60]. In one French study, this prevalence was 7% among 1614 HCV-infected patients [3]. Overall, prevalence of type 2 diabetes mellitus was also higher in patients with than without cirrhosis. Data concerning the effect of antiviral treatment on its occurrence are a matter of debate. A recent study suggested that HCV clearance did not significantly reduce the risk of glucose intolerance in HCV patients [61]. In contrast, another recent study indicated that sustained virologic response caused a two-thirds reduction in the risk of type 2 diabetes development in HCV-positive treated patients [62].

Conclusion

HCV infection is a widespread disease that may affect numerous organs based on its extrahepatic manifestations. Those for which a tight association was demonstrated are less numerous (cryoglobulinemia and associated manifestations, systemic vasculitis, B-cell non-Hodgkin lymphoma, fatigue). In most of these HCV-induced extrahepatic diseases, long-term clearance of HCV is associated with good control of the immune disease. Immunosuppressive drugs, corticosteroids, or plasmapheresis may have some interest in very severe forms.

References

1. Hu YW, Rocheleau L, Larke B, et al. Immunoglobulin mimicry by hepatitis C virus envelope protein E2. *Virology* 2005;332:538–49.

2. Landau DA, Saadoun D, Calabrese LH, Cacoub P. The pathophysiology of HCV induced B-cell clonal disorders. *Autoimmun Rev* 2007;6:581–7.

3. Cacoub P, Poynard T, Ghillani P, et al. Extrahepatic manifestations of chronic hepatitis C. MULTIVIRC Group. Multidepartment virus C. *Arthritis Rheum* 1999;42:2204–12.

4. Monti G, Galli M, Invernizzi F, et al. Cryoglobulinaemias: a multi-centre study of the early clinical and laboratory manifestations of primary and secondary disease. GISC. Italian Group for the Study of Cryoglobulinaemias. *QJM* 1995;88: 115–26.

5. Dupin N, Chosidow O, Lunel F, et al. Essential mixed cryoglobulinemia. A comparative study of dermatologic manifestations in patients infected or noninfected with hepatitis C virus. *Arch Dermatol* 1995;131:1124–7.

6. Leone N, Pellicano R, Ariata Maiocco I, et al. Mixed cryoglobulinaemia and chronic hepatitis C virus infection: the rheumatic manifestations. *J Med Virol* 2002;66:200–03.

7. Lee YH, Ji JD, Yeon JE, et al. Cryoglobulinaemia and rheumatic manifestations in patients with hepatitis C virus infection. *Ann Rheum Dis* 1998;57:728–31.

8. Sene D, Ghillani-Dalbin P, Limal N, et al. Anti-cyclic citrullinated peptide antibodies in hepatitis C virus associated rheumatological manifestations and Sjogren's syndrome. *Ann Rheum Dis* 2006;65:394–7.

9. Cacoub P, Renou C, Rosenthal E, et al. Extrahepatic manifestations associated with hepatitis C virus infection. A prospective multicenter study of 321 patients. The GERMIVIC. Groupe d'Etude et de Recherche en Medecine Interne et Maladies Infectieuses sur le Virus de l'Hepatite C. *Medicine (Baltimore)* 2000;79:47–56.

10. Sene D, Ghillani-Dalbin P, Thibault V, et al. Longterm course of mixed cryoglobulinemia in patients infected with hepatitis C virus. *J Rheumatol* 2004;31:2199–206.

11. Apartis E, Leger JM, Musset L, et al. Peripheral neuropathy associated with essential mixed cryoglobulinaemia: a role for hepatitis C virus infection? *J Neurol Neurosurg Psychiatry* 1996;60:661–6.

12. Migliaresi S, Di Iorio G, Ammendola A, et al. [Peripheral nervous system involvement in HCV-related mixed cryoglobulinemia]. *Reumatismo* 2001;53:26–32.

13. Rieu V, Cohen P, Andre MH, et al. Characteristics and outcome of 49 patients with symptomatic cryoglobulinaemia. *Rheumatology (Oxford)* 2002;41:290–300.

14. Authier FJ, Bassez G, Payan C, et al. Detection of genomic viral RNA in nerve and muscle of patients with HCV neuropathy. *Neurology* 2003;60:808–12.

15. Cacoub P, Maisonobe T, Thibault V, et al. Systemic vasculitis in patients with hepatitis C. *J Rheumatol* 2001;28: 109–18.

16. De Martino L, Sampaolo S, Tucci C, et al. Viral RNA in nerve tissues of patients with hepatitis C infection and peripheral neuropathy. *Muscle Nerve* 2003;27:102–4.

17. Origgi L, Vanoli M, Carbone A, Grasso M, Scorza R. Central nervous system involvement in patients with HCV-related cryoglobulinemia. *Am J Med Sci* 1998;315:208–10.

18. Casato M, Lilli D, Donato G, et al. Occult hepatitis C virus infection in type II mixed cryoglobulinaemia. *J Viral Hepat* 2003;10:455–9.

19. Mazzaro C, Tulissi P, Moretti M, et al. Clinical and virological findings in mixed cryoglobulinaemia. *J Intern Med* 1995;238: 153–60.

20. D'Amico G. Renal involvement in hepatitis C infection: cryoglobulinemic glomerulonephritis. *Kidney Int* 1998;54: 650–71.

21. Beddhu S, Bastacky S, Johnson JP. The clinical and morphologic spectrum of renal cryoglobulinemia. *Medicine (Baltimore)* 2002;81:398–409.

22. Alric L, Plaisier E, Thebault S, et al. Influence of antiviral therapy in hepatitis C virus-associated cryoglobulinemic MPGN. *Am J Kidney Dis* 2004;43:617–23.

23. Tarantino A, Campise M, Banfi G, et al. Long-term predictors of survival in essential mixed cryoglobulinemic glomerulonephritis. *Kidney Int* 1995;47:618–23.

24. Brouet JC, Clauvel JP, Danon F, et al. Biologic and clinical significance of cryoglobulins. A report of 86 cases. *Am J Med* 1974;57:775–88.

25. Pawlotsky JM, Ben Yahia M, Andre C, et al. Immunological disorders in C virus chronic active hepatitis: a prospective case-control study. *Hepatology* 1994;19:841–8.

26. Casato M, Agnello V, Pucillo LP, et al. Predictors of long-term response to high-dose interferon therapy in type II cryoglobulinemia associated with hepatitis C virus infection. *Blood* 1997;90:3865–73.

27. Misiani R, Bellavita P, Fenili D, et al. Interferon alfa-2a therapy in cryoglobulinemia associated with hepatitis C virus. *N Engl J Med* 1994;330:751–6.

28. Dammacco F, Sansonno D, Han JH, et al. Natural interferon-alpha versus its combination with 6-methyl-prednisolone in the therapy of type II mixed cryoglobulinemia: a long-term, randomized, controlled study. *Blood* 1994;84: 3336–43.

29. Zuckerman E, Keren D, Slobodin G, *et al*. Treatment of refractory, symptomatic, hepatitis C virus related mixed cryoglobulinemia with ribavirin and interferon-alpha. *J Rheumatol* 2000;27:2172–8.

30. Naarendorp M, Kallemuchikkal U, Nuovo GJ, Gorevic PD. Longterm efficacy of interferon-alpha for extrahepatic disease associated with hepatitis C virus infection. *J Rheumatol* 2001;28:2466–73.

31. Cacoub P, Lidove O, Maisonobe T, *et al*. Interferon-alpha and ribavirin treatment in patients with hepatitis C virus-related systemic vasculitis. *Arthritis Rheum* 2002;46: 17–3326.

32. Saadoun D, Delluc A, Piette JC, Cacoub P. Treatment of hepatitis C-associated mixed cryoglobulinemia vasculitis. *Curr Opin Rheumatol* 2008;20(1):23–8.

33. Saadoun D, Resche-Rigon M, Thibault V, *et al*. Antiviral therapy for hepatitis C virus-associated mixed cryoglobulinemia vasculitis: a long-term followup study. *Arthritis Rheum* 2006;54:3696–706.

34. McHutchison JG, Everson GT, Gordon SC, *et al*. Telaprevir with peginterferon and ribavirin for chronic HCV genotype 1 infection. *N Engl J Med* 2009;360:1827–38.

35. Hezode C, Forestier N, Dusheiko G, *et al*. Telaprevir and peginterferon with or without ribavirin for chronic HCV infection. *N Engl J Med* 2009;360:1839–50.

36. Sansonno D, De Re V, Lauletta G, *et al*. Monoclonal antibody treatment of mixed cryoglobulinemia resistant to interferon alpha with an anti-CD20. *Blood* 2003;101:3818–26.

37. Roccatello D, Baldovino S, Rossi D, *et al*. Long-term effects of anti-CD20 monoclonal antibody treatment of cryoglobulinaemic glomerulonephritis. *Nephrol Dial Transpl* 2004;19: 3054–61.

38. Saadoun D, Resche Rigon M, Sene D, *et al*. Rituximab plus Peg-interferon-alpha/ribavirin compared with Peg-interferon-alpha/ribavirin in hepatitis C-related mixed cryoglobulinemia. *Blood* 2010;116(3): 326–34

39. Terrier B, Saadoun D, Sene D, *et al*. Efficacy and tolerability of rituximab with or without PEGylated interferon alfa-2b plus ribavirin in severe hepatitis C virus-related vasculitis: a long-term followup study of thirty-two patients. *Arthritis Rheum* 2009;60:2531–40.

40. Sene D, Ghillani-Dalbin P, Amoura Z, *et al*. Rituximab may form a complex with iGmkappa mixed cryoglobulin and induce severe systemic reactions in patients with hepatitis C virus-induced vasculitis. *Arthritis Rheum* 2009;60: 3848–55.

41. Hausfater P, Cacoub P, Assogba U, *et al*. Plasma exchange and interferon-alpha pharmacokinetics in patients with hepatitis C virus-associated systemic vasculitis. *Nephron* 2002; 91:627–30.

42. Monti G, Pioltelli P, Saccardo F, *et al*. Incidence and characteristics of non-Hodgkin lymphomas in a multicenter case file of patients with hepatitis C virus-related symptomatic mixed cryoglobulinemias. *Arch Intern Med* 2005;165: 101–5.

43. Gisbert JP, Garcia-Buey L, Pajares JM, Moreno-Otero R. Prevalence of hepatitis C virus infection in B-cell non-Hodgkin's lymphoma: systematic review and meta-analysis. *Gastroenterology* 2003;125:1723–32.

44. Mazzaro C, Zagonel V, Monfardini S, *et al*. Hepatitis C virus and non-Hodgkin's lymphomas. *Br J Haematol* 1996;94: 544–50.

45. Zuckerman E, Zuckerman T, Levine AM, *et al*. Hepatitis C virus infection in patients with B-cell non-Hodgkin lymphoma. *Ann Intern Med* 1997;127:423–8.

46. Luppi M, Longo G, Ferrari MG, *et al*. Clinico-pathological characterization of hepatitis C virus-related B-cell non-Hodgkin's lymphomas without symptomatic cryoglobulinemia. *Ann Oncol* 1998;9:495–8.

47. Mele A, Pulsoni A, Bianco E, *et al*. Hepatitis C virus and B-cell non-Hodgkin lymphomas: an Italian multicenter case-control study. *Blood* 2003;102:996–9.

48. Silvestri F, Pipan C, Barillari G, *et al*. Prevalence of hepatitis C virus infection in patients with lymphoproliferative disorders. *Blood* 1996;87:4296–301.

49. Saadoun D, Suarez F, Lefrere F, *et al*. Splenic lymphoma with villous lymphocytes, associated with type II cryoglobulinemia and HCV infection: a new entity? *Blood* 2005;105: 74–6.

50. Hermine O, Lefrere F, Bronowicki JP, *et al*. Regression of splenic lymphoma with villous lymphocytes after treatment of hepatitis C virus infection. *N Engl J Med* 2002;347: 89–94.

51. Cacoub P, Ratziu V, Myers RP, *et al*. Impact of treatment on extra hepatic manifestations in patients with chronic hepatitis C. *J Hepatol* 2002;36:812–18.

52. Poynard T, Cacoub P, Ratziu V, *et al*. Fatigue in patients with chronic hepatitis C. *J Viral Hepat* 2002;9:295–303.

53. Buskila D, Shnaider A, Neumann L, *et al*. Musculoskeletal manifestations and autoantibody profile in 90 hepatitis C virus infected Israeli patients. *Semin Arthritis Rheum* 1998; 28:107–113.

54. Pawlotsky JM, Bouvier M, Fromont P, *et al*. Hepatitis C virus infection and autoimmune thrombocytopenic purpura. *J Hepatol* 1995;23:635–9.

55. Hernandez F, Blanquer A, Linares M, *et al*. Autoimmune thrombocytopenia associated with hepatitis C virus infection. *Acta Haematol* 1998;99:217–20.

56. Uygun A, Kadayifci A, Ercin N, *et al*. Interferon treatment for thrombocytopenia associated with chronic HCV infection. *Int J Clin Pract* 2000;54:683–4.

57. Rajan S, Liebman HA. Treatment of hepatitis C related thrombocytopenia with interferon alpha. *Am J Hematol* 2001;68:202–9.

58. Caronia S, Taylor K, Pagliaro L, *et al*. Further evidence for an association between non-insulin-dependent diabetes

mellitus and chronic hepatitis C virus infection. *Hepatology* 1999; 30:1059–63.

59. Arao M, Murase K, Kusakabe A, *et al.* Prevalence of diabetes mellitus in Japanese patients infected chronically with hepatitis C virus. *J Gastroenterol* 2003;38:355–60.

60. Thuluvath PJ, John PR. Association between hepatitis C, diabetes mellitus, and race. A case-control study. *Am J Gastroenterol* 2003;98:438–41.

61. Giordanino C, Bugianesi E, Smedile A, *et al.* Incidence of type 2 diabetes mellitus and glucose abnormalities in patients with chronic hepatitis C infection by response to treatment: results of a cohort study. *Am J Gastroenterol* 2008; 103:2481–7.

62. Arase Y, Suzuki F, Suzuki Y, *et al.* Sustained virological response reduces incidence of onset of type 2 diabetes in chronic hepatitis C. *Hepatology* 2009;49:739–44.

20 Cytopenias: How they Limit Therapy and Potential Correction

Mitchell L. Shiffman

Liver Institute of Virginia, Bon Secours Virginia Health System, Richmond and Newport News, VA, USA

Cytopenias are one of the three most common adverse events associated with peginterferon and ribavirin therapy [1,2], the other two being flu-like symptoms and psychiatric disorders, including insomnia. Peginterferon suppresses the bone marrow production of all three hematologic cell lines [3,4] and ribavirin-induced hemolysis further exacerbates anemia [5,6]. This exacerbates the fatigue associated with peginterferon treatment, contributes to irritability and depression, and is the primary reason many patients discontinue HCV therapy.

Cytopenias can be managed in one of two ways: by reducing the dose of peginterferon and/or ribavirin or by utilizing growth factors. Although the later approach has been shown to reverse cytopenias, it is costly and without any demonstrated benefit to sustained virologic response (SVR) [7–13]. The management of cytopenias during peginterferon and ribavirin therapy has therefore become one of the most confusing and controversial aspects of HCV treatment.

Mechanisms by which Interferon Contributes to Cytopenia

The mechanism by which interferon causes a decline in the neutrophil, platelet, and red cell counts is the result of multiple effects on mature circulating cells, progenitor cells within the bone marrow, and cytokines, which affect the maturation of these cell lines [3]. These effects are summarized in Table 20.1. Interferon has an immediate effect on mature circulating cells, leading to sequestration of neutrophils, platelets, and red cells within the capillary bed. This leads to a 14–38% decline in the platelet and neutrophil counts and a 4% decline in the hemoglobin.

The primary mechanism by which interferon causes cytopenias is by inhibiting maturation and proliferation of bone marrow progenitor cells. This dose-dependent effect leads to a 30–50% decline in the neutrophil and platelet counts and a lesser decline in hemoglobin [3,14]. Under normal circumstances, declines in these cell lines initiate compensatory mechanisms, which stimulate the maturation of bone marrow progenitor cells. However, interferon also inhibits the secretion of thrombopoetin (TPO), granulocyte stimulating factor (GCSF), and erythropoietin (EPO), which stimulate the synthesis of platelets, neutrophils, and red cells, respectively. EPO in turn stimulates the maturation of megakaryocytes [3]. As a result, the degree of thrombocytopenia observed during treatment with peginterferon and ribavirin is somewhat less when compared to peginterferon monotherapy [15].

Interferon and Immune Thrombocytopenia

Interferon-induced immune thrombocytopenia (ITP) is characterized by a precipitous decline in the platelet count, usually to values less than 30 000/mm^3, which typically occurs within 4–8 weeks after initiating interferon therapy [16,17]. This is secondary to an immune response against platelets although anti-platelet antibodies are not always detectable. If interferon-induced ITP is suspected, interferon must be discontinued immediately and the platelet count monitored closely. In some patients, the platelet count will not increase after interferon is discontinued and corticosteroids may need to be instituted. The development of interferon-induced ITP is a contraindication to future interferon therapy, even if the initial episode resolves and the platelet count returns to the pretreatment baseline.

Advanced Therapy for Hepatitis C, First Edition. Edited by Geoffrey W. McCaughan, John G. McHutchison and Jean-Michel Pawlotsky.
© 2012 Blackwell Publishing Ltd. Published 2012 by Blackwell Publishing Ltd.

Table 20.1 Mechanisms by which peginterferon and ribavirin lead to cytopenias.

	Peginterferon	Ribavirin
Mature cells	Sequestration of neutrophils, lymphocytes, platelets, and red cells in peripheral capillary beds	Alters electrolyte transport across red cell membranes. Enhances binding of immunoglobulins to red cell membranes, leading to enhanced phagocytosis within the spleen
Bone marrow precursors	Reduced maturation and production of progenitor cells for all three cell lines	No effect
Cytokines and growth factors	Reduced secretion of growth factors, including GCSF, TPO, and EPO; enhanced secretion of cytokines, which inhibit the proliferation and maturation of bone marrow progenitor cells	Leads to an increase in erythropoietin release, which enhances red cell and platelet production

Mechanisms by Which Ribavirin Contributes to Anemia

Ribavirin is a guanosine analog that is transported into red cells. Once inside the red cell, ribavirin undergoes phosphorylation. Red cells do not contain 5'-nucleotidases or alkaline phosphatase to dephosphorylate ribavirin phosphates. Ribavirin is therefore trapped within red cells; its intracellular concentration rises and after 2–4 weeks exceeds plasma by 60-fold. The continuous phosphorylation of ribavirin depletes red cell ATP and this enhances intracellular oxidative damage and alters red cell membrane activity and function. Ribavirin alters the normal transport of electrolytes across the red cell membrane by affecting the sodium-potassium ATPase and the potassium-chloride co-transporter, and also leads to accumulation of immunoglobulins on the red cell surface. It is unclear if this accumulation of immunoglobulins is secondary to alterations in electrolyte transport, increased oxidative stress, or a separate effect of ribavirin. Red cells with increased membrane -associated immunoglobulins are removed from the circulation by the spleen [18–21].

Within days after administering ribavirin (without interferon) the serum hemoglobin declines. The mean decline over 2–4 weeks is 1–2 g [22]. This leads to a compensatory rise in serum erythropoietin levels. The reticulocyte count then increases and new red cell production blunts the decline in serum hemoglobin.

Management of Neutropenia

The vast majority of patients with chronic HCV have a normal total WBC and neutrophil count at baseline. These counts decline during the initial 2–4 weeks after initiating peginterferon and ribavirin but remain within the limits of normal throughout therapy and return to the pre-treatment baseline 1–4 weeks after treatment has been discontinued [23,24]. Patients with cirrhosis frequently have neutrophil counts that are at or below the lower limits of normal and these decline further during treatment. Many African Americans have essential neutropenia and may therefore also develop significant neutropenia during treatment [25,26].

The current recommendations state that peginterferon should not be initiated if the neutrophil count is below 1500/cc^3, that the dose be reduced if the neutrophil count declines below 750 cells/mm^3 and discontinued if below 500/cc^3 (Table 20.2). In contrast, many physicians with significant experience treating chronic HCV will initiate peginterferon if the neutrophil count is at least 1000/cc^3 and allow this to decline to 500 cells/mm^3 before dose reducing and only discontinue treatment if the neutrophil count cannot be maintained above 250–500/cc^3 or if the patient develops a systemic infection. Previous studies have demonstrated that the risk of developing bacterial infections is not increased in patients who develop neutropenia while receiving peginterferon, even in patients with advanced fibrosis or stable Child-Turcotte-Pugh

Table 20.2 Hematologic parameters to initiate and continue peginterferon and ribavirin therapy.

	Package insert	Author recommendations
Prior to initiating treatment		
Hemoglobin	Women >12 g/dl Men >13 g/dl	Check ferritin and iron saturation and replete if iron deficient All patients >13 m/l
Neutrophils	>1500/cc^3	>1000/cc
Platelets	Peginterferon alfa-2a: >70 000/cc Peginterferon alfa-2b: >90 000/cc	>60 000/cc
Values requiring dose reduction		
Hemoglobin	*Peginterferon alfa-2a* Reduce ribavirin to 600 mg/day if <10 g/dl. In patients with heart disease reduce dose to 600 mg/day if declines by >2 g/dl during any 4-week period. Stop treatment if <8.5 g/dl *Peginterferon alfa-2b* Reduce by 200 mg decrements if <10 g/dl. Stop treatment if <8.5 g/dl	Reduce ribavirin dose by 200 mg decrements every 1–2 weeks to maintain Hb 10 g/dl or if symptomatic regardless of Hb value. May also reduce peginterferon alfa-2a from 180 to 135 mcg/week or peginterferon alfa-2b from 1.5 to 1.0 mcg/kg/week. Stop treatment if <8.5 g/dl
Neutrophils	*Peginterferon alfa-2a* Reduce to 135 mcg/week if <750/cc. Interrupt dosing if <500/cc until increases to >1000/cc and then restart at 90 mcg/week *Peginterferon alfa-2b* Reduce dose by 50% if <750/cc. Stop treatment if <500/cc	Reduce peginterferon alfa-2a to 135 and then 90 mcg/week or peginterferon alfa-2b to 1.0 and then 0.5 mcg/kg/week when neutrophil count declines to 500–750/cc to maintain neutrophil count >500/cc. Stop if cannot maintain neutrophil count >500/cc or if patient develops systemic infection
Platelets	*Peginterferon alfa-2a* Reduce to 90 mcg/week if <50/cc. Stop if <25,000/cc *Peginterferon alfa-2b* Reduce by 50% if <75 000/cc. Stop if <50 000/cc	Reduce peginterferon alfa-2a stepwise to 135 and then 90 mcg/week or peginterferon alfa-2b to 1.0 and then 0.5 mcg/kg/week when <30 000/cc to maintain platelet count above 20 000/cc. Stop if cannot maintain platelet count above 20 000/cc

(CTP) class A cirrhosis [25,27]. In contrast, patients with decompensated cirrhosis and especially those with ascites, patients with HIV co-infection, and liver transplant recipients have an increased rate of severe infections during treatment with peginterferon and ribavirin and this may lead to mortality [28]. Although no formal guidelines currently exist, GCSF should be utilized in these high-risk patients to maintain the absolute neutrophil count above 1000–1500/cc^3. In patients with severe neutropenia at baseline, this may require that GCSF be initiated prior to peginterferon and ribavirin.

GCSF has been shown to increase the total WBC and absolute neutrophil count in patients receiving peginterferon and ribavirin for treatment of chronic HCV

[4,12,13]. GCSF is administered at a dose of 300 mcg 1–3 times weekly. This causes a prompt and significant rise in the total WBC and absolute neutrophil counts. The dose and frequency are then titrated to maintain the absolute neutrophil count in the 1500–2500/cc^3 range. No study has demonstrated that administering GCSF enhances SVR when compared to patients managed by dose reduction.

Management of Thrombocytopenia

Thrombocytopenia is common in patients with chronic HCV and cirrhosis. This is due to a combination of portal hypertension, increased sequestration of platelets within the spleen, a reduction in TPO production, and possibly a direct effect of HCV on megakaryocyte maturation [29–31].

The current recommendations state that peginterferon alfa-2a or -2b should not be initiated if the platelet count is below 75 000 and 90 000, respectively, and that the dose should be reduced if the platelet count declines to less than 50 000/cc^3 and 75 000/cc^3, respectively (Table 20.2). These reflect the cut-off values utilized during the phase III clinical trials for these agents. There is no physiologic or medical rationale why the two interferons should have different threshold values. Many physicians with significant experience treating chronic HCV will initiate treatment as long as the platelet count is at least 50 000–60 000 and allow the platelet count to decline to 25 000–30 000 regardless of the type of interferon utilized before reducing the dose or discontinuing treatment. There is no data to suggest that the risk of bleeding is increased with platelet counts within this range. However, if the platelet count cannot be maintained at or above this value, treatment should be discontinued.

Eltrombopag is an oral small molecule non-peptide that binds to the TPO receptor and enhances the proliferation and differentiation of megakaryocytes. Eltrombopag increases the platelet count in a dose-dependent manner in patients with ITP [32] and cirrhosis secondary to chronic HCV [10]. In this later study, the mean platelet count rose from 55 000 to 151 000 within 28 days after initiating 75 mg/day of eltrombopag, and 95% of patients with a baseline platelet count under 70 000/cc were able to initiate HCV treatment. Following the initiation of peginterferon and ribavirin, the mean platelet count declined by 30% despite continuing eltrombopag. However, 65% of these patients were able to maintain their platelet count above 50 000 and complete at least 12 weeks of peginterferon and ribavirin therapy. Eltrombopag is now approved by the US Food and Drug Administration (FDA) and available for the treatment of ITP. A randomized controlled trial to determine if eltrombopag could enhance SVR in patients with chronic HCV and thrombocytopenia is ongoing. Another synthetic platelet growth factor, romiplastin, has also been approved by the FDA for the treatment of ITP. However, this agent has not been evaluated in patients with chronic HCV and cirrhosis.

Interleukin-11 is also approved by the FDA for the treatment of thrombocytopenia. This agent leads to a marginal increase in the platelet count in patients with chronic HCV, cirrhosis, and thrombocytopenia [9]. However, this agent is associated with significant fluid retention and this leads to edema and ascites in patients with cirrhosis. This agent should therefore not be utilized to treat thrombocytopenia in patients with cirrhosis.

Management of Anemia

The hemoglobin declines in all patients receiving peginterferon and ribavirin [33]. The mean decline is 2–4 g. However, a decline by more than 4 g occurs in up to 20% of patients. It is therefore imperative that all patients have an adequate hemoglobin prior to initiating treatment. The current recommendations state that the hemoglobin should be above 12 and 13 g/dl for women and men, respectively, prior to initiating peginterferon and ribavirin (Table 20.2). However, the risk of developing severe, symptomatic anemia and interrupting or discontinuing treatment is significantly increased if treatment is initiated when the hemoglobin is at or barely above these threshold values. These hemoglobin levels are typically observed in patients with cirrhosis, portal hypertension, gastropathy, and chronic low-grade gastrointestinal blood loss, and in many young to middle-aged women. These patients typically have low iron stores. This reduces the ability of these patients to develop a compensatory reticulocytosis and significantly exacerbates anemia following the initiation of peginterferon and ribavirin. Measuring ferritin and iron saturation and taking several weeks to months to replete iron if necessary is important prior to initiating peginterferon and ribavirin. In patients with chronic low-grade gastrointestinal blood loss and/or those with severe iron deficiency, this may require intravenous iron replacement.

Current recommendations state that the dose of ribavirin be reduced if the hemoglobin declines to less than 10 g/dl and that treatment with both peginterferon and ribavirin be discontinued if the hemoglobin falls below 8.5 g/dl (Table 20.2). However, many patients develop a significant decline in their quality of life, fatigue, and irritability, and become depressed whenever the hemoglobin declines by more than 4 g or to under 12 g/dl [34]. These patients are likely to purposely skip ribavirin doses to lessen the severity of these side effects and frequently do not inform the treating physician or nurse that they have done so. Missing doses of ribavirin significantly reduces cumulative exposure to this drug and may increase the risk of breakthrough and relapse [35]. It is therefore imperative that patients understand that they should not miss doses of ribavirin. However, it is equally important that physicians understand that symptomatic patients need to have their ribavirin dose lowered and that small stepwise reductions in ribavirin dosing, especially in patients who have already become HCV RNA undetectable on treatment, does not increase the risk of breakthrough or relapse.

Several studies have demonstrated that administering epoetin alfa or darbypoetin to patients who develop anemia while being treated with peginterferon and ribavirin will lead to a 2–3 g increase in hemoglobin and an improvement in the quality of life [7,11,13]. Unfortunately, utilizing epoetin alfa to treat anemia in this setting significantly increases the cost of HCV treatment and has not been associated with an increase in SVR even in patients with HIV co-infection [11,36]. Furthermore, epoetin alfa has been reported to cause red cell aplasia in patents with HCV and has been associated with an increased risk of thrombosis and embolic events [37]. As a result, the use of a hematologic growth factor to treat peginterferon- and ribavirin-induced anemia should be strongly discouraged unless the risk benefit ratio has been carefully evaluated and discussed with the patient.

Two recent analyses support the concept that reducing the dose of ribavirin is preferable to adding a hematologic growth factor in patients who develop anemia during treatment with peginterferon and ribavirin. A retrospective review of a large database demonstrated that reducing the ribavirin dose after the patient became HCV RNA undetectable had minimal impact on breakthough, relapse, and SVR [38]. Another retrospective analysis demonstrated that utilizing epoetin alfa in patients who developed anemia after treatment week 8 did not increase SVR when compared to patients whose anemia was managed by dose reduction [39]. In contrast, patients who developed anemia rapidly, within the first 8 weeks after initiating treatment, did have a significant increase in SVR when they received epoetin alfa compared to patients who did not. Anemia which develops rapidly following the initiation of peginterferon and ribavirin is often severe and associated with a marked reduction in quality of life. It is uncommon for these patients to remain on treatment, and premature discontinuation of therapy is associated with a high rate of non-response, breakthrough, and relapse. Utilizing epoetin alfa allows these patients, who are the most sensitive to ribavirin, the opportunity to remain on treatment and achieve SVR.

If utilized, epoetin alfa should be administered at a dose of 60 000 IU once weekly and the dose and frequency titrated to maintain the hemoglobin in the 10–12 g/dl range. The starting dose of darbypoetin is 3 mg/kg every 1–2 weeks.

The Importance of Assessing Response During Therapy

One of the most important aspects in the management of peginterferon and ribavirin treatment is to assess HCV RNA. This provides both the patient and physician information regarding the virologic response and whether it would be appropriate to dose reduce, initiate growth factor support, or discontinue treatment. My practice is to measure HCV RNA at monthly intervals until undetectable and then every 3 months to ensure that breakthrough viremia has not occurred.

Patients who develop profound cytopenias before they become HCV RNA undetectable, particularly when this occurs before treatment week 8, are unlikely to achieve a virologic response if the doses of peginterferon and/or ribavirin are reduced. The best option for such patients is to initiate a hematologic growth factor. However, in many cases these agents either cannot be provided fast enough or the response to the growth factor is not quick enough and peginterferon and/or ribavirin dosing must be interrupted. If this occurs it is probably best to discontinue treatment altogether, allow the cytopenia to resolve, obtain approval from the patient's insurance carrier to utilize a hematologic growth factor and reinitiate treatment at some point in the near future. My preference is to initiate the hematologic growth factor simultaneously with peginterferon and ribavirin if at all possible during re-treatment so as not to risk developing profound cytopenia and having to again discontinue treatment. Alternatively, the growth factor can be initiated as soon as the particular hematologic cell line begins to decline.

Unfortunately, there is a great tendency on the part of many physicians to continue treatment once initiated even in the face of severe cytopenias and after peginterferon and ribavirin dosing has been interrupted. Unfortunately, interrupting treatment leads to non-response, breakthrough, and relapse. Assessing HCV RNA when patients develop cytopenias will help guide treatment decisions. Treatment can be continued if HCV RNA continues to decline and/or remains undetectable despite modification of the peginterferon and/or ribavirin dose. In contrast, treatment should be stopped if the serum HCV RNA level increases or recurs after previously being undetectable.

Patients who develop cytopenias after they have become HCV RNA undetectable are best managed by dose reduction. However, many patients may purposefully skip doses of peginterferon and/or ribavirin to manage the

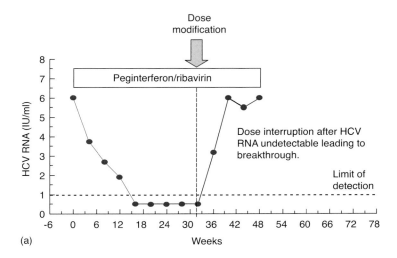

(a)

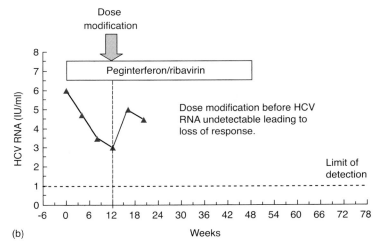

Figure 20.1 Examples from five patients of how HCV RNA could be utilized to help guide the management of cytopenias during treatment with peginterferon and ribavirin. (a) Patient was slow to respond, becoming HCV RNA undetectable between weeks 12 and 24. The patient skipped 1 peginterferon injection and 10 days of ribavirin to combat severe fatigue. He subsequently developed breakthrough. (b) Patient achieved EVR with a 2 log decline in HCV RNA by week 12, but then had a reduction in ribavirin dose from 1200 to 600 mg/day because of anemia and fatigue. This resulted in a loss of the virologic response and a rise in HCV RNA. (c) Patient developed anemia at treatment week 6 and the ribavirin dose was reduced from 1000 to 600 mg/day. The patient went on to become HCV RNA undetectable but developed relapse after discontinuing treatment. (d) Patient achieved a rapid virologic response with undetectable HCV RNA at treatment week 4. The dose of ribavirin was reduced from 1000 to 800 mg/day at treatment week 6 because of anemia. The patient remained HCV RNA undetectable and developed SVR. (e) Patient was slow to respond but became HCV RNA undetectable between weeks 12 and 24. The dose of peginterferon was reduced by 33% and ribavirin by 200 mg/day at treatment week 40 because of severe fatigue. The patient completed 72 weeks of treatment and achieved SVR.

(b)

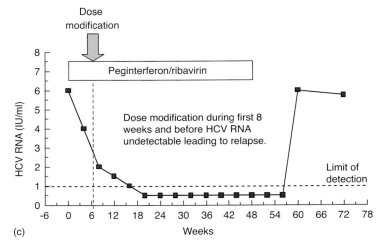

(c)

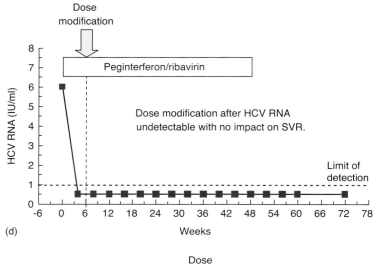

(d)

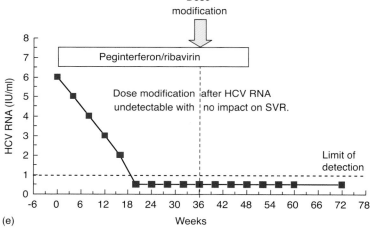

(e)

Figure 20.1 (*Continued*)

side effects of treatment. Missing doses is the single greatest reason for breakthrough viremia. It is therefore best that HCV RNA be assessed when patients are experiencing severe side effects to ensure that breakthrough viremia has not already occurred. HCV RNA should also be assessed 1 month following a physician-recommended dose reduction to ensure that the patient has also not developed breakthrough as a result of this dose modification.

Figure 20.1 provides several examples of how HCV RNA could be utilized to help guide the management of cytopenias. It is apparent that close monitoring of HCV RNA during treatment and intervening with a growth factor can help some but not all patients achieve SVR. How-

ever, the majority of patients are best managed by dose reduction.

Disclosures of Conflicts of Interest

Dr Shiffman is a consultant, speaker, attends advisor meetings for, and has received grant support to conduct clinical trials from Hoffmann-La Roche, Inc; attends advisor meetings for, and has received grant support to conduct clinical trials from Schering-Plough, Biolex, Conatus, Human Genome Sciences, Romark, Valeant, Vertex, and Zymogenetics; receives grant support from Glaxo-SmithKline, Globeimmune, Idenix, and Tibotec; and has attended advisor meetings with BristolMyersSquibb and Pfizer.

References

1. Shiffman ML. Side effects of medical therapy for chronic hepatitis C. *Ann Hepatol* 2004;3:5–10.
2. Russo MW, Fried MW. Side effects of therapy for chronic hepatitis C. *Gastroenterology* 2003;124:1711–19.
3. Peck–Radosavljevic M, Wichlas M, Homoncik–Kraml M, *et al.* Rapid suppression of hematopoiesis by standard or pegylated interferon-alpha. *Gastroenterology* 2002;123: 141–51.
4. Curry MP, Afdhal NH. Use of growth factors with antiviral therapy for chronic hepatitis C. *Clin Liver Dis* 2005;9: 439–51.
5. De Franchesi LD, Fattovich G, Turrini F, *et al.* Hemolytic anemia induced by ribavirin therapy in patients with chronic hepatitis C virus infection: role of membrane oxidative damage. *Hepatology* 2000;31:997–1004.
6. Canonico PG, Kastello MD, Spears CT, *et al.* Effects of ribavirin on red blood cells. *Toxicol Appl Pharmacol* 1984;74: 155–62.
7. Afdhal NH, Dieterich DT, Pockros PJ, *et al.* Epoetin alfa maintains ribavirin dose in HCV-infected patients: a prospective, double-blind, randomized controlled study. *Gastroenterology* 2004;126:1302–11.
8. Van Thiel DH, Faruki H, Friedlander L, *et al.* Combination treatment of advanced HCV associated liver disease with interferon and G-CSF. *HepatoGastroenterology* 1995; 42:907–12.
9. Artz AS, Ershler WB, Rustgi V. Interleukin-11 for thrombocytopenia associated with hepatitis C. *J Clin Gastroenterol* 2001;33:425–6.
10. McHutchison JG, Dusheiko G, Shiffman ML, *et al.* Eltrombopag for thrombocytopenia in patients with cirrhosis associated with hepatitis C. *N Engl J Med* 2007;357: 2227–36.
11. Shiffman ML, Salvatori J, Hubbard S, *et al.* Treatment of chronic hepatitis C virus genotype 1 with peginterferon, ribavirin, and epoetin alpha. *Hepatology* 2007;46: 371–9.
12. Carreno V, Martin J, Pardo M, *et al.* Randomized controlled trial of recombinant human granulocyte macrophage stimulating factor for the treatment of chronic hepatitis C. *Cytokine* 2000;12:165–70.
13. Younossi ZM, Nader FH, Bai C, *et al.* A phase II dose finding study of darbepoetin alpha and filgrastim for the management of anaemia and neutropenia in chronic hepatitis C treatment. *J Viral Hepatitis* 2008;15:370–78.
14. Ernstoff MS, Kirkwood JM. Changes in the bone marrow of cancer patients treated with recombinant interferon alpha-2. *Am J Med* 1984;76:593–6.
15. Fried MW. Side effects of therapy of hepatitis C and their management. *Hepatology* 2002;36:S237–44.
16. Shrestha R, McKinley C, Bilir BM, Everson GT. Possible idiopathic thrombocytopenic purpura associated with natural alpha interferon therapy for chronic hepatitis C infection. *Am J Gastroenterol* 1995;90:1146–7.
17. López Morante AJ, Sáez-Royuela F, Casanova Valero F, Yuguero del Moral L, Martín Lorente JL, Ojeda Giménez C. Immune thrombocytopenia after alpha-interferon therapy in a patient with chronic hepatitis C. *Am J Gastroenterol* 1992;87:809–10.
18. Page T, Connor JD. The metabolism of ribavirin in erythrocytes and nucleated cells. *Int J Biochem* 1990;22: 379–83.
19. Russmann S, Grattagliano I, Portincasa P, *et al.* Ribavirin-induced anemia: mechanisms, risk factors and related targets for future research. *Curr Med Chem* 2006;13:3351–7.
20. Glue P. The clinical pharmacology of ribavirin. *Semin Liver Dis* 1999;19(Suppl 1):17–24.
21. Homma M, Matsuzaki Y, Inoue Y, *et al.* Marked elevation of erythrocyte ribavirin levels in interferon and ribavirin-induced anemia. *Clin Gastroenterol Hepatol* 2004;2:337–9.
22. Bodenheimer HC, Jr., Lindsay KL, Davis GL, *et al.* Tolerance and efficacy of oral ribavirin treatment of chronic hepatitis C: a multicenter trial. *Hepatology* 1997;26:473-7.
23. Manns MP, McHutchinson JG, Gordon SC, *et al.* Peginterferon-alfa-2b plus ribavirin compared with interferon alfa-2b plus ribavirin for initial treatment of chronic hepatitis C: a randomized trial. *Lancet* 2001;358:958–65.
24. Fried MW, Shiffman ML, Reddy KR, *et al.* Combination of peginterferon alfa-2a (40 kd) plus ribavirin in patients with chronic hepatitis C virus infection. *N Engl J Med* 2002;347: 975–82.
25. Soza A, Everhart JE, Ghany MG, *et al.* Neutropenia during combination therapy of interferon alfa and ribavirin for chronic hepatitis C. *Hepatology* 2002;36:1273–9.
26. Jacobson IM, Brown RS, Jr., McCone J, *et al.* Impact of weight-based ribavirin with peginterferon alfa-2b in African Americans with hepatitis C virus genotype 1. *Hepatology* 2007;46:982–90.
27. Heathcote EJ, Shiffman ML, Cooksley WG, *et al.* Peginterferon alfa-2a in patients with chronic hepatitis C and cirrhosis. *N Engl J Med* 2000;343:1673–80.
28. Crippin JS, McCashland T, Terrault N, *et al.* A pilot study of the tolerability and efficacy of antiviral therapy in hepatitis C virus-infected patients awaiting liver transplantation. *Liver Transpl* 2002;8:350–55.
29. Adinolfi LE, Giordano MG, Andreana A, *et al.* Hepatic fibrosis plays a central role in the pathogenesis of thrombocytopenia in patients with chronic viral hepatitis. *Br J Haematol* 2001;113:590–95.
30. Rios R, Sangro B, Herrero I, Quiroga J, Prieto J. The role of thrombopoietin in the thrombocytopenia of patients with liver cirrhosis. *Am J Gastroenterol* 2005;100:1311–16.

31. Bordin G, Ballaré M, Zigrossi P, *et al.* A laboratory and thrombokinetic study of HCV-associated thrombocytopenia: a direct role of HCV in bone marrow exhaustion? *Clin Exp Rheumatol* 1995;13(Suppl 13):S39–S43.

32. Bussel JB, Cheng G, Saleh MN, *et al.* Eltrombopag for the treatment of chronic idiopathic thrombocytopenic purpura. *N Engl J Med* 2007;357:2237–47.

33. Maddrey WC. Safety of combination interferon alfa-2b/ribavirin therapy in chronic hepatitis C-relapsed and treatment-naive patients. *Semin Liver Dis* 1999;19(Suppl 1): 67–75.

34. Pockros PJ, Shiffman ML, Schiff ER, *et al.* Epoetin alfa improves quality of life in anemic HCV-infected patients receiving combination therapy. *Hepatology* 2004; 40:1450–58.

35. Shifman ML. Optimizing the current therapy for chronic hepatitis C virus. Peginterferon and ribavirin dosing and the utility of growth factors. *Clin Liver Dis* 2008;12:487–505.

36. Alvarez D, Dieterich DT, Brau N, *et al.* Zidovudine use but not weight-based ribavirin dosing impacts anaemia during HCV treatment in HIV-infected persons. *J Viral Hepatitis* 2006;13:683–9.

37. Stravitz RT, Chung H, Sterling RK, *et al.* Antibody-mediated pure red cell aplasia due to epoetin alfa during antiviral therapy of chronic hepatitis C. *Am J Gastroenterol* 2005;100: 1415–19.

38. Shiffman ML, Hamzeh FM, Chung RT. Effect of time to response on viral breakthrough and relapse rates in patients infected with hcv genotype 1 and treated with peginterferon alfa-2a plus ribavirin. *Hepatology* 2008;48(Suppl): 862A.

39. Sulkowski M, Shiffman ML, Afdhal N, *et al.* Hemoglobin decline is associated with SVR among HCV genotype 1-infected persons treated with peginterferon/ribavirin: analysis from the IDEAL study. *J Hepatol* 2009;50(Suppl 1): S51.

21 The Problem of Insulin Resistance and its Effect on Therapy

Venessa Pattullo[1,2] and Jacob George[1]

[1] Storr Liver Unit, Westmead Millenium Institute, University of Sydney, Sydney, NSW, Australia
[2] Division of Gastroenterology, Toronto Western Hospital, University Health Network, University of Toronto, Toronto, Canada

Introduction

Convincing epidemiologic data links chronic hepatitis C (CHC) to insulin resistance (IR), with a reported prevalence of 30–60%. IR in hepatitis C virus (HCV) infection is independent of body mass index (BMI) and is associated with higher serum HCV RNA levels [1–3]. Consequently, a high prevalence of type 2 diabetes (T2DM) is observed in both cirrhotic and non-cirrhotic individuals with CHC. Consistent with these observations, improved insulin sensitivity is observed in those who achieve treatment-induced viral clearance, but not in those who fail to respond to therapy [4,5]. Likewise, the greater the degree of IR, the lower the likelihood of treatment-induced viral clearance [6,7]. This chapter will examine the relationship between CHC, IR, and treatment response, and the role of novel approaches to improve insulin sensitivity in order to enhance treatment outcomes.

Defining Insulin Resistance

Insulin resistance is defined as a state in which higher levels of insulin are required to achieve metabolic homeostasis. In insulin-sensitive individuals, insulin reduces hepatic glucose production, increases glucose uptake and glycogen synthesis, and promotes lipid synthesis, while concomitantly inhibiting adipocyte fatty acid (FA) release. Although IR may develop simultaneously in the liver and peripheral tissues (skeletal muscle and adipose tissue), its severity may differ in the various sites [8]. The gold standard for measuring insulin sensitivity is the glucose clamp technique; however, this is a cumbersome test and impractical for use in routine practice [9]. The homeostasis model for assessment of insulin resistance (HOMA-IR) correlates with the hyperinsulinemic euglycemic clamp and quantifies the degree of IR, particularly in the liver. HOMA-IR is calculated with the equation [9]:

HOMA-IR = (mean fasting insulin (mUI/l) × mean fasting glucose (mmol)/22.5.

The World Health Organization (WHO) defines insulin resistance as a HOMA-IR score in the highest quartile of the non-diabetic population, as this is the cutoff value above which healthy patients are discriminated from those at risk of diabetes [10]. This cut-off value may vary from population to population [11], and, in part, accounts for the heterogeneity in the methodology, reporting of insulin resistance prevalence and outcomes in studies of IR in CHC.

Insulin Signaling

Insulin signaling is complex, relying on various phosphorylation cascades (Figure 21.1). Insulin receptor substrate (IRS) is a key molecule in the pathway with tyrosine phosphorylation of IRS-1 and IRS-2 stimulated by insulin binding to the insulin receptor and triggering a cascade of intracellular signals [12]. In response to this cascade, the glucose transport molecule (GLUT) 4 is translocated to the cell membrane on adipocytes and skeletal muscle [12]; the related isoforms GLUT1 and GLUT2 predominantly control glucose transport in liver [13]. In addition to its effects on GLUT translocation, insulin activates the Akt/PKB complex, a central regulator of the function of many cellular proteins that increases glycogen and protein synthesis and cell survival [12].

Advanced Therapy for Hepatitis C, First Edition. Edited by Geoffrey W. McCaughan, John G. McHutchison and Jean-Michel Pawlotsky.
© 2012 Blackwell Publishing Ltd. Published 2012 by Blackwell Publishing Ltd.

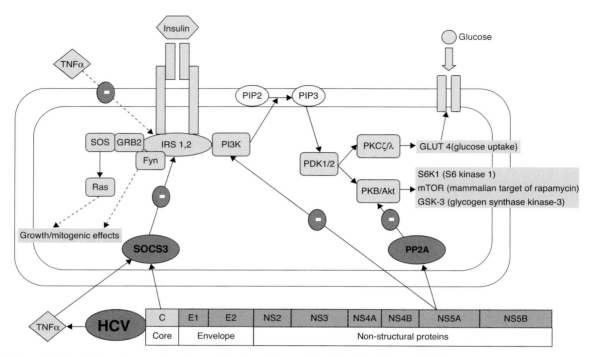

Figure 21.1 Insulin signaling cascade and potential sites of virus-mediated insulin resistance in CHC.

Insulin resistance can occur due to defects at any level of the pathway, but most evidence supports defects at the level of the insulin receptor or IRS molecules resulting from different levels of expression of these molecules, or modulation of the signaling pathway by differential phosphorylation [12]. While tyrosine phosphorylation activates IRS-1, serine phosphorylation inhibits it. There are two isoforms of IRS important in the human liver: IRS-1 and IRS-2. IRS-1 knockout mice are growth retarded and insulin resistant, while IRS-2 knockout mice have T2DM, attesting to the importance of hepatic insulin signaling to the development of T2DM [14].

Molecular Mechanisms of Insulin Resistance in CHC

Evidence for virus-induced IR comes from studies of the outcomes of antiviral treatment in insulin resistant patients with CHC. Insulin sensitivity improves in those achieving viral clearance, but does not improve in nonresponders [6]. However, the pathophysiology of IR in CHC is complex. Altered glucose homeostasis in CHC arises both as a direct consequence of the virus, and indirectly as a consequence of lipid accumulation or inflammation. In addition to representing insulin signaling, Figure 21.1 indicates some of the proposed molecular mechanisms of HCV-induced insulin resistance; further detail about these mechanisms appears in Table 21.1 and reference [15].

Much of the research on HCV-specific mechanisms of IR in CHC focuses on the viral core protein, which is proposed to cause IR in hepatocytes by reducing the level or activity of molecules involved in insulin signaling. Additionally, the HCV non-structural protein 5A (NS5A) is a key mediator in the induction of oxidative stress and inflammation, and may indirectly mediate insulin resistance in CHC.

The role of TNFα and IL-6 as mediators of inflammation-associated IR, and their sequelae (HCV-induced TNFα-mediated up-regulation of the hepatic expression of suppressor of cytokine signaling protein-3 [SOCS3]), is unresolved. However, a large prospective study suggests that virus-specific IR in CHC is likely to be a cytokine-independent effect of the virus to modulate insulin sensitivity [16]. While higher levels of HOMA-IR and the proinflammatory cytokines TNFα and IL-6 were found in HCV-infected subjects compared to healthy controls, they were not associated with the extent of IR on multivariate analysis [16].

Table 21.1 Molecular mechanisms of insulin resistance in chronic hepatitis C.[a]

Molecule	Mechanism
HCV proteins	
HCV core protein	Reduced tyrosine phosphorylation of IRS-1
	Reduced levels of IRS-1 and IRS-2
	Inhibition of peroxisome proliferator-activated receptors (PPARs) α and γ, resulting in accumulation of intrahepatocellular lipid metabolites, leading to decreased insulin receptor kinase activity
	Influence of core protein is genotype dependent:
	– Genotype 3a: IRS-1 degradation through the down-regulation of (PPARγ) and by up-regulating suppressor of cytokine signaling molecules (SOCS).
	– Genotype 1b: serine phosphorylation (i.e., inhibition) of IRS-1 via activation of mTOR or JNK; up-regulation of SOCS
HCV non-structural protein 5A (NS5A)	Activation of nuclear factor-κβ (NF-κβ) via oxidative stress (arising from interaction of NS5A with hepatocyte endoplasmic reticulum) and binding to Toll-like receptor-4 (TLR-4)
	NF-κβ leads to the activation of and the up-regulation of genes involved in the production of tumor necrosis factor alpha (TNFα), interleukin 6 (IL-6), and interleukin 8 (IL-8)
	Up-regulation of protein phosphatase 2A (PP2A) leading to reduced kinase activity of Akt/PKB
Inflammatory cytokines	
TNFα	Serine phosphorylation (i.e. inactivation) of IRS
	Directly interferes with pancreatic β-cell function
	Intracellular lipid accumulation leading to decreased insulin receptor kinase activity:
	– Reduced apolipoprotein B-100 secretion, preventing the formation of very low density lipoproteins (VLDL)
	– Inhibition of lipoprotein lipase (LPL)
IL-6	Inhibition of LPL, resulting in intracellular lipid accumulation
Other molecules	
Suppressor of cytokine signalling-3 (SOCS3)	Promotes the proteosomal degradation of IRS-1
	Reduced tyrosine phosphorylation of IRS-1
	Association with high phosphoenolpyruvate carboxykinase (PEPCK) mRNA, leading to increased gluconeogenesis

[a]This list is not exhaustive. See Serfaty and Capeau for review of this topic [15].

Host Factors Influencing IR

In addition to virus- and inflammation-mediated IR in CHC, hepatic (histological) and host factors may contribute to its development (Figure 21.2).

Hepatic Factors

Insulin resistance is both a cause and a consequence of hepatic fibrosis. Thus, advanced liver fibrosis impairs insulin clearance, resulting in increased serum insulin independent of the insulin secretion status [17]. Alternatively, hyperinsulinemia and hyperglycemia (features of IR and T2DM) may directly promote liver fibrosis by stimula-

tion of hepatic stellate cells, resulting in increased production of connective tissue growth factor and the accumulation of extracellular matrix [18]. Patients with CHC and advanced fibrosis (F2–3) have significantly higher rates of IR compared with patients with mild disease (F0–1) [3]. Conversely, HOMA-IR is an independent predictor of the degree and the rate of fibrosis progression [1].

The relationship between hepatic steatosis and IR is complex, influenced both by host factors and viral genotype. In non-genotype 3 patients, hepatic steatosis appears to arise predominantly from insulin resistance associated with host overweight/obesity. The mean HOMA-IR score of individuals with genotype 3 is similar in patients with

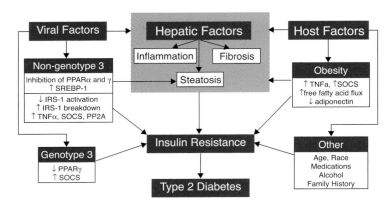

Figure 21.2 Viral, hepatic and host factors influencing insulin resistance in CHC.

and without steatosis [1], further indicating that steatosis in this genotype is not specifically linked with the development of IR in this setting.

Systemic Factors

Clear epidemiologic evidence links obesity to insulin resistance, irrespective of HCV status. Thus, the prevalence of IR among 118 non-cirrhotic patients with CHC at a tertiary referral unit was 38% [2], but in those who were obese (BMI $\geq$ 30, mean 34.2 $\pm$ 3.9 kg/m^2), the rate of IR was 72%. Disrupted lipid and FA homeostasis may be the mechanism through which IR is mediated in obese individuals with CHC [19] as central obesity is associated with increased basal free FA flux relative to lean tissue mass. Additionally, central obesity is now recognized as a low-grade proinflammatory condition as evidenced by elevations in serum levels of inflammatory cytokines including TNFα and IL-6, which may contribute to host-specific IR over and above that due to the virus [20]. Adipose tissue is also capable of producing biologically active proteins such as adiponectin, which when its levels are reduced (as is the case in the obese) has been implicated in the pathogenesis of obesity-induced IR [21]. However, as discussed earlier, clinical studies do not suggest a relationship between adiponectin levels and virus-specific IR in CHC [16].

Effect of IR on Treatment Response

Insulin resistance is independently associated with reduced sustained virologic response (SVR) to pegylated interferon and ribavirin. In genotype 1 patients, SVR was significantly lower in patients with HOMA-IR > 2 compared with patients with HOMA-IR < 2 (32.8% versus 60.5%, $p = 0.007$) [6]. Similarly, in so-called "treatment-responsive" genotype 2 and 3 patients, high HOMA-IR is associated with a reduced response; patients with an SVR had significantly lower HOMA-IR than non-responders (2.5 $\pm$ 0.2 versus 6.1 $\pm$ 1.5; $p = 0.03$) [7]. Further, SVR rates of 94% were achieved in genotype 2 and 3 patients with a HOMA-IR < 2, compared with an SVR rate of only 65% in those with HOMA-IR $\geq$ 2 [7].

The reason for the impaired response to antiviral therapy in the setting of IR is a field of intense study. The SOCS proteins appear to be one common pathway mediating both insulin and interferon signaling. Thus, SOCS-induced proteosomal degradation of IRS-1 leads to impaired insulin signaling, while SOCS 1 and 3 reduce interferon signaling through inhibition of tyrosine phosphorylation of STAT1 [22,23]. In this regard, elevated hepatic SOCS3 has been demonstrated in patients who fail to respond to interferon [22]. While up-regulation of SOCS3 may be in part genotype dependent [24], obese individuals with CHC have increased expression of SOCS3 compared with their lean counterparts, which may account for the higher rate of IR and lower SVR rates in obese patients that is independent of virus genotype [22].

Hyperinsulinemia may likewise indirectly influence interferon alfa signaling. In the ideal situation, binding of pegylated interferon alfa-2 to its extracellular receptor activates Janus kinase (JAK1) and tyrosine kinase (Tyk2) leads to activation of the downstream substrates, signal transducers, and activators of transcription (STAT 1 and STAT2). Translocation of activated STAT into the nucleus and subsequent binding to interferon alfa-2-stimulated response elements in the promoters of interferon alfa-2-stimulated genes then occurs, blocking HCV replication. However, when insulin is added to interferon (mimicking the hyperinsulinemia of insulin resistance), the ability to block HCV replication disappears – experimental evidence suggests that interferon resistance induced by

Table 21.2 Studies examining the impact of insulin sensitizing agents on treatment outcomes in CHC.

Intervention	Patient characteristics	Study design	Outcome
Metformin [26]	$n = 125$ Genotype 1 HOMA > 2	Standard therapy (peginterferon alfa-2a 180 μg/week and ribavirin 1000–1200 mg/day) *plus*: – metformin 425 mg t.i.d. during the first month and 850 mg t.i.d. from week 4 to 48 ($n = 59$) *or* – placebo ($n = 64$)	Metformin patients showed a greater decrease in HOMA-IR (from 4.3 ± 2.2 to 2.6 ± 1.7 versus 4.6 ± 2.7 to 3.8 ± 2.1, $p < 0.001$ No significant difference in: – Early virologic response (EVR), week 12 – Rate of negative HCV PCR at week 24 – Rate of SVR
Pioglitazone [27]	Pioglitazone: BMI > 30, $n = 10$ Control: BMI < 25, $n = 10$ BMI > 30, $n = 10$	Standard therapy with or without pioglitazone (PIO) 30 mg daily beginning 4 weeks prior to antiviral therapy HCV RNA measured days 0, 1, 2, 7, 14, and 28 of therapy	Pioglitazone patients had a greater log decline at each time point compared to patients on standard therapy Rapid virologic response (RVR) occurred in 50% of lean patients, 20% of obese patients receiving standard therapy, and in 60% of patients receiving standard therapy plus pioglitazone
Pioglitazone [28]	$n = 40$ Genotype 1 HOMA-IR > 2.0	Standard antiviral therapy plus: – pioglitazone 30 mg ($n = 20$) *or* – placebo ($n = 20$)	Significant reduction in HOMA-IR in the pioglitazone group In intention-to-treat analysis: – 16 patients on pioglitazone (80%) and 10 patients on placebo (50%) had undetectable HCV RNA at the end of therapy – SVR rates were similar (45%) in both groups
Pioglitazone [29]	$n = 5$ Genotype 1 Prior non-response to IFN/ribavirin	Standard therapy plus pioglitazone 15 mg	3 of 5 patients had an improvement of HOMA-IR score but: – no patient achieved an EVR at week 12 – study terminated due to futility
Pioglitazone [31]	$n = 1$ Genotype 3a Prior non-response to IFN/ribavirin	Pioglitazone 45 mg for 5 months prior to standard therapy Standard therapy plus pioglitazone 45 mg for 48 weeks	HOMA-IR 4.8, improved to 1.3 after 5 months of pioglitazone Obtained SVR
Pioglitazone [32]	$n = 97$ Genotype 4 HOMA-IR > 2.0	Standard therapy (peginterferon alfa-2b 1.5 μg/kg/week, plus daily weight-based ribavirin; 800 mg for < 50 kg, 1000 mg for 50–65 kg, 1200 mg for 65–80 kg and 1400 mg for > 80 kg) *plus*: – pioglitazone 30 mg ($n = 48$) *or* – placebo ($n = 49$)	Significantly higher RVR, ETR, and SVR in pioglitazone group: – RVR 27.08% versus 6.1% ($p = 0.006$) – EVR 68.7% versus 48.97% ($p = 0.06$) – ETR 66.6% versus 44.89% ($p = 0.04$) – SVR 60.4% versus 38.7% ($p = 0.04$)

insulin is mediated by PI3K [25]. The interaction between insulin signaling and interferon signaling is likely to be more complex, involving more than these pathways, and is an area which warrants further investigation.

Management Strategies for CHC in the Setting of IR

As IR is associated with reduced SVR rates, reducing IR can be considered a rational strategy to potentially increase the rate of treatment-induced viral clearance. Both pharmacotherapy and lifestyle intervention have been used with this in mind; however, the outcomes of existing trials have shown limited benefit.

Pharmacotherapy

Insulin sensitizing agents have been used to improve responses to antiviral therapy, with disappointing results to date (Table 21.2). The efficacy of metformin in combination with standard therapy with pegylated interferon and ribavirin was examined in a prospective, randomized, double-blind placebo controlled study (TRIC-1) [26]. While patients who received metformin had a significant reduction in HOMA-IR compared with the placebo group, no significant difference in the rate of SVR compared with non-metformin treated patients was discerned [26].

Pioglitazone, a thiazolidinedione, in combination with pegylated interferon and ribavirin, in non-diabetic treatment-naïve genotype 1 HCV patients improved viral kinetic responses during the first 4 weeks of therapy [27] but has not been shown to enhance SVR rates in genotype 1 CHC [28], nor did it enhance EVR in genotype 1 insulin-resistant CHC non-responders prior to antiviral therapy [29]. The reason for these failures may be that while thiazolidinediones improve insulin sensitivity and induce a decrease in inflammatory mediators through activation of PPARγ, they incompletely inhibit the free fatty acid (FFA) - induced IR mediated by PPARα [32]. Novel thiazolidinediones mediating both PPARγ and PPARα inhibition thus warrant study. However, such drugs are currently limited by their cardiac toxicity. In contrast, a single case report of higher dose pioglitazone prescribed 5 months in advance of antiviral therapy (rather than being introduced concomitantly) was associated with successful reduction in HOMA-IR and SVR [30], suggesting that both the dose and timing of insulin sensitizer prescription may influence treatment outcomes. In genotype 4 infected individuals with IR (HOMA-IR > 2), a randomized controlled trial of pioglitazone 30 mg in combination with pegylated interferon and ribavirin led to significantly higher RVR, ETR, and SVR rates compared with standard therapy [31]. The latter promising findings require validation, but do raise the possibility that co-administration of insulin sensitizers may need to be tailored according to both the degree of IR and the viral genotype.

Diet and Exercise

Owing to their metabolic effects in insulin-resistant subjects, and the current limitations of pharmacotherapy, diet and exercise are obvious adjuncts in insulin resistant and/or obese patients with CHC who are considering antiviral therapy. Weight loss achieved through a combination of diet and exercise improves liver enzymes and histology and reduces insulin levels in patients with both HCV and non-HCV liver disease [33]. Given such data, the impact of a dietary and exercise intervention on IR in patients with CHC needs to be urgently evaluated, and consideration given to its role in enhancing the response to treatment.

Clearly, there are many unanswered questions about the optimal management of insulin resistance in CHC. First and foremost, can reducing insulin resistance enhance antiviral treatment efficacy? Which patients will respond best? Why have current studies given disparate results? Should more potent insulin sensitizing agents be used? When should they be administered, and for how long? Should lifestyle intervention be co-administered with, or used instead of insulin sensitizing agents? What is the role of anti-TNF therapy in CHC since these agents target the pathways mediating both insulin resistance and hepatic inflammation? Will the introduction of novel direct-acting antiviral therapies impact on insulin resistance and the rates of SVR? Although evidence is slowly emerging, until all these questions are answered, reducing insulin resistance to improve treatment response should be considered a theoretical possibility without strong supporting clinical evidence.

Summary

Insulin resistance is a common accompaniment of CHC, mediated by both direct and indirect effects of the virus and host factors such as obesity. The association between insulin resistance and impaired response to antiviral therapy impacts on overall outcomes. Hence, further study into understanding its pathophysiology, and management in the context of CHC, are urgently required.

References

1. Hui JM, Sud A, Farrell GC, et al. Insulin resistance is associated with chronic hepatitis C virus infection and fibrosis progression [corrected]. Gastroenterology 2003;125(6): 1695–704.
2. Soliman W, Kuczynski M, Fantus IG, Heathcote J. The prevalence of insulin resistance in patients with chronic hepatitis C and B (Abstract). Gastroenterology 2008 2008;134(4 Suppl 1):M1771.
3. Moucari R, Asselah T, Cazals-Hatem D, et al. Insulin resistance in chronic hepatitis C: association with genotypes 1 and 4, serum HCV RNA level, and liver fibrosis. Gastroenterology 2008;134(2):416–23.
4. Kawaguchi Y, Mizuta T, Oza N, et al. Eradication of hepatitis C virus by interferon improves whole-body insulin resistance and hyperinsulinaemia in patients with chronic hepatitis C. Liver Int 2009;29(6):871–7.
5. Conjeevaram HS, Wahed AS, Afdhal N, et al. Changes in insulin sensitivity and body weight during and after peginterferon and ribavirin therapy for hepatitis C. Gastroenterology 2011;140(2):469–77.
6. Romero-Gomez M, Del Mar Viloria M, Andrade RJ, et al. Insulin resistance impairs sustained response rate to peginterferon plus ribavirin in chronic hepatitis C patients. Gastroenterology 2005;128(3):636–41.
7. Poustchi H, Negro F, Hui J, et al. Insulin resistance and response to therapy in patients infected with chronic hepatitis C virus genotypes 2 and 3. J Hepatol 2008;48(1):28–34.
8. Vanni E, Abate ML, Gentilcore E, et al. Sites and mechanisms of insulin resistance in non-obese, non-diabetic patients with chronic hepatitis C. Hepatology 2009;50(3):697–706.
9. Matthews DR, Hosker JP, Rudenski AS, et al. Homeostasis model assessment: insulin resistance and beta-cell function from fasting plasma glucose and insulin concentrations in man. Diabetologia 1985;28(7):412–19.
10. Alberti KG, Zimmet PZ. Definition, diagnosis and classification of diabetes mellitus and its complications. Part 1: diagnosis and classification of diabetes mellitus provisional report of a WHO consultation. Diabet Med 1998;15(7): 539–53.
11. Radikova Z, Koska J, Huckova M, et al. Insulin sensitivity indices: a proposal of cut-off points for simple identification of insulin-resistant subjects. Exp Clin Endocrinol Diabetes 2006;114(5):249–56.
12. Sesti G. Pathophysiology of insulin resistance. Best Pract Res Clin Endocrinol Metab 2006;20(4):665–79.
13. Olson AL, Pessin JE. Structure, function, and regulation of the mammalian facilitative glucose transporter gene family. Annu Rev Nutr 1996;16: 235–56.
14. Thirone AC, Huang C, Klip A. Tissue-specific roles of IRS proteins in insulin signaling and glucose transport. Trends Endocrinol Metab 2006;17(2):72–8.
15. Serfaty L, Capeau J. Hepatitis C, insulin resistance and diabetes: clinical and pathogenic data. Liver Int 2009;29(Suppl 2):13–25.
16. Cua IH, Hui JM, Bandara P, et al. Insulin resistance and liver injury in hepatitis C is not associated with virus-specific changes in adipocytokines. Hepatology 2007;46(1):66–73.
17. Petrides AS, Vogt C, Schulze-Berge D, et al. Pathogenesis of glucose intolerance and diabetes mellitus in cirrhosis. Hepatology 1994;19(3):616–27.
18. Ratziu V, Munteanu M, Charlotte F, et al. Fibrogenic impact of high serum glucose in chronic hepatitis C. J Hepatol 2003;39(6):1049–55.
19. Riccardi G, Giacco R, Rivellese AA. Dietary fat, insulin sensitivity and the metabolic syndrome. Clin Nutr 2004;23(4): 447–56.
20. Shoelson SE, Herrero L, Naaz A. Obesity, inflammation, and insulin resistance. Gastroenterology 2007;132(6): 2169–80.
21. Monzillo LU, Hamdy O, Horton ES, et al. Effect of lifestyle modification on adipokine levels in obese subjects with insulin resistance. Obes Res 2003;11(9):1048–54.
22. Walsh MJ, Jonsson JR, Richardson MM, et al. Non-response to antiviral therapy is associated with obesity and increased hepatic expression of suppressor of cytokine signalling 3 (SOCS-3) in patients with chronic hepatitis C, viral genotype 1. Gut 2006;55(4):529–35.
23. Jonsson JR, Barrie HD, O'Rourke P, et al. Obesity and steatosis influence serum and hepatic inflammatory markers in chronic hepatitis C. Hepatology 2008;48(1):80–87.
24. Persico M, Capasso M, Persico E, et al. Suppressor of cytokine signaling 3 (SOCS3) expression and hepatitis C virus-related chronic hepatitis: insulin resistance and response to antiviral therapy. Hepatology 2007;46(4):1009–15.
25. Sanyal AJ, Chand N, Comar K, Mirshahi F. Hyperinsulinemia blocks the inhibition of HCV replication by interferon: a potential mechanism for failure of interferon therapy in subjects with HCV and NASH. Hepatology 2004;40: 179A.
26. Romero-Gomez M, Diago M, Andrade RJ, et al. Treatment of insulin resistance with metformin in naive genotype 1 chronic hepatitis C patients receiving peginterferon alfa-2a plus ribavirin. Hepatology 2009;50(6):1702–8.
27. Elgouhari HM, Cesario KB, Lopez R, Zein NN. Pioglitazone improves early virologic kinetic response to Peg IFN/RBV combination therapy in hepatitis C genotype 1 naïve pts. Hepatology 2008;48(4 Suppl 1):383A.
28. Conjeevaram HS, Burant CF, McKenna B, et al. A randomized, double-blind, placebo-controlled study of PPAR-gamma agonist pioglitazone given in combination with peginterferon and ribavirin in patients with genotype-1 chronic hepatitis C. Hepatology 2008;48(4 Suppl 1):384A.

29. Overbeck K, Genne D, Golay A, Negro F. Pioglita-
    zone in chronic hepatitis C not responding to pegy-
    lated interferon-alpha and ribavirin. *J Hepatol* 2008;49(2):
    295–8.

30. Serfaty L, Fartoux L, Poupon R. Pioglitazone as adjuvant
    therapy in chronic hepatitis C: sequential rather than con-
    comitant administration with pegylated interferon and rib-
    avirin? *J Hepatol* 2009;50(6):1269–71.

31. Khattab M, Emad M, Abdelaleem A, *et al.* Pioglita-
    zone improves virological response to peginterferon alpha-
    2b/ribavirin combination therapy in hepatitis C geno-

32. Dhindsa S, Tripathy D, Sanalkumar N, *et al.* Free fatty
    acid-induced insulin resistance in the obese is not pre-
    vented by rosiglitazone treatment. *J Clin Endocrinol Metab*
    2005;90(9):5058–63.

33. Hickman IJ, Jonsson JR, Prins JB, *et al.* Modest weight loss
    and physical activity in overweight patients with chronic
    liver disease results in sustained improvements in alanine
    aminotransferase, fasting insulin, and quality of life. *Gut*
    2004;53(3):413–19.

type 4 patients with insulin resistance. *Liver Int* 2010;30(3):
    447–54.

22 HIV and Hepatitis C Co-infection

Gail V. Matthews and Gregory J. Dore

Viral Hepatitis Program, National Centre in HIV Epidemiology and Clinical Research, University of New South Wales, Sydney, NSW, Australia

Global Prevalence of HIV/HCV Co-Infection

The global burden of both human immunodeficiency virus (HIV) and hepatitis C virus (HCV) infection is substantial, with significant overlap in the geographical areas and populations most affected. Similar routes of transmission, particularly where a large proportion of HIV cases are acquired through injecting drug use (IDU), can result in extremely high rates of HIV and HCV co-infection. Increasingly recognized is the contribution that sexual HCV transmission among HIV-infected men who have sex with men is making to HIV-HCV co-infection prevalence [1–5].

Natural History of HCV in HIV Co-infection

After acute HCV infection, progression to chronic HCV infection is increased from 70–80% in those not infected with HIV to 85–90% in HIV-infected individuals [6,7]. Individuals with HIV-HCV co-infection have higher HCV RNA levels [8–10], leading to enhanced risk of transmission such as in the perinatal setting [11].

There is convincing evidence that co-infection with HIV worsens the prognosis of HCV-related liver disease: risk of cirrhosis is two-fold higher compared with HCV mono-infected individuals, with limited impact of introduction of highly active antiretroviral therapy (HAART) on this level of risk. The estimated prevalences of cirrhosis after 20 and 30 years infection among HIV-HCV co-infected individuals are 21% and 49%, respectively [12]. HIV-HCV co-infected individuals with cirrhosis have a six-fold higher risk of progression to liver failure [13]. Hepatocellular carcinoma (HCC) risk is also high among HIV-HCV co-infected individuals with cirrhosis, and is associated with shorter duration of HCV infection, younger age at diagnosis, and more aggressive clinical course than in HCV mono-infected individuals [14,15]. Risk factors for liver disease progression in HIV-HCV co-infected individuals include heavy alcohol intake, older age (>25 years) at HCV acquisition, and more advanced HIV disease (CD4 count <200–250 cells/mm^3)[16,17].

The impact of HIV on HCV-related liver disease progression, relatively low HCV treatment uptake among HIV-HCV co-infected populations, and sub-optimal efficacy have meant that in an era of improved antiretroviral therapy (ART) -based HIV control the proportion of deaths attributed to liver disease has increased, particularly in settings where co-infection is common [18–20].

Diagnosis and Monitoring of HCV in HIV Infection

Due to increased HCV prevalence in HIV-infected individuals, and the implications of HIV-HCV co-infection on disease progression, all HIV-infected individuals should be tested for anti-HCV antibody. Thereafter, testing should be repeated based on ongoing risk exposure. Anti-HCV antibody may be negative, despite active HCV viremia, in a small proportion of immunosuppressed patients [21,22] Consideration should therefore be given to HCV RNA testing despite negative anti-HCV antibody in cases of unexplained transaminase elevation, in patients with CD4 counts <200 mm^3, when acute hepatitis C is suspected, or among subjects with a high risk of acquiring HCV (e.g., IDU).

Advanced Therapy for Hepatitis C, First Edition. Edited by Geoffrey W. McCaughan, John G. McHutchison and Jean-Michel Pawlotsky.
© 2012 Blackwell Publishing Ltd. Published 2012 by Blackwell Publishing Ltd.

HIV-HCV co-infected patients should undergo a similar work-up as HCV mono-infected patients, with assessment of HCV genotype, HCV viral load, HBV serology, HBV and HAV vaccination status, and laboratory and clinical assessment of liver disease stage. The role of liver biopsy in HIV-HCV co-infected patients is under re-evaluation, as in HCV mono-infection. The decision to biopsy is made on an individual basis; it is most useful to clarify treatment decisions, for example, in patients with HCV genotype 1 and high viral load who have particularly poor treatment responses. Non-invasive methods of diagnosing and staging liver disease, such as transient elastography (Fibroscan) and the use of algorithms involving serum biochemical markers (e.g., Fibrotest, FIB-4) have been evaluated in HIV-HCV co-infection [23–25]. To date these techniques show promise, particularly in the identification and monitoring of patients with cirrhosis.

All HIV-HCV co-infected individuals with confirmed or suspected cirrhosis should undergo regular (every 6–12 months) monitoring with alfa-fetoprotein and liver ultrasound for HCC, as well as screening for the complications of cirrhosis, such as esophageal varices.

Treatment of HIV-HCV Co-infection

All HIV-infected patients with detectable HCV RNA should undergo further assessment for HCV treatment. The significant morbidity associated with end-stage liver disease (ESLD) from untreated HCV within this population dictates a low threshold for the consideration of HCV treatment [26,27], particularly as treatment outcomes in the co-infected population continue to improve. Factors to be considered prior to treatment include those that are HCV related, those that are HIV related, and those related to psychosocial issues (Table 22.1). HIV-HCV co-infected patients often have complex medical, psychiatric, and social circumstances.

An assessment of likelihood of response to therapy and tolerance of treatment, combined with an assessment of the potential toxicity, is vital to successful treatment. However, few pre-treatment variables are absolute contraindications to treatment. Further, those that are, such as the use of didanosine (which may increase the risk of more serious forms of HAART-related hepatotoxicity and metabolic acidosis), can usually be modified prior to treatment commencement. In an individual in whom HCV treatment is not considered an option, ongoing HCV monitoring and modification of factors that may negatively affect liver disease progression (e.g., drug toxicities, alcohol use, obesity and insulin resistance, uncontrolled HIV infection) should continue.

The goals of HCV treatment in HIV-HCV co-infected patients are similar to those in HCV mono-infected patients. Treatment success is defined by sustained virologic response (SVR), due to its relationship with fibrosis regression [28], reduction in liver disease related morbidity and mortality [29], and durability of non-viremia [30].

Standard HCV treatment in HIV-HCV co-infected patients is with pegylated interferon (Peg-IFN) (alfa-2a or alfa-2b) plus ribavirin [31]. Both forms of Peg-IFN have been studied in large trials in HIV-HCV co-infected populations [32–35], with similar efficacy. Overall SVR rates have been 27–44% (genotype 1 or 4, 14–38%; genotype 2 or 3, 44–73%) (Table 22.2), 10–20% lower than similar large-scale trials in HCV mono-infected populations.

Lower HCV treatment response rates in HIV-HCV co-infected populations are probably related to multiple factors, including higher HCV viral load, immunosuppression, increased toxicity/poorer treatment adherence, and suboptimal dosing of ribavirin. Initially, ribavirin was administered at the lower dose of 800 mg/day, regardless of genotype, largely due to concerns about anemia. This lower dose may have been partly responsible for the particularly poor responses to therapy in genotype 1 high viral load co-infected patients seen in the APRICOT study, where the SVR was only 18%, compared to approximately 60% for patients with genotype 2/3 and genotype 1 low viral load [32]. Subsequent studies have demonstrated that higher doses of ribavirin, based on body weight, can be used safely and are associated with an improvement in SVR [36,37]. The current recommendation for HCV treatment in HIV-HCV co-infection is to utilize the same Peg-IFN and ribavirin dosing strategy as HCV mono-infection, thus using Peg-IFN alfa-2a 180 mcg/week or Peg-IFN alfa-2b 1.5 mcg/kg/week with weight-based ribavirin [38].

Guidelines have recommended 48 weeks of therapy for all genotypes in HIV-HCV co-infection based on the duration of therapy used in the early published trials [31]. However, more recent data indicates that HIV-HCV co-infected patients with genotype 2 or 3 who achieve undetectable HCV RNA at week 4 (rapid virologic response, RVR) and have other associated favorable factors (low baseline HCV viral load, no advanced fibrosis), may be able to shorten therapy to 24 weeks [39,40]. Similarly, extended courses of therapy to 72 weeks have been proposed for individuals with a poor early response to therapy, particularly those with genotype 1 and high

Table 22.1 Variables to consider in pre-treatment assessment.

	Comment
HCV	
Genotype	1 versus non-1 (2, 3, and 4)
	Most important predictor of SVR
Baseline HCV viral load	HCV viral load (greater or less than 400 000 IU/ml)
	predicts SVR, particularly in genotype 1
Liver biopsy	Not required in all cases
	Recommended if risk/benefit of treatment unclear
Non-invasive markers	Role in assessment of liver fibrosis still unclear
(biochemical or radiological)	Not routinely available in many countries
ALT	Normal ALT does not preclude significant fibrosis, and does not constitute a contraindication for treatment
HIV	
CD4	Consider HIV treatment first if CD4 <350 cells/ml
Antiretroviral therapy	Should be stable
	Avoid DDI: absolute contraindication
	AZT/D4T: relative contraindications
	If initiating HAART choose "liver-friendly" regimen
Lipids	Insulin resistance may be associated with poor treatment response
Other factors	
Alcohol intake	Advise abstinence from alcohol during therapy to maximize treatment response
Recreational drugs	Not a contraindication to therapy providing drug use stable
Injecting behavior	Advise about potential for re-infection
Opioid substitution therapy	Not a contraindication to therapy
Social/psychological	
Social support/networks	Important for patient support through treatment
Psychiatric history	History of severe or current depression may be a contraindication to treatment
	Consider role of prophylactic antidepressant in selected patients

ALT, alanine aminotransferase; DDI, didanosine; AZT, zidovudine; D4T, stavudine.
Source: From Matthews GV, Dore G. HIV and hepatitis C coinfection. *J Gastroenterol Hepatol* 2008;23(7 Pt 1):1000–1008.

baseline viral load. A recent response-guided pilot study in sixty HIV-HCV co-infected patients demonstrated that irrespective of genotype, therapy could be shortened to 24 weeks if RVR was achieved, with an SVR rate of 90% in this group [41]. However, in genotype 1 and 4 patients without RVR but complete EVR who were treated with 48 weeks of therapy, the relapse rate was 46%.

As with HCV mono-infection, the negative predictive value of a lack of HCV viral load reduction < 2 logs at week 12 (no EVR) for eventual SVR is high (98–100%) in genotype 1 infection [32], thus supporting cessation of treatment at this time point in non-EVR cases. A lack of HCV viral load reduction to <500 000 IU/ml at week 4

also has a very high negative predictive value for SVR [42], thus allowing earlier consideration of treatment cessation, particularly in those patients with considerable toxicity.

HIV-HCV co-infected individuals require careful monitoring during HCV treatment. Discontinuation and toxicity rates from earlier trials were higher than those seen with HCV mono-infection (the serious adverse event rate in RIBAVIC was 35%). Drug interactions are a particular concern in HIV-HCV co-infected individuals on antiretroviral therapy. Mitochondrial toxicity, lactic acidosis, and hepatic decompensation have been reported in several individuals on the combination of ribavirin and didanosine (DDI) [43,44]. This interaction is thought to

Table 22.2 Results of large randomized clinical trials of Peg-IFN in HIV/HCV co-infected patients.

	APRICOT [32]	RIBAVIC [33]	ACTG5071 [34]	Laguno et al. [35]
n	868	412	133	95
Location	International	France	USA	Spain
Peg-IFN	Alfa-2a	Alfa-2b	Alfa-2a	Alfa-2b
Ribavirin dose (mg)	800	800	600–1000 (escalation over 12 weeks)	800–1200 (weight based)
Treatment duration (weeks)	48	48	48	48 genotypes 1/4 and genotypes 2/3 (HCV viral load >800 000 IU/ml)
				24 genotypes 2/3 (HCV viral load <800 000 IU/ml)
Mean baseline CD4 cells/ml	530	482	474	570
SVR overall (%)	40	27	27	44
– Genotypes 1/4 (%)	29	17	14	38
– Genotypes 2/3 (%)	62	44	73	53
Dose modification for anaemia (%)	16	11	5	13

Source: From Matthews GV, Dore G. HIV and hepatitis C coinfection. *J Gastroenterol Hepatol* 2008;23(7 Pt 1):1000–1008.

arise due to the inhibition of inosine monophosphate dehydrogenase (IMPDH) by ribavirin and a resultant increase in the intracellular concentration, and therefore toxicity, of DDI. This drug combination is therefore contraindicated and DDI should be switched to alternative nucleoside analogs before commencing HCV therapy.

Concerns regarding the synergistic effect of zidovudine (AZT) and ribavirin in accelerating the onset of severe anemia have led to the recommendation that, where possible, AZT should also be substituted with an alternative antiretroviral agent. A recent study confirmed that anemia during HCV therapy in HIV-HCV was attributable to the AZT dose but not the dose of ribavirin [36]. The use of erythropoietin-alfa (EPO) to maintain hemoglobin levels and thus allow maximal RBV dosing has been used in some centers but the high cost of EPO prohibits this from widespread use in most clinics. Peg-IFN-related neutropenia and thrombocytopenia occur during treatment, although at similar rates to HCV mono-infection, and can usually be managed with dose reduction.

Neuropsychiatric effects of Peg-IFN, in particular depression, are common in HIV-HCV co-infected patients [45]. Early and aggressive intervention with counseling, support, and antidepressants are often required and may be essential to maximize treatment completion and success.

Reduction in the absolute CD4 cell count by 10–15% is common during HCV treatment and has been attributed to IFN-induced myelosuppression. Providing the CD4 percentage remains unaffected and HIV RNA titers remain stable, reassurance can be given that the CD4 decline does not reflect deterioration in HIV control. In fact, Peg-IFN has documented anti-HIV activity and it is common to see HIV viremia fall by approximately 0.5–1.0 log during HCV treatment.

Peg-IFN is contraindicated in decompensated cirrhosis. In the APRICOT trial (also observed in RIBAVIC) an unexpected number of cases of hepatic decompensation were observed (approximately 10% of those with baseline cirrhosis); these resulted in death from liver failure in six individuals, which is rarely observed when treating mono-infected patients with HCV-related compensated cirrhosis. In a multivariate analysis, factors predicting decompensation were markers of advanced liver disease and the use of DDI [46]. Peg-IFN should be used cautiously in any HIV-HCV co-infected patient with cirrhosis.

Table 22.3 Similarities and differences between treatment of HIV-positive and HIV-negative individuals.

Similarities
Late relapse after SVR uncommon in either situation
Early virologic responses including RVR and ETR established as effective predictors of SVR in both groups
Strongest baseline predictors of SVR (HCV viral load, genotype) identical in both
Management of interferon-induced cytopenias similar

Differences
SVR rates generally 10–15% lower in HIV-positive individuals
Baseline HCV viral load generally higher in HIV-positive individuals
Extension of therapy to 48 weeks advised for all HIV-positive genotype 3 patients without RVR
Drug interactions more common in HIV-positive especially between ribavirin and nucleoside analogs
Higher rates of pre- and on-treatment depression in HIV-positive individuals
Higher rates of anemia particularly with concurrent zidovudine in HIV-positive individuals

Baseline factors predictive of treatment outcome have been examined in the pivotal HIV-HCV co-infection studies. In APRICOT the strongest predictors of improved SVR were HCV related: genotype (2 and 3 versus 1) and low HCV viral load (<400 000 IU/ml) [47]. Age, body weight, and fibrosis stage had limited impact on treatment outcome. In contrast to HCV factors, HIV factors (HIV viral load, CD4 count) had no significant influence on SVR in APRICOT. This is somewhat surprising but may reflect the small study populations with advanced HIV disease (in APRICOT individuals with CD4 < 100 cells/ml were excluded and relatively few had counts of 100–200). An association has been suggested between higher CD4 percentage (>25%) and SVR, but only reported in genotype 1 patients. Insulin resistance has been identified as a predictor of non-response in HCV mono-infection studies [48] and may be more common in HIV-positive individuals treated with protease inhibitors. Despite this, insulin resistance to date has not been identified as a significant mechanism behind the lower SVR rates in HIV-HCV coinfection [49].

Decisions on HCV treatment should therefore be determined predominantly by HCV-related rather than HIV-related variables, unless the CD4 count is particularly low. Most clinicians would advise treating HIV disease first if the CD4 count is less than 350 cells/mm³. In contrast, for patients with higher CD4 counts it is probably preferable to treat HCV first to avoid issues of drug interactions and HAART hepatotoxicty.

A summary of the similarities and differences in the treatment of HIV-positive and HIV-negative individuals is given in Table 22.3.

Management of Treatment Non-Response and End-Stage Liver Disease

A large proportion of HIV-HCV co-infected patients will fail to achieve SVR or be intolerant or ineligible for current therapeutic options. As with HCV mono-infection, the primary management aim for these patients is to minimize the risk of progression to cirrhosis, or if cirrhosis is present, to actively screen for and manage complications of ESLD (ascites, esophageal varices, and HCC).

Prevention of fibrosis progression can be optimized in a number of ways. Successful HIV control with suppression of HIV viremia and CD4 count restoration or maintenance slows fibrosis progression [50]. Exposure to other co-factors for fibrosis, such as alcohol or hepatotoxic drugs, should be minimized. Treatment with Peg-IFN/RBV itself results in histologic improvement and limitation/reversal of fibrosis progression, and although this benefit is maximal in subjects who achieve SVR, an effect is also often seen in those without SVR. In large HIV-HCV trials, between 15% and 43% of individuals without SVR (including non-responders and relapsers) have shown histologic improvement with decreased necroinflammation on follow-up biopsy [33,34].

Survival after the first episode of hepatic decompensation is shortened in HIV-HCV co-infected patients, with a median survival of only 16 months [51]. For HIV-HCV co-infected patients with ESLD, the only effective treatment option is liver transplantation. Transplantation for HIV-HCV co-infected individuals has gradually become more widespread in developed countries in recent years [52–54]. Since the advent of HAART, short-term survival post-transplantation has been similar in HIV-HCV co-infected and HCV mono-infected patients. The main cause of death is aggressive post-transplant HCV re-infection and cirrhosis.

The long-term outcome following liver transplantation of individuals with HIV-HCV co-infection compared to HCV mono-infection remains uncertain. Loss of HIV control and AIDS-related opportunistic infections are unusual, although generally HIV-HCV co-infected individuals with advanced HIV disease (CD4 count <150/mm^3 or active opportunistic infections) are excluded from transplantation. Furthermore, a higher proportion of HIV-HCV co-infected individuals with ESLD die while on the transplant waiting list, probably related to both more rapid liver disease progression and HIV-related complications.

New Directions in Therapy

New therapies with direct HCV antiviral activity are currently in development. Broadly, these agents fall into two groups, the HCV protease inhibitors and the HCV polymerase inhibitors. Both appear highly effective in reducing HCV viremia in phase I and II studies [55,56], but their optimal role in the treatment of HCV infection remains to be defined. It is likely that their use will be complicated by issues of both resistance and toxicity. As yet, these agents have not been tested in HIV-HCV co-infected populations, and potential drug interactions with antiretroviral therapies, including drug toxicity and the effects of ritonavir-boosting, are unknown. However, their future availability is likely to further increase therapeutic options for the clinical management of HIV-HCV co-infection.

References

1. Gambotti L, Batisse D, Colin-de-Verdiere N, et al. Acute hepatitis C infection in HIV positive men who have sex with men in Paris, France, 2001–2004. *Euro Surveill* 2005;10(5):115–17.
2. Gilleece YC, Browne RE, Asboe D, et al. Transmission of hepatitis C virus among HIV-positive homosexual men and response to a 24-week course of pegylated interferon and ribavirin. *J Acquir Immune Defic Syndr* 2005;40(1):41–6.
3. Gotz HM, van Doornum G, Niesters HG, et al. A cluster of acute hepatitis C virus infection among men who have sex with men: results from contact tracing and public health implications. *AIDS* 2005;19(9):969–74.
4. Matthews GV, Hellard M, Kaldor J, et al. Further evidence of HCV sexual transmission among HIV-positive men who have sex with men: response to Danta et al. *AIDS* 2007;21(15):2112–13.
5. Fierer DS, Uriel AJ, Carriero DC, et al. Liver fibrosis during an outbreak of acute hepatitis C virus infection in HIV-infected men: a prospective cohort study. *J Infect Dis* 2008;198(5):683–6.
6. Thomas DL, Astemborski J, Rai RM, et al. The natural history of hepatitis C virus infection: host, viral, and environmental factors. *JAMA* 2000;284(4):450–56.
7. Mehta SH, Cox A, Hoover DR, et al. Protection against persistence of hepatitis C. *Lancet* 2002;359(9316):1478–83.
8. Cribier B, Rey D, Schmitt C, et al. High hepatitis C viraemia and impaired antibody response in patients coinfected with HIV. *AIDS* 1995;9(10):1131–6.
9. Thomas DL, Shih JW, Alter HJ, et al. Effect of human immunodeficiency virus on hepatitis C virus infection among injecting drug users. *J Infect Dis* 1996;174(4):690–95.
10. Sherman KE, O'Brien J, Gutierrez AG, et al. Quantitative evaluation of hepatitis C virus RNA in patients with concurrent human immunodeficiency virus infections. *J Clin Microbiol* 1993;31(10):2679–82.
11. Polis CB, Shah SN, Johnson KE, Gupta A. Impact of maternal HIV coinfection on the vertical transmission of hepatitis C virus: a meta-analysis. *Clin Infect Dis* 2007;44(8):1123–31.
12. Thein HH, Yi Q, Dore GJ, Krahn MD. Natural history of hepatitis C virus infection in HIV-infected individuals and the impact of HIV in the era of highly active antiretroviral therapy: a meta-analysis. *AIDS* 2008;22(15):1979–91.
13. Graham CS, Baden LR, Yu E, et al. Influence of human immunodeficiency virus infection on the course of hepatitis C virus infection: a meta-analysis. *Clin Infect Dis* 2001;33(4):562–9.
14. Brau N, Xiao P, Naqvi Z, et al. Hepatocellular carcinoma in 40 HIV/HCV coinfected versus 50 HCV-monoinfected patients. North American HCC in HIV Study Group. Paper presented at 3rd IAS Conference on HIV pathogenesis and treatment, 24–27 July, 2005, Rio de Janeiro, Brazil.
15. Puoti M, Bruno R, Soriano V, et al. Hepatocellular carcinoma in HIV-infected patients: epidemiological features, clinical presentation and outcome. *AIDS* 2004;18(17):2285–93.
16. Benhamou Y, Bochet M, Di M, V, et al. Liver fibrosis progression in human immunodeficiency virus and hepatitis C virus coinfected patients. The Multivirc Group. *Hepatology* 1999;30(4):10548.
17. Mohsen AH, Easterbrook PJ, Taylor C, et al. Impact of human immunodeficiency virus (HIV) infection on the progression of liver fibrosis in hepatitis C virus infected patients. *Gut* 2003;52(7):1035–40.

18. Bica I, McGovern B, Dhar R, *et al.* Increasing mortality due to end-stage liver disease in patients with human immunodeficiency virus infection. *Clin Infect Dis* 2001;32(3): 492–7.

19. Soriano V, Garcia-Samaniego J, Valencia E, *et al.* Impact of chronic liver disease due to hepatitis viruses as cause of hospital admission and death in HIV–infected drug users. *Eur J Epidemiol* 1999;15(1):1–4.

20. Rosenthal E, Poiree M, Pradier C, *et al.* Mortality due to hepatitis C-related liver disease in HIV-infected patients in France (Mortavic 2001 study). *AIDS* 2003;17(12): 1803–9.

21. Ragni MV, Ndimbie OK, Rice EO, *et al.* The presence of hepatitis C virus (HCV) antibody in human immunodeficiency virus-positive hemophilic men undergoing HCV "seroreversion". *Blood* 1993;82(3):1010–15.

22. Sherman KE, Rouster SD, Chung RT, Rajicic N. Hepatitis C virus prevalence among patients infected with human immunodeficiency virus: a cross-sectional analysis of the US Adult AIDS Clinical Trials Group. *Clin Infect Dis* 2002;34(6):831–7.

23. Macias J, Giron-Gonzalez JA, Gonzalez-Serrano M, *et al.* Prediction of liver fibrosis in human immunodeficiency virus/hepatitis C virus coinfected patients by simple noninvasive indexes. *Gut* 2006;55(3):409–14.

24. Myers RP, Benhamou Y, Imbert-Bismut F, *et al.* Serum biochemical markers accurately predict liver fibrosis in HIV and hepatitis C virus co-infected patients. *AIDS* 2003;17(5):721–5.

25. de Ledinghen V, Douvin C, Kettaneh A, *et al.* Diagnosis of hepatic fibrosis and cirrhosis by transient elastography in HIV/hepatitis C virus-coinfected patients. *J Acquir Immune Defic Syndr* 2006;41(2):175–9.

26. Puoti M, Spinetti A, Ghezzi A, *et al.* Mortality for liver disease in patients with HIV infection: a cohort study. *J Acquir Immune Defic Syndr* 2000;24(3):211–17.

27. Salmon-Ceron D, Lewden C, Morlat P, *et al.* Liver disease as a major cause of death among HIV infected patients: role of hepatitis C and B viruses and alcohol. *J Hepatol* 2005;42(6):799–805.

28. Barreiro P, Labarga P, Martin-Carbonero L, *et al.* Sustained virological response following HCV therapy is associated with non-progression of liver fibrosis in HCV/HIV-coinfected patients. *Antivir Ther* 2006;11(7): 869–77.

29. Berenguer J, Alvarez-Pellicer J, Martin PM, *et al.* Sustained virological response to interferon plus ribavirin reduces liver-related complications and mortality in patients coinfected with human immunodeficiency virus and hepatitis C virus. *Hepatology* 2009;50(2):407–13.

30. Soriano V, Maida I, Nunez M, *et al.* Long-term follow-up of HIV-infected patients with chronic hepatitis C virus infection treated with interferon-based therapies. *Antivir Ther* 2004;9(6):987–92.

31. Soriano V, Puoti M, Sulkowski M, *et al.* Care of patients with hepatitis C and HIV co-infection. *AIDS* 2004;18(1):1–12.

32. Torriani FJ, Rodriguez-Torres M, Rockstroh JK, *et al.* Peginterferon alfa-2a plus ribavirin for chronic hepatitis C virus infection in HIV-infected patients. *N Engl J Med* 2004;351(5):438–50.

33. Carrat F, Bani-Sadr F, Pol S, *et al.* Pegylated interferon alfa-2b vs standard interferon alfa-2b, plus ribavirin, for chronic hepatitis C in HIV-infected patients: a randomized controlled trial. *JAMA* 2004;292(23):2839–48.

34. Chung RT, Andersen J, Volberding P, *et al.* Peginterferon alfa-2a plus ribavirin versus interferon alfa-2a plus ribavirin for chronic hepatitis C in HIV-coinfected persons. *N Engl J Med* 2004;351(5):451–9.

35. Laguno M, Murillas J, Blanco JL, *et al.* Peginterferon alfa-2b plus ribavirin compared with interferon alfa-2b plus ribavirin for treatment of HIV/HCV co-infected patients. *AIDS* 2004;18(13):F27–36.

36. Alvarez D, Dieterich DT, Brau N, *et al.* Zidovudine use but not weight-based ribavirin dosing impacts anaemia during HCV treatment in HIV-infected persons. *J Viral Hepatitis* 2006;13(10):683–9.

37. Nunez M, Miralles C, Berdun MA, *et al.* Role of weight-based ribavirin dosing and extended duration of therapy in chronic hepatitis C in HIV-infected patients: the PRESCO trial. *AIDS Res Hum Retroviruses* 2007;23(8):972–82.

38. Soriano V, Puoti M, Sulkowski M, *et al.* Care of patients coinfected with HIV and hepatitis C virus: 2007 updated recommendations from the HCV-HIV International Panel. *AIDS* 2007;21(9):1073–89.

39. Crespo M, Esteban JI, Ribera E, *et al.* Utility of week-4 viral response to tailor treatment duration in hepatitis C virus genotype 3/HIV co-infected patients. *AIDS* 2007;21(4):477–81.

40. Soriano V, Puoti M, Sulkowski M, *et al.* Care of patients coinfected with HIV and hepatitis C virus: 2007 updated recommendations from the HCV-HIV International Panel. *AIDS* 2007;21(9):1073–89.

41. Van den Eynde E, Crespo M, Esteban JI, *et al.* Response-guided therapy for chronic hepatitis C virus infection in patients coinfected with HIV: a pilot trial. *Clin Infect Dis* 2009;48(8):1152–9.

42. Payan C, Pivert A, Morand P, *et al.* Rapid and early virological response to chronic hepatitis C treatment with IFN alpha2b or PEG-IFN alpha2b plus ribavirin in HIV/HCV co-infected patients. *Gut* 2007;56(8):1111–16.

43. Lafeuillade A HG, Chapadaud S. Increased mitochondrial toxicity with ribavirin in HIV/HCV coinfection. *Lancet* 2001;357: 280-81.

44. Fleischer R, Boxwell D, Sherman KE. Nucleoside analogues and mitochondrial toxicity. *Clin Infect Dis* 2004;38(8):e79–80.

45. Laguno M, Blanch J, Murillas J, *et al.* Depressive symptoms after initiation of interferon therapy in human immunod-

eficiency virus-infected patients with chronic hepatitis C. *Antivir Ther* 2004;9(6):905–9.

46. Mauss S, Valenti W, DePamphilis J, *et al.* Risk factors for hepatic decompensation in patients with HIV/HCV coinfection and liver cirrhosis during interferon-based therapy. *AIDS* 2004;18(13):F21–25.

47. Dore GJ, Torriani FJ, Rodriguez-Torres M, *et al.* Baseline factors prognostic of sustained virological response in patients with HIV-hepatitis C virus co-infection. *AIDS* 2007;21(12):1555–9.

48. Romero-Gomez M, Del Mar Viloria M, Andrade RJ, *et al.* Insulin resistance impairs sustained response rate to peginterferon plus ribavirin in chronic hepatitis C patients. *Gastroenterology* 2005;128(3):636–41.

49. Merchante N, Rivero A, de Los Santos-Gil I, *et al.* Insulin resistance is associated with liver stiffness in HIV/HCV-coinfected patients. *Gut* 2009;58(12):1654–60.

50. Quirishi N, Kreuzberg C, Luchters G, *et al.* Effect of antiretroviral therapy on liver-related mortality in patients with HIV and hepatitis C virus coinfection. *Lancet* 2003;362: 1708–13.

51. Pineda JA, Romero-Gomez M, Diaz-Garcia F, *et al.* HIV coinfection shortens the survival of patients with hepatitis C virus–related decompensated cirrhosis. *Hepatology* 2005;41(4):779–89.

52. Neff GW, Bonham A, Tzakis AG, *et al.* Orthotopic liver transplantation in patients with human immunodeficiency virus and end-stage liver disease. *Liver Transpl* 2003;9(3):239–47.

53. Ragni MV, Belle SH, Im K, *et al.* Survival of human immunodeficiency virus-infected liver transplant recipients. *J Infect Dis* 2003;188(10):1412–20.

54. Rufi G, Barcena R, Vargas V, Valdivieso A, *et al.* Orthotopic liver transplantation in 15 HIV-1-infected recipients: evaluation of Spanish experience in the HAART era (2002–2003). *Paper presented at 11th Conference on Retroviruses and Opportunistic Infections, 2004, San Francisco, CA.*

55. McHutchison JG, Everson GT, Gordon SC, *et al.* Telaprevir with peginterferon and ribavirin for chronic HCV genotype 1 infection. *N Engl J Med* 2009;360(18):1827–38.

56. Hezode C, Forestier N, Dusheiko G, *et al.* Telaprevir and peginterferon with or without ribavirin for chronic HCV infection. *N Engl J Med* 2009;360(18):1839–50.

23 HCV and Racial Differences

Andrew J. Muir

Duke Clinical Research Institute, Duke University Medical Center, Durham, NC, USA

Introduction

The past decade has seen remarkable advances in our understanding of hepatitis C virus (HCV) infection. One of the interesting yet concerning findings has been the variation observed in prevalence and response to infection among different racial and ethnic groups. As we approach a new era with the introduction of direct antivirals, this chapter will review current prevalence and treatment outcomes according to race and ethnicity.

Epidemiology

The World Health Organization estimates that 2.2% of the world's population or 170 million people are infected with HCV [1]. These prevalence estimates are limited by incomplete data and varied approaches in select populations, but the highest rates are in the African and Eastern Mediterranean regions [2]. Reports from China, which has one fifth of the world's population, have suggested disease prevalence of 3.2% for HCV [3]. In India, which also has one fifth of the world's population, the epidemiology of HCV has not been systematically studied, and screening programs in blood donors have reported wide ranges in prevalence of HCV infection [4]. Egypt has reported the highest seroprevalence rate from a systematic screening program at 22% [5].

In the United States, with its mixture of racial and ethnic groups, the National Health and Nutrition Examination Survey (NHANES) has provided HCV prevalence statistics. NHANES is conducted by the National Center for Health Statistics of the Centers for Disease Control and Prevention. The sample includes non-institutionalized civilians throughout the United States. The most recent NHANES report from 1999 through 2002 found that 1.6% or an estimated 4.1 million people had antibodies to HCV with 1.3% or an estimated 3.2 million with viremia and chronic infection [6]. Overall, prevalence was higher in men and in non-Hispanic blacks (3.0%) compared to non-Hispanic whites (1.5%) and Mexican Americans (1.3%). The differences in race and ethnicity mainly occurred in people over age 40. Among the group 40 to 49 years of age, 9.4% of non-Hispanic blacks had HCV antibodies compared to 3.8% of non-Hispanic whites ($p < 0.001$). Non-Hispanic black men between 40 and 49 years had the highest prevalence at 13.6%.

Minority groups also have increased mortality related to HCV. Using US census data and other national mortality statistics resources, Wise *et al.* found that mortality rates from HCV increased 123% from 1995 to 2004 (from 1.09 per 100 000 persons to 2.44 per 100 000) [7]. The increases were greater among non-Hispanic blacks (170%) and Native Americans (241%) compared to non-Hispanic whites (124%) and Hispanics (84%).

These statistics highlight the need for increased identification and treatment of patients with HCV infection. A recent study from Philadelphia suggests that underrepresented minorities were less likely to receive HCV testing [8]. In this retrospective study of 4407 patients in 4 primary care sites, only 55% of all patients who admitted history of injection drug use were tested for HCV. African Americans were more likely to have the risk factor documented than whites (79% versus 68%, $p < 0.0001$) in the history, but minorities were less likely to be tested for HCV than whites in the presence of a known risk factor (23% versus 35%, $p = 0.004$).

Treatment

The decision to treat a patient with HCV infection can be complex and take into account a number of factors, including stage of disease, genotype, co-morbidities that are contraindications to treatment, side effects, and

Advanced Therapy for Hepatitis C, First Edition. Edited by Geoffrey W. McCaughan, John G. McHutchison and Jean-Michel Pawlotsky.
© 2012 Blackwell Publishing Ltd. Published 2012 by Blackwell Publishing Ltd.

patient preferences. Studies in American veterans suggest that members from different racial and ethnic groups may not be offered HCV treatment in similar rates to whites. In their multicenter VA cohort, Cheung et al. found that Latino veterans were more likely than Caucasian veterans to meet HCV treatment criteria and to be considered by health care providers as eligible for HCV therapy, but Latino and Caucasian veterans underwent therapy at similar rates (20.9% and 19.2%, respectively) [9]. In a retrospective cohort study of eight Veterans Affairs medical centers in the northwest United States, medical records from 4263 HCV-infected patients were studied [10]. When compared to whites, African Americans were less likely to receive antiviral treatment (OR 0.38; 95% CI 0.23, 0.63). Topics such as patient eligibility for treatment, patient preferences, or potential provider biases were not examined and will be important to understand how to help more patients receive treatment.

African Americans

The first sign of differences in HCV treatment response among racial groups came in African Americans. Reddy et al. performed a retrospective analysis from multicenter trial databases of patients treated with consensus interferon or interferon alfa-2b, and African Americans had lower sustained virologic response (SVR) rates compared to whites (2% versus 12%) [11]. McHutchison et al. addressed the same question from multicenter trial databases of patients treated with interferon alfa alone or in combination with ribavirin, and African Americans had a significantly lower overall SVR rate than Caucasian patients (11% versus 27%, $p = 0.01$) [12]. African Americans had a significantly higher rate of genotype 1 infection compared to whites (88% versus 65%). Analysis of genotype 1 patients indicated no statistical difference in SVR between African Americans and whites, suggesting that the previous observations were due to the genotype frequency and not race.

In the past several years, multiple prospective trials have been conducted in patients receiving peginterferon alfa and ribavirin. These studies have consistently demonstrated lower SVR rates among African Americans. Muir et al. treated 100 African Americans and 100 Caucasians with peginterferon alfa-2b and ribavirin [13]. The study population was 98% genotype 1, and African Americans had significantly lower SVR rates than Caucasians (19% versus 52%, $p < 0.001$). Using peginterferon alfa-2a and ribavirin, Jeffers et al. reported SVR of 26% for African Americans and 39% for whites [14]. VIRAHEP-C was a multicenter NIH study that enrolled 196 African Americans and 205 Caucasians to receive peginterferon alfa-2a and ribavirin. SVR rates are presented in Figure 23.1 and occurred in 28% of African Americans and 50% of Caucasians ($p < 0.0001$) [15]. This collection of studies confirmed that response rates among African Americans are lower. More recently, the WIN-R trial highlighted the importance of the dose of ribavirin. The WIN-R trial was a large multicenter study that investigated differences in response to HCV treatment with peginterferon alfa-2b used in combination with either flat dose (800 mg) ribavirin or weight-based doses (800–1400 mg) of ribavirin. In the subgroup analysis of African American patients, SVR rates were higher (21% versus 10%; $p = 0.0006$) in the weight-based group than in the flat-dose group [16].

The most recent report on this topic came from the IDEAL trial, which enrolled 3070 total patients, including 570 African Americans with genotype 1 HCV infection, and randomized them to a standard (1.5 mcg/kg) or low

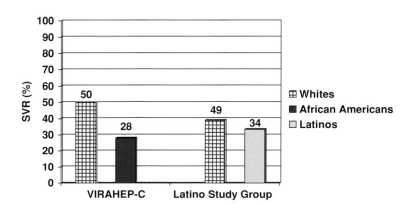

Figure 23.1 Sustained virologic rates in major prospective trials.

Table 23.1 Virologic response for African Americans and non-African Americans in the IDEAL trial [17].

Virologic response	Peg-IFN alfa-2b 1.5 mcg/kg plus ribivarin (%)		Peg-IFN alfa-2b 1.0 mcg/kg plus ribivarin (%)		Peg-IFN alfa-2a plus ribivarin (%)	
	AA	Non-AA	AA	Non-AA	AA	Non-AA
End of treatment	32	58	21	56	45	69
Relapse (%)	26	23	16	20	37	31
SVR (%)	23	44	17	43	26	44

AA, African American.

dose (1.0 mcg/kg) of peginterferon alfa-2b and ribavirin or peginterferon alfa-2a and ribavirin [17]. The side effect profiles were similar among the treatment groups and among the African Americans and non-African Americans. SVR rates are summarized in Table 23.1 and reveal similar SVR rates except for perhaps a lower response for the African Americans treated with the lower dose of peginterferon alfa-2b [18].

Genotype 2 and 3 infection is less common in African Americans, and the reported outcomes suggest higher SVR rates for African Americans compared to genotype 1. In a prospective study at US Veterans Affairs medical centers, patients received interferon alfa-2b three times weekly plus ribavirin. SVR rates were 50.0% for African Americans and 36.5% for non-African Americans ($p = 0.47$) [19]. A recent single-center cohort included patients receiving either standard interferon or peginterferon along with ribavirin [20]. SVR rates were lower for African Americans compared to whites (57% versus 82%, $p = 0.012$) but again appear higher than SVR rates reported for African Americans with genotype 1 infection.

Latinos

In the initial report on ethnic variation in HCV treatment response by Reddy *et al.*, SVR rates to treatment with consensus interferon or interferon alfa-2b were reported [11]. Latinos had similar SVR rates to non-Latino Caucasians (10% versus 12%). Subsequently, Hepburn *et al.* presented their cohort of patients receiving daily interferon alfa-2b and weight-based doses of ribavirin for 48 weeks, and the SVR rate appeared higher for Caucasians (39%) than for Latinos (23%), although this was not statistically different

in this small study [21]. Most recently, the Latino Study Group presented the results from their multicenter, open-label, non-randomized, prospective study of 269 Latino and 300 non-Latino whites with genotype 1 HCV infection [22]. Patients received peginterferon alfa-2a and ribavirin (1000/1200 mg per day) for 48 weeks. The SVR rate was higher in non-Latino whites than Latinos (49% versus 34%, $p < 0.001$) (see Figure 23.1). Baseline differences included greater BMI and cirrhosis in the Latino group, but the regression analysis demonstrated that Latino background was an independent predictor of SVR.

Asians

In a variety of studies of different treatment regimens, Asians with HCV infection appear to have higher SVR rates than other racial and ethnic groups. The early study by Reddy *et al.* reported an SVR rate of 30%, which was three times greater than in whites [11]. Subsequent studies have also reported higher SVR rates in Asians. Missiha *et al.* compared Asians and Caucasians taking peginterferon alfa-2a and fixed-dose ribavirin (800 mg daily) [23]. In this study, 67% of Asians and 45% of Caucasians achieved SVR ($p = 0.0022$). On multivariable logistic regression, Asian race, viral genotype, BMI, severity of fibrosis, and treatment adherence were independently associated with SVR. A recent randomized trial in Taiwan of 308 treatment-naïve genotype 1 patients examined a different question by looking at shorter duration of therapy. Patients received 24 or 48 weeks of treatment with peginterferon alfa-2a and ribavirin. Patients who received 48 weeks of therapy had significantly higher SVR rates compared to those who received 24 weeks of therapy (76% versus 56%; $p < 0.001$). The findings are notable for both the high response overall and a relatively high SVR rate with only 24 weeks of treatment [24].

Genetics of HCV Treatment Response

To better understand predictors of HCV treatment response, a recent genome-wide association study was conducted using the patients from the IDEAL trial [17]. Of the 3070 patients in IDEAL, 1671 patients provided consent for collection of their DNA and were genotyped using the Illumina Human610-quad Bead Chip. The number of Asian American patients was small, and this group was not studied as a distinct group in the analysis but included in the group of "other" racial groups. In order to enrich the number of African American patients, patients from an earlier prospective study of treatment with Peg-IFN alfa-2b were also included [5]. The analysis was then performed on 1137 patients who were compliant with therapy. This analysis identified a single nucleotide polymorphism (SNP) upstream from *IL28B* that strongly predicts HCV treatment response [25]. Patients with the CC genotype at the polymorphism site were much more likely to achieve SVR than patients with the TT or CT genotypes. Patients of European ancestry with the CC genotype had SVR rates greater than 80%. African American patients with the CC genotype had higher rate of SVR (53.3%) than patients of European ancestry with TT genotype (33%, $p < 0.05$). The authors estimated that this polymorphism explained approximately half the difference in SVR rates observed between African Americans and Caucasians. Two subsequent studies have now confirmed the association of the region near the *IL28B* with HCV treatment response [26,27]. The mechanism of this difference in the genome is under investigation. *IL28B* is a member of the interferon lambda family, and interferon lambda compounds have antiviral activity against HCV [28]. A commercially available diagnostic test for this polymorphism is available.

Future Directions

With the emergence of direct antiviral medications in the next few years, it will be important to see how the addition of these medications impacts treatment responses in the different racial and ethnic groups. The early studies with telaprevir, which is an NS3/4A protease inhibitor, have been encouraging. One of the initial studies treated 12 genotype 1 patients with triple combination of telaprevir, peginterferon alfa-2a, and ribavirin for 28 days [29]. Of the 12 patients, 10 were Latino, and all 12 patients had undetectable HCV RNA at 12 weeks. In the recently reported PROVE1 study of combination therapy with telapre-

vir, peginterferon alfa-2a, and ribavirin, patients received 12 weeks of triple combination and then different groups received 0, 12, or 36 more weeks of peginterferon alfa-2a and ribavirin [30]. When combining the telaprevir arms, the African American patients had higher rates of SVR with telaprevir (8/18, 44%) compared to the control group (1/9, 11%). These numbers need validation in larger studies but do suggest improved response rates for patients from all racial and ethnic backgrounds in the future.

Summary

With its global presence, HCV infects a diverse array of racial and ethnic groups. Estimates of infection vary widely around the world and may be related to prevalence patterns but also methodology of individual studies. Despite changes and refinements in regimens over the years, patterns of variation have emerged with lower response rates among people of African and Latino descent but higher response rates among Asians. Understanding these differences will be important and helpful as we try to improve response rates for all patients.

References

1. Shepard CW, Finelli L, Alter MJ. Global epidemiology of hepatitis C virus infection. *Lancet Infect Dis* 2005;5(9): 558–67.
2. Global Burden of Hepatitis C Working Group. Global burden of disease (GBD) for hepatitis C. *J Clin Pharmacol* 2004; 44(1):20–29.
3. Xia GL, Liu CB, Cao HL *et al.* Prevalence of hepatitis B and C virus infections in the general Chinese population: results from a nationwide cross-sectional seroepidemiologic study of hepatitis A, B, C, D, and E virus infections in China, 1992, *Int Hepatol Commun* 1996;5:62–73.
4. Mukhopadhyaya A. Hepatitis C in India. *J Biosci* 2008;33(4): 465–73.
5. Frank C, Mohamed MK, Strickland GT, *et al.* The role of parenteral antischistosomal therapy in the spread of hepatitis C virus in Egypt. *Lancet* 2000;355:887–91.
6. Armstrong GL, Wasley A, Simard EP, *et al.* The prevalence of hepatitis C virus infection in the United States, 1999 through 2002. *Ann Intern Med* 2006;144(10):705–14.
7. Wise M, Bialek S, Finelli L, *et al.* Changing trends in hepatitis C-related mortality in the United States, 1995–2004. *Hepatology* 2008;47(4):1128–35.
8. Trooskin SB, Navarro VJ, Winn RJ, *et al.* Hepatitis C risk assessment, testing and referral for treatment in urban

primary care: role of race and ethnicity. *World J Gastroenterol* 2007;13(7):1074–8.

9. Cheung RC, Currie S, Shen H, *et al.* Chronic hepatitis C in Latinos: natural history, treatment eligibility, acceptance, and outcomes. *Am J Gastroenterol* 2005;100:2186–93.

10. Rousseau CM, Ioannou GN, Todd-Stenberg JA, *et al.* Racial differences in the evaluation and treatment of hepatitis C among veterans: a retrospective cohort study. *Am J Public Health* 2008;98(5):846–52.

11. Reddy KR, Hoofnagle JH, Tong MJ, *et al.* Racial differences in responses to therapy with interferon in chronic hepatitis C. *Consensus Interferon Study Group.* Hepatology 1999;30: 787–93.

12. McHutchison JG, Poynard T, Pianko S, *et al.* The impact of interferon plus ribavirin on response to therapy in black patients with chronic hepatitis C. *Gastroenterology* 2000; 119: 1317–23.

13. Muir AJ, Bornstein JD, Killenberg PG. Peginterferon alfa-2b and ribavirin for the treatment of chronic hepatitis C in blacks and non-Hispanic whites. *N Engl J Med* 2004;350: 2265–71.

14. Jeffers LJ, Cassidy W, Howell CD, *et al.* Peginterferon alfa-2a (40kd) and ribavirin for black American patients with chronic HCV genotype 1. *Hepatology* 2004;39:1702–8.

15. Conjeevaram HS, Fried MW, Jeffers LJ *et al.* Peginterferon and ribavirin treatment in African American and Caucasian American patients with hepatitis C genotype 1. *Gastroenterology* 2006;131(2):470–77.

16. Jacobson IM, Brown RS, Jr., McCone J, *et al.* Impact of weight-based ribavirin with peginterferon alfa-2b in African Americans with hepatitis C virus genotype 1. *Hepatology* 2007;46(4):982–90.

17. McHutchison JG, Lawitz EJ, Shiffman ML, *et al.* Peginterferon alfa-2b or alfa-2a with ribavarin for treatment of hepatitis C infection. *N Engl J Med* 2009;361:580–93.

18. McCone J, Hu KW, McHutchison JG, *et al.* Sustained virologic response and predictors of response in African American patients in the ideal (Individualized Dosing Efficacy Versus Flat Dosing to Assess Optimal Pegylated Interferon Therapy) Phase 3b Study. *Hepatology* 2008;48(4 Suppl): 430A.

19. Brau N, Bini EJ, Currie S, *et al.* Black patients with chronic hepatitis C have a lower sustained viral response rate than non-blacks with genotype 1, but the same with genotypes 2/3, and this is not explained by more frequent dose reductions of interferon and ribavirin. *J Viral Hepatitis* 2006; 13(4):242–9.

20. Shiffman ML, Mihas AA, Millwala F, *et al.* Treatment of chronic hepatitis C virus in African Americans with genotypes 2 and 3. *Am J Gastroenterol* 2007;102(4):761–6.

21. Hepburn MJ, Hepburn LM, Cantu NS, *et al.* Differences in treatment outcome for hepatitis C among ethnic groups. *Am J Med* 2004;117:163–8.

22. Rodriguez-Torres M, Jeffers LJ, Sheikh MY, *et al.* Peginterferon alfa-2a and ribavirin in Latino and non-Latino whites with hepatitis C. *N Engl J Med* 2009;360(3):257–67.

23. Missiha S, Heathcote J, Arenovich T, *et al.* Impact of Asian race on response to combination therapy with peginterferon alfa-2a and ribavirin in chronic hepatitis C. *Am J Gastroenterol* 2007;102(10):2181–8.

24. Liu CH, Liu CJ, Lin CL, *et al.* Pegylated interferon-alpha-2a plus ribavirin for treatment-naive Asian patients with hepatitis C virus genotype 1 infection: a multicenter, randomized controlled trial. *Clin Infect Dis* 2008;47(10):1260–69.

25. Ge D, Fellay J, Thompson AJ, *et al.* Genetic variation in *IL28B* predicts hepatitis C treatment-induced viral clearance. *Nature* 2009;461(7262):399-401.

26. Suppiah V, Moldovan M, Ahlenstiel G, *et al.* IL28B is associated with response to chronic hepatitis C interferon-alpha and ribavirin therapy. *Nat Genet* 2009;41:1100–04.

27. Tanaka Y, Nishida N, Sugiyama M, *et al.* Genome-wide association of IL28B with response to pegylated interferon-alpha and ribavirin therapy for chronic hepatitis C. *Nat Genet* 2009;41:1105–09.

28. Kotenko SV, Gallagher G, Baurin VV, *et al.* IFN-lambdas mediate antiviral protection through a distinct class II cytokine receptor complex. *Nat Immunol* 2003;4(1): 69–77.

29. Rodriguez-Torres M, Lawitz E, Muir A, *et al.* Current status of subjects receiving peginterferon alfa-2a and ribavirin follow-on therapy after 28-day treatment with the hepatitis C protease inhibitor telaprevir (VX-950), PEG-IFN, and RBV. *Hepatology* 2006;44(4 Suppl 1):532A.

30. McHutchison JG, Everson GT, Gordon SC, *et al.* Telaprevir with peginterferon and ribavirin for chronic HCV genotype 1 infection. *N Engl J Med* 2009;360(18):1827–38.

24 HCV and the Pediatric Population

Kathleen B. Schwarz

Johns Hopkins Pediatric Liver Center, Baltimore, MD, USA

Epidemiology and Natural History

In the National Health and Nutrition Evaluation Survey (NHANES) conducted between 1988 and 1994 in a cross-sectional cohort representative of the US population, the prevalence of antibody to HCV (anti-HCV) among children ages 6 to 11 years was 0.2% and among adolescents ages 12 to 19 years 0.4%. Using these prevalence rates one could estimate 132 000 children and adolescents with anti-HCV in the United States [1]. The rate of chronic hepatitis C was likely to be less since only about half of antibody-positive subjects are infected. Recently it has been estimated that between 23 048 and 42 296 children in the United States are chronically infected with HCV and that 7200 new cases occur annually [2]. Maternal-child transmission rates are 4–7% from viremic mothers with HCV RNA > 10^6 cpm and/or HIV co-infection being risk factors for transmission [3] and maternal HLA-*DRB1*04* conferring protection against transmission [4]. Children generally exhibit a low rate of spontaneous viral clearance; in a large prospective study only 14% of children cleared the virus over a 10-year follow-up with most clearance occurring in the first five years of observation [5,6].

HCV is an uncommon but important cause of liver disease in children, most of whom acquire the infection by vertical transmission [7]. The European Paediatric Hepatitis C Virus Network recently found that 20% of vertically infected newborns recovered from infection, 50% developed mild chronic HCV infection without symptoms, and 30% developed symptomatic or progressive disease [8]. Although chronic hepatitis C appears to run a more benign course in children than adults [9] significant histologic liver disease, including cirrhosis, can occur during childhood [10]. Liver transplantation has been performed in a small number of children and ado-lescents in the US [11] and cirrhosis may rarely progress to hepatocellular carcinoma [12]. Furthermore, chronic hepatitis C rarely resolves spontaneously, so that children with the infection become adults who may develop cirrhosis and liver cancer after decades of infection.

Clinical Trials: Past, Present, and Future

The optimal approach to therapy of hepatitis C in children and adolescents was originally derived from controlled trials in adults. However, in the past decade a number of pediatric trials have been reported. Standard interferon and ribavirin have been shown to yield response rates somewhat better than those in adults [13–15]. There are only pilot data on peginterferon alfa-2a monotherapy in young children [16]. Based on results from an uncontrolled trial, the combination of peginterferon alfa-2b plus ribavirin was recently approved for use in children in the United States [17]. The PEDS-C trial, a prospective randomized placebo-controlled trial of peginterferon alfa-2a plus ribavirin or placebo, showed that sustained virologic response (SVR) with combination therapy was clearly superior to results with peginterferon alone [18]. Table 24.1 summarizes these pediatric clinical trials.

Gonzalez-Peralta *et al.* performed the large multicenter multinational trial leading to FDA approval of interferon alfa-2b plus ribavirin [19]. In the phase I trial, three doses of ribavirin were tested: 8, 12, and 15 mg/kg/day (maximum 1200 mg/day) orally given twice daily along with interferon 3 MIU/m^2 (maximum 6 MIU) subcutaneously thrice weekly. The highest ribavirin dose was most effective and was used for the phase III trial, in which both drugs were given for 48 weeks with a follow-up of 24 weeks off therapy. Inclusion criteria in the phase III trial included children with chronic HCV infection ages 3

Advanced Therapy for Hepatitis C, First Edition. Edited by Geoffrey W. McCaughan, John G. McHutchison and Jean-Michel Pawlotsky.
© 2012 Blackwell Publishing Ltd. Published 2012 by Blackwell Publishing Ltd.

Table 24.1 Summary of pediatric clinical trials.

Agent and reference	Treated (n)	Control (n)	SVR non-1[c] (%)	SVR G1 (%)	Comment
Interferon monotherapy, review of 19 trials [20]	366	105	70	27	
Interferon/ribavirin [19]	118	0	84	46	Multi-center
Peg-IFN alfa-2a 8y [16]	14	0	0	46	PK, 2-
Peg-IFN alfa-2b/ribavirin [17]	62	0	93	48	Multi-center
Peg-IFN alfa-2a/ribavirin [18]	59[a]	55[b]	80	47	PEDS C

[a]Received Peg-IFN alfa-2a plus ribavirin. [b]Received Peg-IFN alfa-2a plus placebo. [c]Sustained virologic response, non-1 genotype.

to 16 years at study entry who were treatment naïve and had compensated liver disease. In the trial, 46% (54/118) of the children achieved an SVR, which was significantly higher in children with HCV genotype 2/3 (84%) than in those with HCV genotype 1 (36%). Adverse events (largely anemia and/or neutropenia) led to dose modification in 37 (31%) and discontinuation in 8 (7%). Interestingly, the average hemoglobin drop (1.75 g/dl) was less than that for adults treated with comparable doses of ribavirin (2.5 g/dl) [13]. Neutropenia, which was the most common serious adverse event, usually responded to dose reduction. Although 50% of children experienced neuropsychiatric side effects, these were generally mild to moderate and were transient. However, there was less depression (13%) than in adults treated with combination therapy (36%) [14]. Flu-like side effects (headache, fever, fatigue, anorexia), presumably attributable to interferon, were observed in the majority. There was on-treatment impairment of both linear and ponderal growth with improvement post-discontinuation of therapy. Baseline viral load ≥ 2M cpm in children with genotype 1 was associated with a lower SVR (26%) versus those with lower viral load (48%). Multiple dose pharmacokinetics of both interferon and ribavirin were similar to results in adults. In general, the combination of interferon plus ribavirin was considered to meet standards of safety and efficacy, resulting in FDA approval of the therapy for children 3–18 years of age.

In an open-labeled, uncontrolled pilot study with 62 children and adolescents (age 2–17 years), the combination of weekly peginterferon alfa-2b at a dose of 1.5 μg/kg body weight with ribavirin (15 mg/kg/day) for 48 weeks was associated with an SVR in 22 (48%) of 46 patients with genotype 1, 13 (100%) of 13 with genotype 2 or 3, and in 1 of 2 with genotype 4 [17]. In this study, 83% had leukopenia but most did not require dose

reduction; 10% developed antithyroid antibodies. Pretreatment alanine aminotransferase (ALT) values did not influence the response. In the small number of children with non-1 genotype, treatment for 24 versus 48 weeks did not influence the excellent response. In general, the therapy was well tolerated and this treatment is now FDA approved for children 3–18 years of age.

Thus, in summary, in the past decade there have been a number of multicenter studies of various therapeutic agents in treatment-naïve children with chronic HCV and compensated liver disease. Although these studies have resulted in the development of two FDA-approved therapies, SVR rates for the large number of children with genotype 1 remain around 50%, suggesting that much more work needs to be done to develop safe and effective therapies for children with persistent infection despite treatment.

There are a number of considerations to be taken into account for future clinical trials of newer antiviral agents in children. For example, as noted by Karnsakul et al. [21], although telaprevir appears to be a promising agent in conjunction with peginterferon and ribavirin, drug-induced rash occurred with median time 73 days (range 8–88 days) after the start of treatment, and severe rash and pruritus were a common indication to discontinue telaprevir in 12 of 175 patients with all telaprevir-based regimens [22]. A good design for a pediatric trial might be a lead-in 60-day period of telaprevir or placebo plus peginterferon/ribavirin since telaprevir would be likely tolerated in the first 60 days after the administration of this medication. The drugs could then be discontinued in those who do not respond or achieve viral response ≥ 2 log₁₀ IU/ml decline in HCV RNA from pre-treatment baseline at 60 days of the treatment to avoid these side effects. This type of approach could be used to maximize benefit to pediatric subjects who would respond while minimizing toxicity in those who would not. As the side effect profiles of other promising antiprotease and antipolymerase drugs are characterized in adults with HCV, we will be better equipped to tailor pediatric trials accordingly.

The PEDS-C trial was instructive as to other considerations necessary for the design of clinical trials for children with HCV. Careful studies of the effect of therapies on growth and development as well as health-related quality of life and neurocognitive function are essential [23]. Siblings should be excluded from any controlled trial to eliminate the bias of both similar HCV virus and similar compliance, and perhaps other genetic modifiers of disease. Ideally, therapies would either be parenteral or oral, available in a liquid suspension. If a tablet or capsule is necessary, then the child must demonstrate the ability to swallow a look-alike placebo in the presence of the medical team. Since ribavirin is embryotoxic and teratogenic [24], patients and families must be carefully instructed in the use of two methods of birth control, and pregnancy tests must be done repeatedly at each visit. Children must be screened carefully for evidence of depression at enrollment and throughout the trial using an instrument such as the Childhood Depression Inventory [25]. During the trial there must be frequent laboratory monitoring of neutropenia, anemia, and the development of autoantibodies as well as the HCV RNA and liver panels.

Special Treatment Considerations for Pediatric Populations

There are several special considerations when one contemplates treating the child with chronic HCV. These considerations include the as-yet unresolved question as to whether or not treatment should be considered at all, the list of rare conditions for which there is little or no data to guide therapy, and then the "bottom line" of what to do at the present time when caring for a child with chronic HCV.

The controversies regarding whether or not to treat children with uncomplicated HCV were vigorously discussed at a Single Topic Conference of the American Association for the Study of Liver Diseases in 2006 [26]. They are summarized in Table 24.2. Nonetheless, the recently updated AASLD Guidelines for HCV recommended consideration of treatment of children with compensated uncomplicated liver disease secondary to HCV who are >2 years of age [27] using the same indications as described for adults. There is no evidence at the present time for use of hematopoietic agents during therapy, and antidepressants would be indicated only on an individual basis. Whether or not to perform a liver biopsy in a child in whom therapy is contemplated is another decision to be individualized.

There are some pediatric conditions in which the child with HCV has other comorbidities and there are

Table 24.2 Rationale for and against treatment.

In favor of treatment	In favor of deferring treatment
Patient benefits	
Prevent disease progression	Avoid unpleasant therapy
Eliminate social stigma	Wait until more effective therapy
Improve tolerance	Wait for better predictors of disease progression
Avoid neurocognitive sequelae	
Drug delivery considerations	
Improve compliance	Improve compliance with better tolerated drugs
Utilize parental supervision	
Public health benefits	
Decrease disease burden	Avoid expensive therapy
Decrease health care costs	Avoid monitoring costs
Use less drug	
Avoid liver disease costs	
Avoid loss of employment	

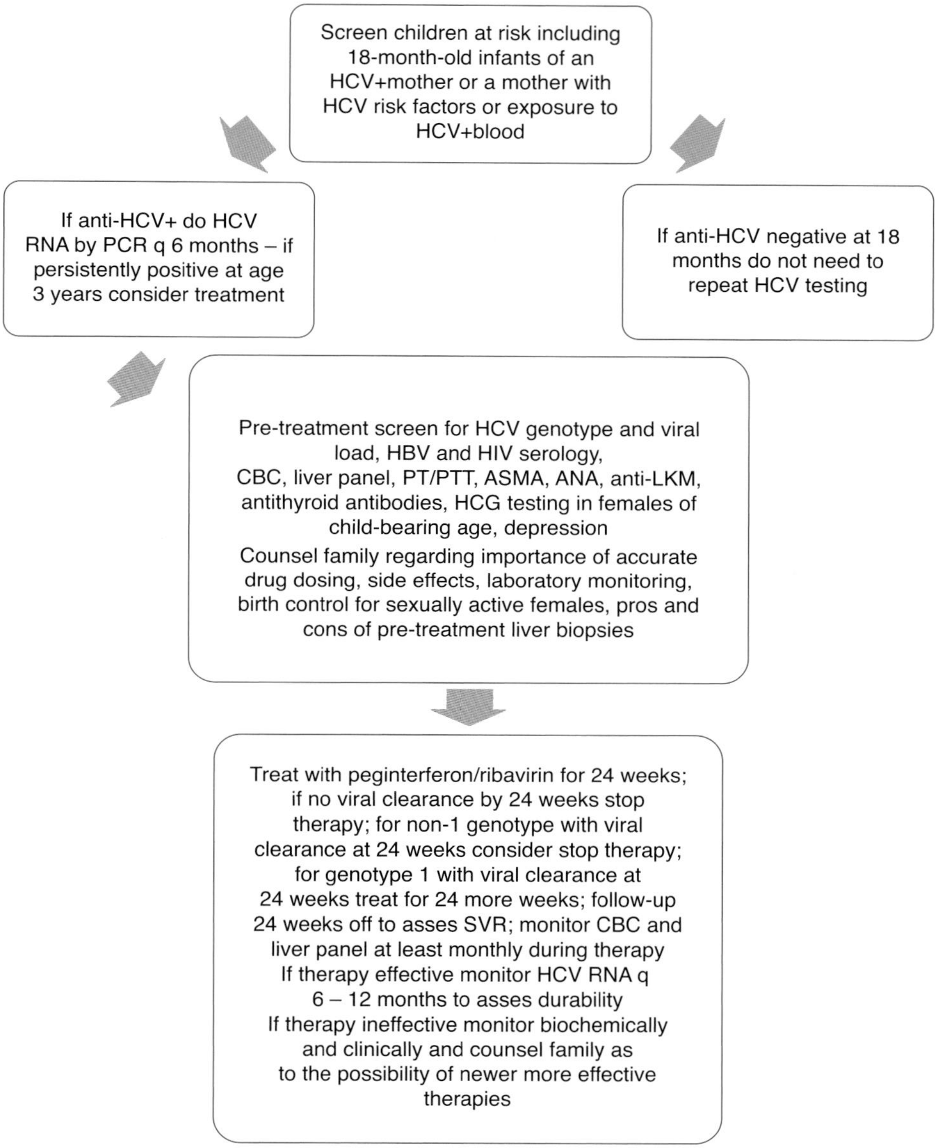

Screen children at risk including 18-month-old infants of an HCV+mother or a mother with HCV risk factors or exposure to HCV+blood

If anti-HCV+ do HCV RNA by PCR q 6 months – if persistently positive at age 3 years consider treatment

If anti-HCV negative at 18 months do not need to repeat HCV testing

Pre-treatment screen for HCV genotype and viral load, HBV and HIV serology, CBC, liver panel, PT/PTT, ASMA, ANA, anti-LKM, antithyroid antibodies, HCG testing in females of child-bearing age, depression
Counsel family regarding importance of accurate drug dosing, side effects, laboratory monitoring, birth control for sexually active females, pros and cons of pre-treatment liver biopsies

Treat with peginterferon/ribavirin for 24 weeks; if no viral clearance by 24 weeks stop therapy; for non-1 genotype with viral clearance at 24 weeks consider stop therapy; for genotype 1 with viral clearance at 24 weeks treat for 24 more weeks; follow-up 24 weeks off to asses SVR; monitor CBC and liver panel at least monthly during therapy
If therapy effective monitor HCV RNA q 6 – 12 months to asses durability
If therapy ineffective monitor biochemically and clinically and counsel family as to the possibility of newer more effective therapies

Figure 24.1 Recommended treatment algorithm. See Schwarz *et al.* [32] for further details.

only scattered reports to help guide therapeutic considerations, necessitating reliance on adult data, in which larger numbers of subjects have been treated. Although caution has been utilized in prescribing ribavirin to thalassemics receiving peginterferon for HCV, a recent report noted improved SVR when ribavirin was added to the therapy. However ribavirin-treated subjects had increased transfusion requirements. Age under 18 years

was a good prognostic factor predicting response to therapy [28]. There are no published trials for children with HIV/HCV or HCV/HBV co-infection. However, there is data demonstrating that HIV/HCV co-infected children have higher morbidity than do HIV mono-infected children [29], suggesting cautious consideration of treatment. One very small report suggested that children with HCV and chronic renal failure might have some benefit from interferon monotherapy [30]. In one large single-center experience with pediatric renal transplants, the presence of HCV infection did not have a negative impact on outcome, suggesting that treatment of the infection in this population may not be indicated with present therapies [31]. Children who undergo liver transplantation for end-stage liver disease secondary to HCV tend to do poorly, with high rates of HCV recurrence and graft loss [11]. Better management strategies are clearly needed for this unfortunate group of pediatric patients.

Thus, treatment of early disease for children with HCV should be strongly considered before cirrhosis and liver failure ensues in that small group of children destined to have a poor outcome during childhood. One reasonable approach is the algorithm summarized in Figure 24.1.

References

1. Alter MJ, Kruszon-Moran D, Nainan OV, *et al.* The prevalence of hepatitis C virus infection in the United States, 1988 through 1994. *New Engl J Med* 1999;341(8):556–62.

2. Jhaveri R, Grant W, Kauf TL, McHutchison J. The burden of hepatitis C virus infection in children; estimated direct medical costs over a ten-year period. *J Pediatr* 2006: 148; 353–8.

3. Roberts EA, Yeung L. Maternal-infant transmission of hepatitis C virus infection. *Hepatology* 2002;36(5 Suppl 1):S106–13.

4. Bevilacqua E, Fabris A, Floreano P, *et al.* Genetic factors in mother-to-child transmission of HCV infection. *Virology* 2009;390(1):64–70.

5. Chen ST, Ni YH, Chen PJ, *et al.* Low viraemia at enrollment in children with chronic hepatitis C favours spontaneous viral clearance. *J Viral Hepatitis* 2009;16(11):796–801.

6. Bortolotti F, Verucchi G, Camma C, *et al.* Long-term course of chronic hepatitis C in children: from viral clearance to end-stage liver disease. *Gastroenterology* 2008;134(7):1900–1907.

7. Davison SM, Kelly DA. Management strategies for hepatitis C virus infection in children. *Paediatr Drugs* 2008;10(6):357–65.

8. European Paediatric Hepatitis C Virus Network. Three broad modalities in the natural history of vertically acquired hepatitis C virus infection. *Clin Infect Dis* 2005;41(1):45–51.

9. Murray KF, Finn LS, Taylor SL, *et al.* Liver histology and alanine aminotransferase levels in children and adults with chronic hepatitis C infection. *J Pediatr Gastroenterol Nutr* 2005;41(5):634–8.

10. Goodman ZD, Makhlouf HR, Liu L, *et al.* Pathology of chronic hepatitis C in children: liver biopsy findings in the Peds-C Trial. *Hepatology* 2008;47(3):836–43.

11. Barshes NR, Udell IW, Lee TC, *et al.* The natural history of hepatitis C virus in pediatric liver transplant recipients. *Liver Transpl* 2006;12(7):1119–23.

12. Gonzalez-Peralta RP, Langham MR, Jr., Andres JM, *et al.* Hepatocellular carcinoma in 2 young adolescents with chronic hepatitis C. *J Pediatr Gastroenterol Nutr* 2009;48(5): 630–35.

13. McHutchison JG, Gordon SC, Schiff ER, *et al.* Interferon alfa-2b alone or in combination with ribavirin as initial treatment for chronic hepatitis C. Hepatitis Interventional Therapy Group. *N Engl J Med* 1998;339(21):1485–92.

14. Masci P, Bukowski RM, Patten PA, *et al.* New and modified interferon alfas: preclinical and clinical data. *Curr Oncol Rep* 2003;5(2):108–13.

15. Poynard T, Marcellin P, Lee SS, *et al.* Randomised trial of interferon alpha2b plus ribavirin for 48 weeks or for 24 weeks versus interferon alpha2b plus placebo for 48 weeks for treatment of chronic infection with hepatitis C virus. International Hepatitis Interventional Therapy Group (IHIT). *Lancet* 1998;352(9138):1426–32.

16. Schwarz KB, Mohan P, Narkewicz MR, *et al.* Safety, efficacy and pharmacokinetics of peginterferon alpha2a (40 kd) in children with chronic hepatitis C. *J Pediatr Gastroenterol Nutr* 2006;43(4):499–505.

17. Wirth S, Pieper-Boustani H, Lang T, *et al.* Peginterferon alfa-2b plus ribavirin treatment in children and adolescents with chronic hepatitis C. *Hepatology* 2005;41(5):1013–18.

18. Schwarz KB, Gonzalez-Peralta RB, Murray KF. The combination of ribavirin and peginterferon is superior to peginterferon and placebo for children and adolescents with chronic hepatitis C. *Gastroenterology* 2011;140(2):450–58.

19. Gonzalez-Peralta RP, Kelly DA, Haber B, *et al.* Interferon alfa-2b in combination with ribavirin for the treatment of chronic hepatitis C in children: efficacy, safety, and pharmacokinetics. *Hepatology* 2005;42(5):1010–18.

20. Jacobson KR, Murray K, Zellos A, Schwarz KB. An analysis of published trials of interferon monotherapy in children with chronic hepatitis C. *J Pediatr Gastroenterol Nutr* 2002;34(1):52–8.

21. Karnsakul W, Alford MK, Schwarz KB. Managing pediatric hepatitis C: current and emerging treatment options. *Ther Clin Risk Manag* 2009;5(3):651–60.

22. Hezode C, Forestier N, Dusheiko G, *et al.* Telaprevir and peginterferon with or without ribavirin for chronic HCV infection. *N Engl J Med* 2009;360(18):1839–50.

23. Murray KF, Rodrigue JR, Gonzalez-Peralta RP, *et al.* Design of the PEDS-C trial: pegylated interferon +/- ribavirin for children with chronic hepatitis C viral infection. *Clin Trials* 2007;4(6):661–73.

24. Mahadevan U. Gastrointestinal medications in pregnancy. *Best Pract Res Clin Gastroenterol* 2007;21(5):849–77.

25. Reynolds WM, Anderson G, Bartell N. Measuring depression in children: a multimethod assessment investigation. *J Abnorm Child Psychol* 1985;13(4):513–26.

26. Shneider BL, Gonzalez-Peralta R, Roberts EA. Controversies in the management of pediatric liver disease: hepatitis B, C and NAFLD: summary of a single topic conference. *Hepatology* 2006;44(5):1344–54.

27. Ghany MG, Strader DB, Thomas DL, *et al.* Diagnosis, management, and treatment of hepatitis C: an update. *Hepatology* 2009;49(4):1335–74.

28. Inati A, Taher A, Ghorra S, *et al.* Efficacy and tolerability of peginterferon alpha-2a with or without ribavirin in thalassaemia major patients with chronic hepatitis C virus infection. *Br J Haematol* 2005;130(4):644–6.

29. Shivraj SO, Chattopadhya D, Grover G, *et al.* Role of HCV coinfection towards disease progression and survival in HIV-1 infected children: a follow-up study of 10 years. *J Trop Pediatr* 2006;52(3):206–11.

30. Szczepanska M, Tobis A, Schneiberg B, *et al.* Treatment of chronic hepatitis with interferon in children with kidney diseases. *Pol Merkur Lekarski* 2005;18(103):22–8.

31. Mir S, Erdogan H, Serdaroglu E, *et al.* Pediatric renal transplantation: single center experience. *Pediatr Transpl* 2005;9(1):56–61.

32. Schwarz KB, Gonzalez-Peralta RP, Murray KF, Molleston JP, Haber BA, Jonas MM, Rosenthal P, Mohan P, Balistreri WF, Narkewicz MR, Smith L, Lobritto S, Rossi S, Valsamakis A, Goodman Z, Robuck PR, Barton BA – Peds C Clinical Research Network. The combination of ribavirin and peginterferon is superior to peginterferon and placebo for children and adolescents with chronic hepatitis C., *Gastroenterology.* 2011 Feb;140(2):450–458.e1. Epub 2010 Oct 28.

25 New Horizons: IL28, Direct-acting Antiviral Therapy for HCV

Alexander J. Thompson,[1,2,3] John G. McHutchison,[4] and Geoffrey W. McCaughan[5]

[1]St. Vincent's Hospital Melbourne, University of Melbourne, Melbourne, VIC, Australia
[2]Victorian Infectious Diseases Reference Laboratory (VIDRL), North Melbourne, VIC, Australia
[3]Department of Gastroenterology and Duke Clinical Research Institute, Duke University, Durham, NC, USA
[4]Gilead Sciences, Inc., Foster City, CA, USA
[5]A.W. Morrow Gastroenterology and Liver Center, Centenary Institute, Royal Prince Alfred Hospital, University of Sydney, Sydney, NSW, Australia

Introduction

The global prevalence of chronic hepatitis C virus (HCV) infection is estimated at 130–170 million [1]. These individuals are at risk for the long-term complications of cirrhosis, liver failure, and hepatocellular carcinoma. Chronic hepatitis C (CHC) is the leading cause of death from liver disease and the most common indication for liver transplantation in Western countries [2] (UNOS database, http://optn.transplant.hrsa.gov/organDatasource/about.asp?display=Liver). Although the incidence of new infections has decreased in the past decade, it is predicted that the number of patients presenting for management of their HCV-related morbidity will continue to increase over the next 10–20 years, as the infected population pool ages [3,4]. HCV infection is curable and therefore such complications may be prevented by successful antiviral therapy.

The current standard-of-care (SOC) for the treatment of CHC is combination therapy with pegylated interferon alfa (Peg-IFN) and ribavirin (RBV) for 24–48 weeks. Unfortunately the treatment is only effective in 50% of individuals infected with genotype 1 HCV, the most common HCV genotype. In addition, Peg-IFN and RBV therapy is expensive and associated with considerable treatment-related toxicity, and many patients are not able to access treatment, either for financial reasons or because treatment is contraindicated. There is a need for therapies that are more effective, and better tolerated, to increase treatment uptake and achieve meaningful progress in dealing with the HCV epidemic.

For the past decade therapeutic development has been focused on the discovery of compounds that target specific steps in the viral life cycle, or direct-acting antiviral agents (DAAs) (Table 25.1). The development of the genotype 1 HCV subgenomic replicon system [9–11] and the definition of the crystal structure of the non-structural HCV proteins [12–16] have enabled structure-based drug design and high throughput screening of candidate HCV inhibitors for high in vitro antiviral activity [17].

Inhibitors of the following steps in the HCV life cycle are currently at various stages of clinical development: viral entry, HCV RNA translation and post-translational processing, HCV replication, and viral assembly and release. Potent antiviral effects have been demonstrated but, as predicted by the HIV and HBV experience, monotherapy has been complicated by the rapid selection of drug-resistant variants. Thus, a common theme in the development of agents has been that combination therapy with Peg-IFN and RBV will continue to be important for the medium term, to increase antiviral efficacy and limit the selection of drug-resistant mutants. HCV non-structural (NS) 3 protease inhibitors are the most advanced candidates, and two agents, telaprevir and boceprevir, have just completed phase III development programs. These agents, used in triple therapy combination regimens with Peg-IFN and RBV, will represent a major therapeutic advance for patients chronically infected with genotype 1 HCV. This chapter will review and summarize the current literature on direct-acting antiviral agents in development for the treatment of CHC.

Advanced Therapy for Hepatitis C, First Edition. Edited by Geoffrey W. McCaughan, John G. McHutchison and Jean-Michel Pawlotsky.
© 2012 Blackwell Publishing Ltd. Published 2012 by Blackwell Publishing Ltd.

Table 25.1 Direct acting antiviral agents in development.

(a) DAAs target different steps in the HCV viral life cycle

Life cycle step	Target	Agent	Phase of development
Viral entry	HCV receptor	HCV immunoglobulin (polyclonal)	Phase II
	HCV receptor	HCV-AB 68/65 (monoclonal)	Phase II
HCV RNA translation	HCV RNA – 5′-UTR	AVI-4065 (antisense)	Halted
		ISIS14803 (antisense)	Halted
	IRES/R40/eIF3 complex	VGX-410C (small molecule inhibitor)	Halted
	Liver-specific microRNA-122 (miR122) [5–8]	SPC3649	Phase I
Post-translational processing	NS3/4A protease – Linear inhibitors	Telaprevir	Phase III
		Bocepreveir	Phase III
		SCH900518 (narlapreivr)	On hold
	NS3/4A protease – Macrocyclic inhibitors	TMC435	Phase II
		R7227 (danoprevir, ITMN-191)	Phase II
		BMS-650032	Phase II
		MK-7009 (vaniprevir)	Phase II
		GS-9256	Phase II
		BI-201335	Phase II
		ACH-1625	Phase II
		VX-500	Phase I
		ABT-450	Phase I
	NS3-NS4A interaction	ACH-806 (GS-9132)	Halted
HCV replication	NS5b polymerase (i) NI (target catalytic site)	RG7128 (mericitabine)	Phase II
		PSI-7977	Phase II
		IDX184	Phase II
		R1626	Halted
		Valopicitabine (NM283)	Halted
		MK-0608	Halted
	(ii) NNI (target allosteric sites)	VCH-759	Phase II
		ANA598	Phase II
		GS 9190 (tegobuvir)	Phase II
		BI207127	Phase II
		PF-00868554 (filibuvir)	Phase II
		PSI-9799	Phase II
		BMS-791325	Phase II
		A-837093	Phase I
		GSK625433	Phase I
		ABT-333	Phase I
		VCH-916	Phase I
	NS5A inhibitors	BMS-790052	Phase II
		A-831	Phase I
	Cyclophilin inhibitors	DEB025 (alisporivir)	Phase II
		NIM-811	Phase II
		SCY-635	Phase II

Table 25.1 (*Continued*)

Viral assembly/release	Glucosidase inhibitor	Celgosivir	Phase II
	Imino sugar – glucosidase inhibitor	UT-231B	Halted
(b) IFN-free combination regimens currently in development			
Combination	RG7128 (mericitabine)	RG7227 (danoprevir)	Phase II
	BMS-790052	BMS-650032	Phase II
	Telaprevir	Vx-222	Phase II
	BI-201335	BI-207127	Phase II
	GS-9256	GS-9190 (tegobuvir)	Phase II
	PSI-7851	PSI-938	Phase I

NS3/4A Protease Inhibitors

The HCV NS3 protein is required for viral replication. NS3 consists of an amino-terminal serine protease and a carboxy-terminal helicase/nucleoside triphosphatase domain [18]. With its co-factor NS4A, the NS3 serine protease is necessary for post-translational cleavage of the HCV NS elements at the NS3/4A, NS4A/B, NS4B/5A, and NS5A/B junctions, releasing NS proteins that are necessary for assembly of the viral replication complex. The NS3 serine protease has more recently been shown to also cleave IPS-1 [19–21] and TRIF [22] to inhibit IRF-3 phosphorylation and IFN-β induction via the RIG-I and TLR3 pathways, respectively. The NS3 helicase is thought to have a role in viral replication by unwinding the viral RNA [18]. Inhibitors of the NS3/4A protease therefore have a direct effect to inhibit viral replication, and in addition may stimulate the innate antiviral immune response by restoring intracellular IFN signaling. The first NS3/4A protease inhibitor to enter clinical trials was BILN 2061 in 2002/3. Treatment of patients with genotype 1 CHC for two days resulted in a greater than 2 $\log_{10}$ reduction in all subjects at higher doses [23,24]. Unfortunately, clinical development was halted after cardiac toxicity was observed in animal models [25]. Proof-of-concept had been established, however, and there are now multiple NS3 protease inhibitors that have entered clinical development. Two linear protease inhibitors, telaprevir and boceprevir, successfully completed phase III programs in 2010.

Telaprevir

Telaprevir (TVR) is a linear peptidomimetic inhibitor of the HCV NS3/4A protease with potent antiviral effect against genotype 1 HCV. As for other protease inhibitors, the antiviral effect appears to be relatively specific for genotype 1 HCV [26]. In early phase Ib development, 14 days of TVR monotherapy at 750 mg 8 hourly was associated with maximal median viral load reduction of 4.4 $\log_{10}$ IU/ml. Resistant variants were rapidly selected, however, and viral breakthrough was noted in a significant number of patients during the second week of treatment. Viral breakthrough during telaprevir therapy has since been associated with a number of characteristic single- or double-point mutations in the catalytic region of the enzyme – see below [27]. Combination therapy with Peg-IFN and RBV was subsequently found to have synergistic antiviral effect, with median viral load reductions at day 14 of up to 5.5 $\log_{10}$ IU/ml [28], and to reduce the emergence of TVR-resistant variants. A critical role for both Peg-IFN and RBV in combination therapy was established in the PROVE2 study, the European phase II study that included a TVR plus Peg-IFN treatment arm [29]. Virologic breakthrough was significantly higher than in the triple therapy arms (24% compared to 2%) [30]). Phase III development programs for both treatment-naïve and treatment-experienced patients were completed in 2010. The two phase III studies in treatment-naïve patients have recently been presented in abstract form at peer-reviewed meetings.

The ADVANCE study enrolled 1088 treatment-naïve patients infected with genotype 1 HCV [31]. Treatment arms were: (i) TVR, 750 mg q8h plus Peg-IFN alfa-2a and RBV for 12 weeks, followed by additional weeks of Peg-IFN alfa-2a and RBV (T12PR); (ii) TVR, 750 mg q8h, plus Peg-IFN alfa-2a and RBV for 8 weeks, followed by additional weeks of Peg-IFN alfa-2a and RBV (T8PR); or (iii) Peg-IFN alfa-2a and RBV for 48 weeks (control arm). Patients treated with TVR who achieved an extended rapid viral response (eRVR) received a total of 24 weeks of therapy while those who did not received a total of 48 weeks of therapy. "eRVR" was defined by undetectable HCV RNA at weeks 4 and 12 of therapy (undetectable HCV RNA was <25 IU/ml using a sensitive real-time polymerase chain reaction [RT-PCR] assay). Patients were required to stop TVR treatment if HCV RNA was >1000 IU/ml at week 4. The sustained virologic response (SVR) rates in the T12PR (75%) and T8PR (69%) treatment arms were significantly higher than with control (44%, $p < 0.0001$). The rates of eRVR were 58%, 57%, and 8% for the T12PR, T8PR, and control arms; SVR rates following an eRVR were then 89%, 83% with 24 weeks total treatment in the TVR arms, compared to 97% in the control arm. Therefore, almost 60% of TVR-treated patients were treated for 24 weeks total (Table 25.2). SVR rates were 2-fold higher in patients with advanced liver disease (bridging fibrosis/cirrhosis), and in African Americans, comparing the TVR-treatment arms to control. Virologic failure in TVR treatment arms was defined as HCV RNA > 1000 IU/ml at week 4 or at week 12, or HCV RNA detectable (≥ 25 IU/ml) at weeks 24–48. Virologic failure occurred in 8% of the T12PR patients and 13% of the T8PR patients. Failures during TVR therapy were associated with the detection by population sequencing of resistant viral variants (see below); resistant variants were detectable in <50% of failures occurring after TVR was stopped. Relapse rates were low in TVR-treatment arms (9% versus 9% versus 28% for T12PR and T8PR compared to control in patients with undetectable HCV RNA at the end of treatment).

The ILLUMINATE study was a phase III open-label study that confirmed the equivalence of 24 versus 48 weeks of total TVR-based triple therapy for treatment-naïve patients with genotype 1 HCV who achieved on-treatment eRVR [32]. This study enrolled 540 patients and treated them with TVR, 750 mg q8h, plus Peg-IFN and RBV for 12 weeks, followed by Peg-IFN plus RBV for 24–48 weeks. The rate of eRVR (undetectable HCV RNA at weeks 4 and 12, again defined as < 25 IU/ml) was 65%, and eRVR was achieved by 322 patients, who

were randomized at week 20 to continue receiving Peg-IFN and RBV for 24 or 48 weeks of total treatment. In these patients, the SVR rate did not differ according to treatment duration of 24 or 48 weeks (92% versus 87.5%, respectively). Those not achieving eRVR (118 patients) were treated with Peg-IFN and RBV for 48 weeks total and the SVR rate was 64%. Another 100 patients stopped therapy prior to randomization at week 20 ($n = 62$ for adverse event [AE], $n = 12$ for virologic failure, $n = 26$ for other reasons) and in this group the SVR rate was 23%. Relapse rates were low in the eRVR populations receiving either 24 or 48 weeks total treatment (6% versus 3%).

The REALIZE study was a phase III study investigating the use of TVR-based triple therapy compared to 48 weeks of Peg-IFN plus RBV in 662 treatment-experienced patients. The study included prior relapsers, partial responders, and null responders (null response defined as a $< 2 \log_{10}$ IU/ml reduction in HCV RNA at week 12 of Peg-IFN plus RBV therapy). Patients in the active treatment arms were treated with (i) 12 weeks of TVR (750 mg, q8h), Peg-IFN, and RBV, followed by 36 weeks of Peg-IFN and RBV alone, or (ii) a 4-week lead-in of Peg-IFN and RBV followed by 12 weeks of TVR (750 mg, q8h), Peg-IFN, and RBV, followed by 32 weeks of Peg-IFN and RBV alone [29]. Increased rates of SVR were observed with TVR treatment in all patient categories (relapsers, SVR = 83% / 88% vs 24%; partial responders 59% / 54% vs 15% and null responders 29% / 33% vs 5%, P < 0.001 vs Peg-IFN and RBV control). There was no SVR benefit associated with the use of lead-in Peg-IFN and RBV. Response-guided therapy was not evaluated.

Telaprevir therapy is associated with additional toxicity. In both phase II and phase III studies, adverse events were more common with TVR-treatment arms than the control arms. Pruritis and rash (including severe rash), gastrointestinal symptoms (nausea, diarrhea), and anemia were more common with TVR therapy. Discontinuation rates due to adverse events were 7%, 8%, and 4% in the T12PR, T8PR, and control arms, respectively. Adverse events from the ADVANCE study are summarized in Table 25.2.

The development of TVR has therefore been instructive. TVR is a potent inhibitor of genotype 1 HCV. Despite potent antiviral efficacy, the rapid emergence of drug resistance limits monotherapy and therefore combination with Peg-IFN/RBV will be required. The phase III data confirm that triple therapy regimens will significantly increase SVR rates for patients infected with genotype 1 HCV, and that over 50% of treatment-naïve patients will only require 24 weeks of treatment. There is some additional cost in

Table 25.2 Summary results from the abstract presentations of the recent phase III studies investigating (a) telaprevir and (b,c) boceprevir.

(a) Telaprevir – ADVANCE trial (treatment-naïve)		T12PR $n = 363$	T8PR $n = 364$	PR48 $n = 361$
SVR (%)		75	69	44
RVR[a] (%)		68	66	9
eRVR[b] (%)		58	57	8
SVR (%)	eRVR	89	83	97
	No eRVR	54	50	39
SVR (%)	Metavir F0-2	78	73	47
	Metavir F3-4	62	53	33
SVR (%)	White	75	70	46
	Black	62	58	25
	Hispanic	74	66	39
Relapse		9	9	28
Virologic failure[c]		8	13	NA
Adverse event[d]	Pruritus	50	45	36
	Rash	37	35	24
	Severe rash	6	3	1
	Nausea	43	40	31
	Diarrhea	28	32	22
	Hb < 10g/dl	36	40	14
	Hb < 8.5g/dl	9	9	2
Discontinuation	Any adverse event	10	10	7
	Severe rash	7	5	1
	Anemia[e]	4	2	0

[a] RVR = undetectable HCV RNA at week 4 of treatment (< 25 IU/ml).
[b] eRVR = extended RVR = undetectable HCV RNA at week 4 and week 12 of treatment (<25 IU/ml).
[c] HCV RNA > 1000 IU/ml at week 4 or week 12 or detectable HCV RNA weeks 24–48.
[d] ≥10% more frequent in TVR arms.
[e] Erythropoietin (EPO) not permitted.

(b) Boceprevir SPRINT-2 study (treatment-naïve) (two cohorts per protocol: non-black ($n = 938$), black ($n = 159$)			BOC-PR28/PR48 (RGT) $n = 368$	BOC-PR48 $n = 366$	PR48 $n = 363$
SVR (%)		Non-black	67	68	40
		Black	42	53	23
SVR (%) according to week 4	≥1 $\log_{10}$IU/ml	Non-black	82	82	52
		Black	67	61	46
reduction in HCV RNA (lead-in)	<1 $\log_{10}$IU/ml	Non-black	29	39	5
		Black	25	31	0
SVR (%) according to RVR (week 8)	RVR[a]	Non-black	89	91	86
		Black	78	82	75
	Non-RVR	Non-black	37	43	31
		Black	32	28	21

(Continued)

Table 25.2 (*Continued*)

(b) Boceprevir SPRINT-2 study (treatment-naïve) (two cohorts per protocol: non-black ($n = 938$), black ($n = 159$))		BOC-PR28/PR48 (RGT) $n = 368$	BOC-PR48 $n = 366$	PR48 $n = 363$
Relapse	Non-black	9	8	23
	Black	12	17	14
Discontinuation due to stopping rule[b]	Non-black	8	9	27
	Black	17	15	46
Adverse events[c]	Dysgeusia	37	43	18
	Hb 8.5–10.0 g/dl	45	41	26
	Hb < 8.5 g/dl	5	9	4
	EPO use	43	43	24
	ANC 500–750/mm^3	24	25	14
	ANC <500/mm^3	6	8	4
Discontinuation	Any adverse event	12	16	16
	Anemia[d]	2	2	1

[a]Week 8 RVR (week 4 of BOC therapy).
[b]detectable HCV RNA at week 24.
[c]More common with BOC therapy.
[d]EPO permitted.
Rates of RVR were not presented, sub-analyses according to fibrosis stage were not presented.

(c) Boceprevir RESPOND-2 study (treatment-experienced)		BOC-PR32/PR48 (RGT) $n = 162$	BOC-PR48 $n = 161$	PR48 $n = 80$
SVR (%)		59	66	21
SVR (%) according to previous response	Relapser	69	75	29
	Non-responder[a]	40	52	7
SVR (%) according to week 4 reduction in HCV RNA (lead-in)	$\geq 1 \log_{10}$IU/ml	73	79	25
	$<1 \log_{10}$IU/ml	33	34	0
SVR (%) according to RVR (week 8)	RVR	86	88	100
	Non-RVR	40	43	12
Relapse		15	12	32
Discontinuation	Any adverse event	8	12	3
	Anemia[b]	3	0	0

[a]Null responders were excluded (defined as < 2 log reduction in HCV RNA at week 12 of previous treatment with Peg-IFN and RBV). Despite this, 26% of patients had a < 1 $\log_{10}$ decline in HCV RNA at the end of the week 4 lead-in, which has been shown to correlate well with < 2 log reduction at week 12.
[b]EPO not permitted.

terms of increased toxicity; it is hoped that with greater experience these will be able to be better managed.

Boceprevir

Boceprevir (BOC, formerly SCH 503034) is a second linear HCV NS3/4A protease inhibitor. In phase I development, 14 days of BOC monotherapy at 400 mg t.i.d. produced a maximal mean HCV RNA reduction of 2.06 $\log_{10}$ IU/ml in genotype 1 HCV non-responders [34]. Antiviral effect in combination with Peg-IFN was subsequently found to be additive, achieving a mean maximal reduction of viral load of 2.88 ± 0.22 $\log_{10}$ IU/ml at 14 days. As for TVR, monotherapy was associated with the rapid selection of resistant variants. Resistance and virologic breakthrough were limited by combination with Peg-IFN and RBV. The key point of distinction of the BOC development program was the use of a lead-in phase of 4 weeks of Peg-IFN and RBV prior to the introduction of BOC. Other points of difference were a longer duration of BOC therapy, and the use of Peg-IFN alfa-2b rather than Peg-IFN alfa-2a in the triple therapy backbone. The results of phase III studies in treatment-naïve and -experienced patients have recently been presented [35,36].

SPRINT-2 was an international phase III study that randomized 1097 treatment-naïve genotype 1 patients to a 4 week lead-in phase of Peg-IFN alfa-2b plus RBV treatment, followed by: (i) BOC plus Peg-IFN alfa-2b plus RBV for 44 weeks (BOC-48); (ii) response-guided therapy (RGT): BOC plus Peg-IFN alfa-2b plus RBV for 24 weeks, with an additional 20 weeks of Peg-IFN alfa-2b plus RBV only if HCV RNA was detectable during weeks 8–24; or (iii) Peg-IFN alfa-2b plus RBV plus placebo for 44 weeks. The BOC dose was 800 mg, p.o., t.i.d., the Peg-IFN alfa-2b was dosed at 1.5 μg/kg, SC, weekly, and RBV dose was weight-based (600–1400 mg/day). Patients with detectable HCV RNA at week 24 were discontinued for futility. Non-black ($n = 938$) and black ($n = 159$) patients were enrolled and analyzed separately as per protocol. Results are summarized in Table 25.2. In the non-black patients, the rate of SVR in the 48-week BOC-arm (69%) and the RGT-BOC arm (67%) were significantly higher than PR alone (40%). BOC was associated with higher rates of SVR in black subjects also. Of the non-black subjects, 47% had persistently undetectable HCV RNA from weeks 8 to 24 of treatment and were eligible for short duration therapy (28 weeks). RGT was associated with a similar rate of SVR compared to the 48-week BOC regimen, and this is likely to become the licensed protocol.

The second phase III BOC study, RESPOND-2, enrolled treatment-experienced patients. This included prior non-responders (defined as subjects who had previously attained a ≥ 2 log drop in HCV RNA at week 12 of SOC therapy, but who never reached undetectable levels) and relapsers. Prior null responders (< 2 log drop in HCV RNA at week 12) were excluded. Genotype 1 patients ($n = 403$) were randomized 1:2:2 to receive a 4-week lead-in phase of Peg-IFN alfa-2b plus RBV treatment, followed by either: (i) BOC 800 mg, p.o. t.i.d. plus Peg-IFN alfa-2b plus RBV for 44 weeks (BOC-48); (ii) RGT: BOC 800 mg p.o. t.i.d. plus Peg-IFN alfa-2b plus RBV for 32 weeks, with an additional 12 weeks of Peg-IFN alfa-2b plus RBV only if HCV RNA was detectable at week 8; or (iii) Peg-IFN alfa-2b plus RBV plus placebo for 44 weeks. All patients with detectable HCV-RNA at week 12 were discontinued for futility. The rate of SVR in the 48-week BOC arm (66%) and the RGT arm (59%) were significantly higher than PR alone (21%) (results are summarized in Table 25.2). There was no significant difference in SVR rate between the 48-week BOC and RGT treatment arms, and approximately 45% of patients were eligible for shorter treatment in the RGT arm. Rates of SVR were higher in relapsers compared to prior non-responders.

Lead-in dosing was intended to minimize the development of drug resistance by achieving steady state concentrations of both Peg-IFN alfa-2b and RBV prior to the introduction of boceprevir. Although there is no evidence that lead-in therapy is associated with an increase in overall SVR rate, it does allow a "real-time" assessment of IFN sensitivity, and the virologic decline < 1 $\log_{10}$ IU/ml at week 4 in both SPRINT-2 and RESPOND-2 was strongly associated with SVR rate, largely due to selection of resistant NS3 variants and virologic breakthrough. In SPRINT-2, SVR rate in non-blacks who attained ≥ 1 $\log_{10}$ decline in HCV RNA after week 4 lead-in was 82% in both BOC treatment arms, compared to 29% and 39% of patients in the RGT and 48-week BOC arms if < 1 $\log_{10}$ decline [35]. BOC resistance variants were detected in 41% of BOC-treated patients with < 1 $\log_{10}$ IU/ml decline at the end of the lead-in phase in SPRINT-2, compared to 4% of patients achieving ≥ 1 $\log_{10}$ decline [35]. In RESPOND-2, the SVR rates were 79%, 73%, and 25% for the 48-week BOC arm, the RGT arm, and SOC if the virologic decline was ≥ 1 $\log_{10}$ IU/ml after the week-4 lead-in, compared to 34%, 33%, and 0% if < 1 $\log_{10}$ decline [36]. BOC-resistance variants were detected more commonly if virologic decline was < 1 $\log_{10}$ during the lead-in phase (32% and 28% versus 6% and 8% in the 48-week and RGT arms). RESPOND-2 also showed that IFN sensitivity may decline over time; despite excluding null responders, 26%

of patients had a $< 1 \log_{10}$ decline in HCV RNA at week 4 [36]. Therefore, the week-4 lead-in may have clinical utility for individualizing therapy according to IFN sensitivity.

The major added toxicities of BOC therapy are anemia and dysgeusia (Table 25.2). In SPRINT-2, anemia (Hb $<$ 10 g/dl) occurred in 49% of patients treated with BOC-containing regimens compared to 29% of controls. There was no increased rate of discontinuation due to anemia, but the use of growth factors was permitted and erythropoietin (EPO) therapy was common (43% of patients treated with BOC, compared to 24% of patients treated with control). Dysgeusia occurred in 43% and 37% of patients in the BOC-48 and RGT arms, compared to 18% in the control arm. Serious AEs were reported in 12%, 11%, and 9% of subjects in the BOC-48, RGT, and control arms, dose modifications due to AEs in 35%, 40%, and 26%, and discontinuations due to AEs in 16%, 12%, and 16%. Anemia and dysgeusia were also more common, and occurred at similar rates with BOC use, in RESPOND-2. Moderate neutropenia was also more common with BOC treatment in RESPOND-2 (absolute neutrophil count [ANC] 500–750/mm^3 occurred in 27% and 25% of patients in the BOC-48 and RGT arms, compared to 13% in the control arm; there was no difference in rates of ANC < 500 mm^3), suggesting that BOC may be associated with bone marrow; suppression.

Other HCV NS3/4A Protease Inhibitors

A number of other protease inhibitors are in phase I–II clinical programs. The most advanced are all macrocyclic protease inhibitors: TMC435, RG7227 (danoprevir, formerly ITMN-191), GS-9256, MK-7009 (vaniprevir), MK-5172, BMS-650032, and BI201335. At high doses, RG7227 has been associated with grade 4 ALT rises. RG7227 is metabolized through cytochrome P450 3A4, and the use of ritonavir boosting to minimize drug exposure is now being explored. The goals for development of these next-generation agents will be greater antiviral potency, reduced duration of therapy, high genetic barrier to resistance, and minimal toxicity.

ACH-806

ACH-806 (GS-9132) was an inhibitor of the binding of NS4A to the NS3 protease and inhibited polyprotein processing by preventing the formation of the active proteinase complex. Five days of monotherapy led to a 0.9 $\log_{10}$ reduction in HCV RNA in a phase I study [37].

Although clinical development was subsequently halted because of concerns regarding proximal renal tubular toxicity, this study provided proof of concept for an alternate molecular target for inhibition of the NS3/4A protease complex, without cross-resistance to the peptidomimetic inhibitors.

NS5B Polymerase Inhibitors

The NS5B RNA-dependent RNA polymerase (RdRp) catalyzes the synthesis of the complementary minus-strand RNA, and the subsequent synthesis of the genomic plus-strand HCV RNA. It is therefore a key enzyme involved in HCV replication, and as mammalian cells do not express an equivalent enzyme, highly selective targeting is possible. Both nucleos(t)ide and non-nucleos(t)ide polymerase inhibitors (NI/NNI) are currently in the pipeline, though no polymerase inhibitors are currently in phase III trials. NIs bind to the NS5B catalytic site and act as chain terminators, whereas NNIs cause allosteric inhibition of the active site. The NS5B active site is relatively invariant between different HCV genotypes, and also poorly tolerant to amino acid substitutions. As a general rule, NIs therefore have broader HCV genotypic activity, and the selection of resistant variants is restricted due to the negative effect of active-site mutations on viral fitness. In contrast, all NNIs in development have been optimized against genotype 1b NS5B and have less activity against other genotypes. Mutations at the allosteric binding sites have less impact on viral fitness and therefore the selection of NS5B-resistant HCV variants is more common with NNI therapy.

NS5B Nucleos(t)ide Inhibitors

RG7128 (mericitabine) is the oral prodrug of PSI-6130, a cytidine nucleoside analog. It is the most advanced NI in clinical development. In a dose-escalating phase Ib trial, a dose-dependent decrease in HCV RNA was observed in genotype 1 prior non-responders. After 14 days of treatment, a maximum mean decline of 2.72 $\log_{10}$ IU/ml occurred at the highest dose of 1500 mg b.i.d. [38]. No virologic rebound was observed. The drug was well tolerated as monotherapy and no serious AEs were reported in any study arm. In treatment-naïve genotype 1 patients, the combination of RG7128 (1500 mg, b.i.d.) with Peg-IFN and RBV achieved a reduction in HCV RNA of approximately 5 $\log_{10}$ IU/ml at 4 weeks, translating to an RVR rate of 85% (versus -2 $\log_{10}$ IU/ml and 10% in the SOC control arm) [39]. No virologic rebound was observed during RG7128 treatment to 4 weeks. Importantly, RG7128 was generally well tolerated in combination with Peg-IFN and RBV; grade 3/4 hematological toxicity was rare and not different to the control arm (5% versus 10%). Headache (65% versus 40%), fatigue (40% versus 20%), and chills (35% versus 20%) were all more common than control; all were classed as mild AEs. Preliminary resistance testing did not identify any variants to week 4. The combination of a potent antiviral effect and satisfactory toxicity profile make RG7128 an attractive agent. RG7128 was used in combination with the protease inhibitor RG7227 in the first IFN-free DAA treatment regimen [40] (INFORM-1, see below). In addition, RG7128 is now moving into a phase IIb program treating patients with genotypeS 2 and 3 HCV, on the basis of *in vitro* and early clinical data supporting efficacy [41].

Other NI

Unfortunately the development of a number of promising NIs has been limited by drug toxicity. R1626 was stopped because of an unacceptably high rate of severe leukopenia, and valopicitabine because of gastrointestinal toxicity. The development of MK-0608 was abandoned for undisclosed reasons. The development of IDX-184 was interrupted when the program was placed on hold by the FDA due to concerns regarding hepatotoxicity. This hold has recently been removed and phase II studies are planned [42].

NS5B Non-Nucleos(t)ide Inhibitors

Non-nucleos(t)ide inhibitors (NNIs) target the NS5B RdRp at a secondary allosteric site, separate from the enzyme catalytic site. Binding to the allosteric site leads to conformational changes to the active site, inhibiting replication. Four allosteric sites, A–D, have been identified so far, and there are multiple agents that have entered clinical development. In contrast to the NIs, which appear to have a high genetic barrier to the development of drug resistance, virologic breakthrough has been observed to occur rapidly during NNI monotherapy. As a general rule, NNIs have shown moderate antiviral effect, and are relatively specific for genotype 1 HCV. Candidates that are now in phase II development include VCH-759, ANA598, GS 9190 (tegobuvir), BI207127, PF-00868554 (filibuvir), PSI-9799, and BMS-791325.

NS5A Inhibitors

The exact function of the NS5A protein remains unclear: it is necessary for viral replication and important for the production of infectious virus particles, yet is not known to have enzymatic activity [43]. Goa and colleagues have recently identified a potent NS5A inhibitor using a chemical genetics screening strategy designed to focus on new targets beyond NS3-4A, NS5B, or the virus's helicase [44]. BMS-790052 displayed potent activity against all HCV genotypes *in vitro*. Mean half maximal effective concentrations (EC_{50}) ranged from 9 pM and 50 pM for the HCV replicon genotypes 1b and 1a, up to 146 pM for the genotype 3a replicon, making it the most potent inhibitor of HCV replication publicly identified to date. Replicon combination studies demonstrated additive-synergistic activity of BMS-790052 with IFN and RBV, as well as inhibitors of the NS3 protease and NS5B polymerase (NI/NNI). In proof-of-concept single ascending dose-finding studies of healthy volunteers and chronic hepatitis C patients, BMS-790052 was orally bio-available and the plasma half-life ranged from 10 to 14 hours, suggesting that once daily dosing will be feasible. In genotype 1 HCV-infected patients, mean HCV RNA declines of 1.8 (0.2–3.0), 3.2 (2.9–4.0), and 3.3 (2.7–3.6) $\log_{10}$ IU/ml were observed at 24 hours following single doses of 1, 10, and 100 mg of the drug. BMS-790052 has now entered phase IIa development in combination with Peg-IFN and RBV. BMS-790052 is also being studied in combination with an NS3 protease inhibitor (BMS-650032) [45]. Twenty-one patients with previous null response to Peg-IFN/RBV were randomized to BMS-790052 60 mg, p.o., daily plus BMS-650032 600 mg, p.o., twice daily, or BMS-790052 and BMS-650032 plus Peg-IFN and RBV. In this difficult-to-treat group, 46% of patients in the combination DAA arm without Peg-IFN and RBV attained a complete week-12 response, and virologic breakthrough occurred in 55% of patients. In contrast, 90% of patients treated with quadruple therapy had undetectable serum HCV RNA at week 12 and no viral breakthrough was observed.

Cyclophilin Inhibitors

Cyclophilins are cellular isomerases that augment HCV replication. The exact mechanism remains unclear, but they have been shown to interact with both the NS5A protein and the NS5B RdRp [46]. Cyclophilin A appears to be particularly important for promoting HCV replication. The cyclophilin inhibitor cyclosporine A has been known to have an anti-HCV effect *in vitro* for a number of years but clinical use has been limited by its immunosuppressive effects [47–49]. DEB025 (alisporivir, formerly Debio-025) is a novel cyclophilin inhibitor that does not bind calcineurin and is less immunosuppressive. A dose-finding study compared DEB025 plus peginterferon combination with either DEB025 or Peg-IFN monotherapy [50]. Patients treated with high-dose DEB025 plus Peg-IFN experienced a mean HCV RNA decline of 4.8 $\log_{10}$ IU/ml at day 29, a very significant reduction when compared with only 2.5 and 2.2 $\log_{10}$ IU/ml drops in the Peg-IFN /placebo and high-dose DEB025 monotherapy groups, respectively. Notably, the drug was active against all genotypes and resistant viral mutants were not detected. The cyclophilin inhibitors appear to have a high barrier to resistance, consistent with the drug target being a cellular enzyme. Treatment was associated with reversible hyperbilirubinemia, the clinical significance of which remains unclear. Phase II studies have now been initiated in both genotype 1 HCV (treatment-naïve and treatment-experienced parallel programs) and genotype 2/3 HCV. Two other cyclophilin inhibitors, NIM811 and SCY-625, have more recently advanced to phase II development [47,51,52].

Other DAA Targets

Alpha-glucosidase I is a host enzyme that is involved in glycoprotein processing. Inhibition leads to HCV envelope protein misfolding, interfering with viral assembly and release. Celgosivir and its active metabolite castanospermine both inhibit alpha-glucosidase I [53]. Monotherapy resulted in a modest antiviral effect. In a 12-week randomized phase II trial, only 2 of 35 patients who completed therapy had peak HCV RNA reductions of more than 1 $\log_{10}$ IU/ml [54]. In a genotype 1 non-responder population, the addition of celgosivir 400 mg daily to Peg-IFN $\pm$ RBV led to an increase in antiviral efficacy at 12 weeks compared to Peg-IFN alfa and RBV alone: a > 2 $\log_{10}$ IU/ml reduction in HCV RNA was observed in 45% (5/12) versus 10% (1/10) control [55]. The development of celgosivir has been discontinued.

Other steps in the HCV viral life cycle are being targeted. These include anti-HCV antibodies (both polyclonal immunoglobulin and monoclonal antibodies), currently in phase II development as viral entry inhibitors for the prevention or treatment of post-transplant HCV recurrence; small molecule entry inhibitors; inhibitors of the HCV RNA translation machinery (antisense oligonucleotides, ribozymes, nucleic acid-based strategies [siRNA, shRNA]); and small molecule inhibitors of HCV IRES function and polyprotein translation [3].

Other Novel Therapeutic Approaches

A number of other novel therapeutic approaches are being developed in parallel to the DAA. These include new interferon alfa formulations, a liver-targeting prodrug of RBV (taribavirin [viramidine]), therapeutic vaccines and other novel immunomodulators, nitazoxanide, intravenous silibinin, vitamin D, and statin therapy.

Novel Interferon-Based Therapies

IFN lambda (IFNλ1 or IL29) belongs to the type 3 IFN family (IFNλ1/2/3 or IL29, IL28A, and IL28B, respectively). Type 3 IFN mediates antiviral activity through the common IFNλ receptor that is distinct from the IFNα receptor. Unlike the IFNα receptor, which is expressed by all cells, expression of the IFNλ receptor is believed to be restricted to epithelial cells, including hepatocytes. The IFNλ receptor is not expressed by most hemopoietic cells. This restricted receptor distribution offers the potential for less toxicity. Type 3 IFN have antiviral activity against HCV and HBV *in vitro* [56,57]. A pegylated formulation of IL29 (Peg-IFNλ) is currently in phase II development. It appears to have similar antiviral efficacy to type 1 IFN, with less toxicity, particularly hematological toxicity [58]. The discovery of the association between *IL28B* polymorphism and Peg-IFN and RBV treatment response has driven great interest in this agent. Whether *IL28B* polymorphism is associated with outcome of Peg-IFNλ therapy is unclear, although preliminary data suggest an association [59].

Albinterferon alfa-2b (albIFNα) is a recombinant polypeptide composed of IFN alfa-2b genetically fused to human albumin. The rationale for development of albIFNα was to increase SVR rates by maximizing drug exposure and to improve convenience with a less frequent dosing schedule. AlbIFNα has been shown to retain the antiviral properties of IFNα *in vitro* [60]. In phase I/II dose-ranging studies albIFNα was found to have an extended half-life of ~144 hours, and displayed dose-dependent antiviral activity in both treatment-naïve and -experienced patients [61,62]. In phase III development albIFNα, used 2 weekly, demonstrated non-inferiority to

Peg-IFN in both genotype 1 and genotype 2/3 HCV, with a similar side effect profile [63,64]. However, at high doses, albIFNα has been associated with cough and dyspnea, and commercial development of albinterferon has been placed on hold [65].

Alternate IFN-based strategies are designed to enhance the pharmacokinetics of IFNα, such as Locteron, a recombinant interferon alfa-2b encapsulated in a biodegradable polymeric drug delivery system for controlled release that allows 2 weekly dosing [66]. Belerofon, another slow-release IFN preparation, has a single amino acid mutation that lowers sensitivity to protease-mediated degradation without compromising antiviral efficacy *in vitro*. Belerofon, in both injectable and oral formulations, has entered phase I investigation. Omega IFN is a member of the type 1 IFN family distinct from IFNα. It is being tested for anti-HCV effect using an implantable infusion pump, intended to deliver a continuous and consistent dose of drug over a period of months.

Taribavirin (TBV, Viramidine)

Taribavirin (TBV, formerly viramidine) is a liver-targeting prodrug of RBV designed to limit the red cell toxicity of RBV. Although TBV caused less anemia in a phase III study (Hb < 10 mg/dl, 5% versus 24%, $p = 0.0001$), it did not meet the non-inferiority virologic endpoint when compared with RBV (SVR rate 38% versus 52%) [67,68]. In a post hoc analysis, high-dose exposure to TBV (>18 mg/kg) was associated with higher rates of SVR, comparable to RBV. Consequently, a phase IIb study of weight-based TBV versus weight-based RBV was performed in the US. Treatment-naïve patients ($n = 278$) with genotype 1 HCV infection were stratified according to body weight and randomized to receive 20, 25, or 30 mg/kg/day of TBV, plus Peg-IFN alfa-2b 1.5 μg/kg/week, compared with weight-based RBV (800, 1000, 1200, or 1400 mg/day) plus Peg-IFN alfa-2b. Taribavirin at all doses produced similar SVR rates to RBV, but was associated with less anemia in the lower dose arms (percentage of patients with Hb < 10 mg/dL was 13.4% and 15.7% in patients receiving 20 and 25 mg/kg/day TBV, versus 32.9% receiving RBV, $p < 0.05$) [69]. Gastrointestinal events (in particular diarrhea) were more common with TBV, but were generally mild and not dose-limiting. The future for TBV is not clear at present and a new phase III program is yet to commence. Taribavirin might be an attractive substitute for RBV in combination DAA regimens that are associated with additive anemia.

Therapeutic Vaccines and Immunomodulators

There continues to be interest in the development of therapeutic vaccines. GI-5005 is a recombinant yeast (*Saccharomyces cerevisiae*) genetically modified to express HCV NS3 and core proteins. GI-5005 is designed to stimulate NS3- and core-specific cytotoxic T cell responses. The development of HCV-specific cellular immunity, with moderate antiviral effect (maximal viral load reduction 1.4 $\log_{10}$ IU/ml), was observed in a number of the phase I trial participants [70]. In phase II development SVR GI-5005, used in combination with Peg-IFN and RBV, was observed to increase SVR rate and augment HCV-specific T cell responses, with the greatest incremental benefit observed in patients carrying the poor responder *IL28B* genotype, suggesting that GI-5005 may augment response in those with unfavorable IL28B variants [71,72]. A number of additional vaccine strategies are in early phase development, including DNA vaccines, T cell vaccines, dendritic cell immunotherapy [73,74], and more traditional peptide-based strategies.

Other novel immune-based strategies under development include the TLR9 ligand IMO-2125 [the TLR9 ligand CPG10101 and the TLR7 ligand isatoribine (ANA245) have previously been abandoned]; bavituximab, a monoclonal antibody directed against aminophospholipid (a phospholipid selectively expressed on the surface of virus-infected cells); and oglufanide and SCV-07, two synthetic dipeptides with immunomodulatory activity.

Drug Resistance

HCV has a high replication rate (10^{10-12} virions/day), an error-prone RdRp, and lacks a proofreading mechanism. The virus therefore exists as a highly diverse quasispecies and resistant mutants may co-exist in the absence of drug therapy. Typically these mutations involve a cost to replication fitness and are present at low concentration compared to the dominant wildtype (WT) virus, but resistant variants have been described as the predominant quasispecies in treatment-naïve patients [75,76]. In the setting of DAA monotherapy, drug-resistant mutations are selected within days. Resistance mutations have been identified for all of the NS3/NS5B and NS5A inhibitors studied to date, and occur as the result of amino acid mutations in the NS3/NS5B/NS5A proteins producing conformational changes that interfere with drug-target interaction. The limited data to date suggest that most of these mutations remain sensitive to type 1 IFN therapy *in vitro* and *in vivo*, meaning that combination therapy of DAA plus a Peg-IFN and RBV backbone is required and effective in patients who are sensitive to type 1 IFN. However, functional monotherapy in prior non-responders to SOC, or in patients who carry the *IL28B* poor responder allele, remains a concern, with virologic breakthrough and emergence of DAA resistant variants occurring in >35% of these patients in the phase III studies of the NS3 protease inhibitors [35,36]. Resistance to emerging DAA therapies has recently been the topic of a number of comprehensive review articles and will not be discussed in great detail here [77,78]. The medium- to long-term clinical significance of DAA-resistant variants is unclear. It is not known whether these DAA-resistant variants are archived in the liver, or what implication they may have for salvage antiviral therapy or disease progression.

Telaprevir-resistance mutations have been classified by *in vitro* phenotypic analysis as associated with low-level (T54A, V36A/M, R155K/T) or high-level (A156T/V, V36M + R155K, V36M + A156T) resistance [27]. All have reduced fitness compared to WT virus *in vitro*, with the most resistant viruses bearing the A156V/T mutations also being the least fit [27]. WT virus again becomes dominant after withdrawal of TVR therapy, though resistant mutants may remain detectable for months to years (R155 variants have been noted to persist for up to 3 years posttreatment [27,79]). Boceprevir has been associated with similar NS3 variants, consistent with cross-resistance and a class effect. There is an important difference in the risk of NS3 protease inhibitor resistance according to the HCV genotype 1a/b. Selection of the R155K/T variant requires two nucleotide substitutions in subtype 1b, but only one substitution in 1a. Resistance and virologic breakthrough were more common in genotype 1a patients treated with TVR or BOC in phase II/III studies.

The NI RG7128 appears to have a high genetic barrier to resistance. Selection of resistant variants *in vivo* has not been reported. The NS5B mutation S282T has been selected with RG7128 treatment in replicon studies. Resistance mutations have been identified for all the allosteric NNI candidates in clinical development. The barrier to resistance is lower than for NI, and monotherapy has been associated with rapid selection of resistance variants in the NS5B region. The amino acid positions have been specific for the allosteric binding site of the respective drugs.

The major resistant variants identified for the NS5A inhibitor BMS-790052 in pre-clinical studies for HCV-1b were L31V and Y93H, both located in domain 1. For HCV-1a, the major variants identified were M28T and Q30H/R in addition to mutations at residues L31 and Y93

(domain 1). Higher levels of resistance were associated with substitutions on the HCV genotype 1a background; however the EC_{50} of the most resistant 1a variant, L31V, was ~ 20 nM, levels readily achievable *in vivo*. Clinical data is limited, although virologic breakthrough was common by week 12 in patients treated with combination BMS-790052 and the NS3 protease inhibitor BMS-650032.

Cyclophilin inhibitors appear to have a high genetic barrier to resistance. Despite the drug target being a cellular enzyme, viral resistance has been described *in vitro*. HCV replicon studies have identified a low frequency and level of resistance to cyclophilin-binding drugs mediated by amino acid substitutions in three viral proteins: NS5A, NS5B, and NS3. NS5A mutations have the largest impact on resistance, including R318W and D320E in domain 2 [46,80]). They do not appear to be cross-resistant with BMS-790052.

Combination Strategies

It is hoped that in the future IFN-free combination DAA regimens will be developed. These will need to include multiple potent agents targeting different steps in the HCV viral life cycle, and that are not cross-resistant. The first study to combine DAAs in an IFN-free regimen was the INFORM-1 study [40]. In this dose-escalation study, the NI RG7128 was combined with the NS3 protease inhibitor RG7227 for 13 days. At maximal dose, a median HCV RNA reduction of 5.1 log_{10} IU/ml was observed. No virologic resistance was reported, although one patient experienced a 1.4 log virologic rebound from nadir on the last day of treatment. No resistant mutations were identified by population sequencing, although clonal analysis identified an RG7227-resistance mutation (NS3_F43S). RG7128 appears to have a high barrier to resistance, and the data suggest that combination therapy was able to restrict breakthrough of NS3 resistant variants, which are rapidly selected during RG7227 monotherapy. There are at least six combinations DAAs regimens currently being evaluated (Table 25.1b). Preliminary analyses of two studies are worth particular comment. The NS5A inhibitor BMS-790052 is being studied in combination with the NS3 protease inhibitor BMS-650032 [45]. Twenty-one patients with previous null response to Peg-IFN/RBV were randomized to BMS-790052 plus BMS-650032 or BMS-790052 and BMS-650032 plus Peg-IFN and RBV for 12 weeks. In this difficult-to-treat group, 46% of patients in the combination DAA arm without Peg-IFN and RBV attained a complete week-12 response,

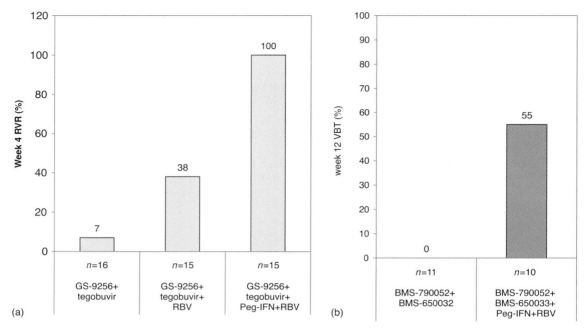

Figure 25.1 Interferon-free DAA therapy has been complicated by disappointing virologic response rates due to the selection of antiviral resistance. Both Peg-IFN and RBV appear to play important roles. (a) Week 4 RVR rates in patients treated with GS-9256 and tegobuvir (GS-9190) alone or in combination with RBV, or Peg-IFN plus RBV [81]. (b) Twenty-one patients with previous null response to Peg-IFN and RBV were randomized to BMS-790052 plus BMS-650032 or BMS-790052 and BMS-650032 plus Peg-IFN and RBV for 12 weeks. Virologic breakthrough (VBT) was higher in patients in the combination DAA arm without Peg-IFN and RBV; no viral breakthrough was observed in the setting of quadruple therapy [45].

and virologic breakthrough occurred in 55% of patients. In contrast, 90% of patients treated with quadruple therapy had undetectable serum HCV RNA at week 12 and no viral breakthrough was observed (Figure 25.1). In a second combination study, 46 treatment-naïve patients were randomized to 4 weeks of treatment with one of three arms: (i) a combination of the protease inhibitor GS-9256 and NNI polymerase inhibitor GS-9190 (tegobuvir); (ii) GS-9256 plus GS-9190 plus weight-based RBV; or (iii) GS-9256 plus GS-9190 plus Peg-IFN plus weight-based RBV. Despite a median decline in HCV RNA of 4.1 $\log_{10}$ IU/ml at day 7, on-treatment resistance was identified in the majority of GS-9256 plus GS-9190 treated patients. RBV therapy was associated with increased virologic response and reduced resistance. The greatest virologic response occurred with quadruple therapy, with no resistance identified. The rates of complete virologic suppression (≤ 25 IU/ml) at week 4 were 7%, 38%, and 100% for dual, triple, and quadruple therapy, respectively (Figure 25.1) [81]. Therefore, despite the encouraging results

of the INFORM-1 study, Peg-IFN and RBV look like they will remain an important and necessary part of combination DAA regimens for the next decade. Although no single point mutation has been identified that confers resistance to different classes of DAA, it appears from this data that a single HCV genome can select mutations against multiple agents. It has recently been estimated that to prevent resistance IFN-free DAA treatment will require combinations with a genetic barrier to resistance of four or more mutations [82].

IL28B Polymorphism

Genetic variation in the region of the *IL28B* gene on chromosome 19 has recently been identified to be the strongest baseline predictor of virologic response to treatment with Peg-IFN and RBV therapy in genotype 1 HCV [83–85]. Patients carrying the good response variant have markedly increased phase I kinetics on-treatment [86]. Differences in allele frequency according to genetic ancestry (Asian versus Caucasian versus African) explain much of the disparity in SVR rates that are observed between ethnic groups [83]. So far the data generated applies to current SOC (pegylated interferon and ribavarin) outcomes. The data predict a two-fold increase in SVR for favorable *IL28* alleles but are not strong enough to make definitive yes or no answers on whom to treat. Such testing however is likely to be incorporated into future treatment algorithms.

As yet there is little data that has considered the relationship between *IL28B* genotype and response to DAA triple therapy regimens. Only one study has examined *IL28B* genotype and TVR triple therapy [68]. In this small Japanese population, including both treatment-naïve and- experienced patients, subjects were treated with TVR plus Peg-IFN and RBV of variable duration. *IL28B* genotype remained strongly associated with treatment outcome, although interpretation was limited by the study design. More recent data in abstract form suggests that DAAs attenuate, but do not overcome, the *IL28B* effect in patients carrying poor response variants [70]. The benefit of DAA combination over SOC in patients carrying the good response variant is not clear. This will be an important question for cost-effectiveness analysis. Finally, *IL28B* genotype is relevant to the early phase development of novel DAAs. It is important that small early phase DAA studies stratify subjects according to *IL28B* genotype, to avoid confounding by mismatch for the good response variant between treatment arms [87].

Unresolved Issues

A number of important questions are yet to be addressed. There is little information about which patients are most likely to benefit from DAA combination strategies, considering both efficacy and cost effectiveness – should DAA be used in all patients, or individualized according to baseline characteristics, including *IL28B* genotype and liver fibrosis stage, or on-treatment response (failure to achieve a week-4 rapid virologic response)? There are a number of key patient subgroups in which there is limited or no experience: advanced cirrhotics with decompensated liver disease, liver transplant recipients with HCV recurrence, renal dialysis patients, and patients with hereditary anemias. Post-registration studies addressing the use of TVR and BOC in these groups are expected. TVR and BOC are relatively specific for genotype 1 HCV. A number of the newer classes of agent appear to have broader HCV genotype activity, including the NS5B NI, the NS5A inhibitors,

and the cyclophilin inhibitors, and clinical studies investigating their use in non-genotype 1 HCV poor responders to Peg-IFN and RBV are needed.

Summary and Conclusions

Chronic hepatitis C is an important cause of liver-related morbidity and mortality. The current standard-of-care treatment, Peg-IFN and RBV, has limited efficacy for genotype 1 HCV and is poorly tolerated by many patients. More effective strategies are needed. The development and introduction of direct-acting acting viral agents is an important advance. Candidates targeting a number of different steps in the HCV life cycle are currently in development and include inhibitors of the HCV NS3 protease, NS5B polymerase, and NS5A protein. Important lessons have been learned in the development process concerning the risks of monotherapy, drug resistance, treatment-limiting toxicities, and the continuing role for Peg-IFN and RBV. The most advanced agents are the NS3 protease inhibitors telaprevir and boceprevir, which have now completed phase III development. Triple therapy regimens including Peg-IFN and RBV will significantly increase rates of SVR and allow many patients to receive shortened duration therapy. Next generation agents will need to offer greater potency, high genetic barrier to resistance, and fewer side effects, with the goal of combination in IFN-free regimens. The future challenge will be to wisely and cost-effectively assimilate these new drugs into treatment algorithms, in the face of a rapidly evolving therapeutic landscape.

Authors' Declaration of Personal Interests

Alex Thompson has served as a speaker and an advisory board member for Roche Pharmaceuticals; Merck, Inc. He has served as an Advisory Board member for Johnson and Johnson. He has received a travel grant from Gilead Pharmaceuticals. He is a co-applicant of a patent related to the *IL28B* discovery.

John McHutchison is an employee of Gilead Pharmaceuticals. He is a co-applicant of a patent related to the *IL28B* discovery.

Geoff McCaughan has served on Advisory Boards for Roche Pharmaceuticals, Australia; Merck, Inc. Australia; Johnson and Johnson, Australia; and Gilead Australia.

References

1. Lavanchy D. The global burden of hepatitis C. *Liver Int* 2009;29(Suppl 1):74–81.
2. Kim WR. The burden of hepatitis C in the United States. *Hepatology* 2002;36(5 Suppl 1):S30–34.
3. Pawlotsky JM, Chevaliez S, McHutchison JG. The hepatitis C virus life cycle as a target for new antiviral therapies. *Gastroenterology* 2007;132(5):1979–98.
4. Davis GL. Chronic hepatitis C and liver transplantation. *Rev Gastroenterol Disord* 2004;4(1):7–17.
5. Shan, Y, *et al.* Reciprocal effects of micro-RNA-122 on expression of heme oxygenase-1 and hepatitis C virus genes in human hepatocytes. *Gastroenterology* 2007;133(4):1166–74.
6. Randall, G, *et al.* Cellular cofactors affecting hepatitis C virus infection and replication. *Proc Natl Acad Sci USA* 2007;104(31):12884–9.
7. Pedersen, I.M, *et al.* Interferon modulation of cellular microRNAs as an antiviral mechanism. *Nature* 2007;449(7164):919–22.
8. Jopling, C.L, *et al.* Modulation of hepatitis C virus RNA abundance by a liver-specific MicroRNA. *Science* 2005;309(5740):1577–81.
9. Lohmann V, Körner F, Koch J, *et al.* Replication of subgenomic hepatitis C virus RNAs in a hepatoma cell line. *Science* 1999;285(5424):110–13.
10. Lohmann V, Körner F, Dobierzewska A, Bartenschlager R. Mutations in hepatitis C virus RNAs conferring cell culture adaptation. *J Virol* 2001;75(3):1437–49.
11. Blight KJ, Kolykhalov AA, Rice CM. Efficient initiation of HCV RNA replication in cell culture. *Science* 2000;290(5498):1972–4.
12. Lesburg CA, Cable MB, Ferrari E, *et al.* Crystal structure of the RNA-dependent RNA polymerase from hepatitis C virus reveals a fully encircled active site. *Nat Struct Biol* 1999;6(10):937–43.
13. Bressanelli, S, Tomei L, Roussel A, *et al.* Crystal structure of the RNA-dependent RNA polymerase of hepatitis C virus. *Proc Natl Acad Sci USA* 1999;96(23):13034–9.
14. Love RA, Parge HE, Wickersham JA, *et al.* The crystal structure of hepatitis C virus NS3 proteinase reveals a trypsin-like fold and a structural zinc binding site. *Cell* 1996;87(2):331–42.
15. Kim JL, Morgenstern KA, Lin C, *et al.* Crystal structure of the hepatitis C virus NS3 protease domain complexed with a synthetic NS4A cofactor peptide. *Cell* 1996;87(2):343–55.
16. Yan Y, Li Y, Munshi S, *et al.* Complex of NS3 protease and NS4A peptide of BK strain hepatitis C virus: a *2.2 A resolution structure in a hexagonal crystal form. Protein Sci* 1998;7(4):837–47.
17. Kato T, Date T, Miyamoto M, *et al.* Efficient replication of the genotype 2a hepatitis C virus subgenomic replicon. *Gastroenterology* 2003;125(6):1808–17.
18. Thimme R, Lohmann V, Weber F. A target on the move: innate and adaptive immune escape strategies of hepatitis C virus. *Antiviral Res* 2006;69(3):129–41.
19. Foy E, Li K, Wang C, *et al.* Regulation of interferon regulatory factor-3 by the hepatitis C virus serine protease. *Science* 2003;300(5622):1145–8.
20. Foy E, Li K, Sumpter R, Jr., Loo YM, *et al.* Control of antiviral defenses through hepatitis C virus disruption of retinoic acid-inducible gene-I signaling. *Proc Natl Acad Sci USA* 2005;102(8):2986–91.
21. Loo YM, Owen DM, Li K, *et al.* Viral and therapeutic control of IFN-beta promoter stimulator 1 during hepatitis C virus infection. *Proc Natl Acad Sci USA* 2006;103(15):6001–6.
22. Li K, Foy E, Ferreon JC, *et al.* Immune evasion by hepatitis C virus NS3/4A protease-mediated cleavage of the Toll-like receptor 3 adaptor protein TRIF. *Proc Natl Acad Sci USA* 2005;102(8):2992–7.
23. Hinrichsen H, Benhamou Y, Wedemeyer H, *et al.* Short-term antiviral efficacy of BILN 2061, a hepatitis C virus serine protease inhibitor, in hepatitis C genotype 1 patients. *Gastroenterology* 2004;127(5):1347–55.
24. Lamarre D, Anderson PC, Bailey M, *et al.* An NS3 protease inhibitor with antiviral effects in humans infected with hepatitis C virus. *Nature* 2003;426(6963):186–9.
25. Reiser M, Hinrichsen H, Benhamou Y, *et al.* Antiviral efficacy of NS3-serine protease inhibitor BILN-2061 in patients with chronic genotype 2 and 3 hepatitis C. *Hepatology* 2005;41(4):832–5.
26. Foster GR, Hezode C, Bronowicki J-P, *et al.* Activity of telaprevir alone or in combination withpeginterferon alfa-2a and ribavirin in treatment-naive genotype 2 and 3 hepatitis C patients: final results of study C209. *J Hepatol* 2010;52 (Suppl 2):S27.
27. Sarrazin C, Kieffer TL, Bartels D, *et al.* Dynamic hepatitis C virus genotypic and phenotypic changes in patients treated with the protease inhibitor telaprevir. *Gastroenterology* 2007;132(5):1767–77.
28. Forestier N, Reesink HW, Weegink CJ, *et al.* Antiviral activity of telaprevir (VX-950) and peginterferon alfa-2a in patients with hepatitis C. *Hepatology* 2007;46(3):640–48.
29. Zeuzem S, Andreone P, Pol S, *et al.* REALIZE trial final results: telaprevir-based regimen for genotype 1 hepatitis C virus infection in patients with prior null response, partial response or relapse to peginterferon/ribavirin. *J Hepatology* 2011;54:(abs 5).
30. Zeuzem S, Hezode C, Ferenci P, *et al.* Telaprevir in combination with peginterferon-alfa-2a with or without ribavirin in the treatment of chronic hepatitis C: final results of the PROVE2 study. *Hepatology* 2008;48(4 (Suppl 1)):418A.
31. Jacobson IM, McHutchison JG, Dusheiko GM, *et al.* Telaprevir in combination with peginterferon and ribavirin in genotype 1 HCV treatment-naïve patients: final results of the phase 3 ADVANCE study. *Hepatology* 2010;52(Suppl 1):211.

32. Sherman KE, Flamm SL, Afdhal NH, *et al.* Telaprevir in combination with peginterferon alfa-2a and ribavirin for 24 or 48 weeks in treatment-naïve genotype 1 HCV patients who achieved an extended rapid viral response: Final results of the phase 3 ILLUMINATE Study. *Hepatology* 2010;52(Suppl 1):LB-2.

33. http://investors.vrtx.com/releasedetail.cfm?ReleaseID= 505239.

34. Zeuzem S, Sarrazin C, Rouzier R, *et al.* Anti-viral activity of SCH 503034, a HCV protease inhibitor, administered as monotherapy in hepatitis C genotype-1 (HCV-1) patients refractory to pegylated interferon (peg-IFN-α). *Hepatology* 2005;42(S1):A94.

35. Poordad F, McCone J, Bacon B, *et al.* Boceprevir combined with peginterferon alfa-2b/ribavirin for treatment-naive patients with HCV genotype 1: SPRINT-2 final results. *Hepatology* 2010;52(Suppl 1):LB4.

36. Bacon BR, Gordon SC, Lawitz EJ, *et al.* HCV RESPOND-2 final results: High sustained virological response among genotype 1 previous non-responders and relapsers to peginterferon/ribavirin when retreated with boceprevir plus PEGINTRON (peginterferon alfa-2b)/ribavirin. *Hepatology* 2010;52(Suppl 1):216A.

37. Pottage JC, Lawitz E, Mazur D, *et al.* Short-term antiviral activity and safety of ACH-806 (GS-9132), an NS4A antagonist, in HCV genotype 1 infected individuals. *J Hepatol* 2008;46(Suppl 1):S294–5.

38. Reddy R, Rodriguez-Torres M, Gane E, *et al.* Antiviral activity, pharmacokinetics, safety, and tolerability of R7128, a novel nucleoside HCV RNA polymerase inhibitor, following multiple, ascending, oral doses in patients with HCV genotype 1 infection who have failed prior interferon therapy. *Hepatology* 2007;46(4 Suppl 1):862A–863A.

39. Lalezari J, Gane E, Rodriguez-Torres M, *et al.* Potent antiviral activity of the HCV nucleoside polymerase inhibitor R7128 with PEG-IFN and ribavirin: interim results of R7128 500 mg bid for 28 days. *J Hepatol* 2008;48(Suppl 2):S29.

40. Gane EJ, Roberts SK, Stedman CA, *et al.* Oral combination therapy with a nucleoside polymerase inhibitor (RG7128) and danoprevir for chronic hepatitis C genotype 1 infection (INFORM-1): a randomised, double-blind, placebo-controlled, dose-escalation trial. *Lancet* 2010;376(9751):1467–75.

41. Gane EJ, Rodriguez-Torres M, Nelson DR, *et al.* Antiviral activity of the HCV nucleoside polymerase inhibitor R7128 in HCV genotype 2 and 3 prior nonresponders: interim results of R7128 1,500 mg bid with PEG-IFN and ribavirin for 28 days. *Hepatology* 2008;48(Suppl 1):LB10.

42. Standring, D, *et al.* Potent Antiviral Activity of 2nd Generation HCV Nucleotide Inhibitors, IDX102 and IDX184, in HCV-infected Chimpanzees. *J Hepatol* 2008;48(Suppl 2):S30 (A67).

43. Tellinghuisen, TL, Foss KL, Treadaway J. Regulation of hepatitis C virion production via phosphorylation of the NS5A protein. *PLoS Pathog* 2008;4(3):e1000032.

44. Gao M, Nettles RE, Belema M, *et al.* Chemical genetics strategy identifies an HCV NS5A inhibitor with a potent clinical effect. *Nature* 2010;465(7294):96–100.

45. Lok AS, Gardiner DF, Lawitz E et al. Combination therapy with BMS-790052 and BMS-650032 alone or with pegIFN/RBV results in undetectable HCV RNA through 12 weeks of therapy in HCV genotype 1 null responders. *Hepatology* 2010;52(2 Suppl 1):LB8.

46. Coelmont L, Hanoulle X, Chatterji U, *et al.* DEB025 (Alisporivir) inhibits hepatitis C virus replication by preventing a cyclophilin A induced cis-trans isomerisation in domain II of NS5A. *PLoS One*; 5(10):e13687.

47. Ma S, Boerner JE, TiongYip C, *et al.* NIM811, a cyclophilin inhibitor, exhibits potent in vitro activity against hepatitis C virus alone or in combination with alpha interferon. *Antimicrob Agents Chemother* 2006;50(9):2976–82.

48. Nakagawa M, Sakamoto N, Tanabe Y, *et al.* Suppression of hepatitis C virus replication by cyclosporin A is mediated by blockade of cyclophilins. *Gastroenterology* 2005;129(3):1031–41.

49. Watashi K, Ishii N, Hijikata M, *et al.* Cyclophilin B is a functional regulator of hepatitis C virus RNA polymerase. *Mol Cell* 2005;19(1):111–22.

50. Flisiak R, Feinman SV, Jablkowski M, *et al.* Efficacy and safety of increasing doses of the cyclophilin inhibitor DEBIO 025 in combination with pegylated interferon alpha-2a in treatment naive chronic HCV patients. *J Hepatol* 2008;48(Suppl 1):S62.

51. Lawitz E, Godofsky E, Rouzier R, *et al.* Safety, pharmacokinetics, and antiviral activity of the cyclophilin inhibitor NIM811 alone or in combination with pegylated interferon in HCV-infected patients receiving 14 days of therapy. *Antiviral Res* 2011;89(3):238–45.

52. Goto K, Watashi K, Murata T, *et al.* Evaluation of the anti-hepatitis C virus effects of cyclophilin inhibitors, cyclosporin A, and NIM811. *Biochem Biophys Res Commun* 2006;343(3):879–84.

53. Whitby K, Taylor D, Patel D, *et al.* Action of celgosivir (6 O-butanoyl castanospermine) against the pestivirus BVDV: implications for the treatment of hepatitis C. *Antivir Chem Chemother* 2004;15(3):141–51.

54. Yoshida E, Kunimoto D, Lee SS, *et al.* Results of a phase 2 dose ranging study of orally administered celgosivir as monotherapy in chronic hepatitis C genotype 1 patients. *Gastroenterology* 2006;130: A784.

55. Kaita K, Yoshida E, Kunimoto D, *et al.* Ph II proof of concept study of celgosivir in combination with peginterferon alfa-2b and ribavirin in chronic hepatitis C genotype 1 nonresponder patients. *J Hepatol* 2007;46(Suppl 1):S56.

56. Robek MD, Boyd BS, Chisari FV. Lambda interferon inhibits hepatitis B and C virus replication. *J Virol* 2005;79(6):3851–4.

57. Marcello T, Grakoui A, Barba-Spaeth G, *et al.* Interferons alpha and lambda inhibit hepatitis C virus replication with

distinct signal transduction and gene regulation kinetics. *Gastroenterology* 2006;131(6):1887–98.

58. Muir AJ, Shiffman ML, Zaman A, *et al.* Phase 1b study of pegylated interferon lambda 1 with or without ribavirin in patients with chronic genotype 1 hepatitis C virus infection. *Hepatology* 2010;52(3):822–32.

59. Muir AJ, Lawitz E, Ghalib RH, *et al.* Pegylated interferon lambda (PEG-IFN-λ) phase 2 dose-ranging, active-controlled study in combination with ribavirin (RBV) for treatment-naïve HCV patients (genotypes 1, 2, 3 or 4): safety, viral response, and impact of IL-28B host genotype through week 12. *Hepatology* 2010;52(2 Suppl 1):821.

60. Liu C, Zhu H, Subramanian GM, *et al.* Anti-hepatitis C virus activity of albinterferon alfa-2b in cell culture. *Hepatol Res* 2007;37(11):941–7.

61. Bain VG, Kaita KD, Yoshida EM, *et al.* A phase 2 study to evaluate the antiviral activity, safety, and pharmacokinetics of recombinant human albumin-interferon alfa fusion protein in genotype 1 chronic hepatitis C patients. *J Hepatol* 2006;44(4):671–8.

62. Balan V, Nelson DR, Sulkowski MS, *et al.* A phase I/II study evaluating escalating doses of recombinant human albumin-interferon-alpha fusion protein in chronic hepatitis C patients who have failed previous interferon-alpha-based therapy. *Antivir Ther* 2006;11(1):35–45.

63. Zeuzem S, Sulkowski MS, Lawitz EJ, *et al.* Albinterferon alfa-2b was not inferior to pegylated interferon-alpha in a randomized trial of patients with chronic hepatitis C virus genotype 1. *Gastroenterology* 2010;139(4):1257–66.

64. Nelson DR, Benhamou Y, Chuang WL, *et al.* Albinterferon Alfa-2b was not inferior to pegylated interferon-alpha in a randomized trial of patients with chronic hepatitis C virus genotype 2 or 3. *Gastroenterology* 2010;139(4):1267–76.

65. Subramanian GM, Fiscella M, Lamousé-Smith A, *et al.* Albinterferon alpha-2b: a genetic fusion protein for the treatment of chronic hepatitis C. *Nat Biotechnol* 2007;25(12):1411–19.

66. Dzyublyk I, Yegorova T, Moroz L, *et al.* Phase 2a study to evaluate the safety and tolerability and anti-viral of 4 doses of a novel, controlled-release interferon alfa-2b (Locteron) given every 2 weeks for 12 weeks in treatment-naive patients with chronic hepatitis C (genotype 1). *Hepatology* 2007;46(4 Suppl 1):863A.

67. Benhamou Y, Pockros P, Rodriguez-Torres M, *et al.* The safety and efficacy of viramidine plus pegIFN alfa-2b versus ribavirin plus pegIFN alfa-2b in therapy-naïve patients infected with HCV: phase 3 results (VISER1). *J Hepatol* 2006;44(Suppl 2):S273.

68. Marcellin P, Lurie Y, Rodriguez-Torres M, *et al.* The safety and efficacy of taribavirin plus pegylated interferon alfa2a versus ribavirin plus pegylated interferon alfa2a in therapy naive patients infected with HCV: phase 3 results. *J Hepatol* 2007;46(Suppl 1):S7.

69. Poordad F, Lawitz E, Shiffman ML, *et al.* Virologic response rates of weight-based taribavirin versus ribavirin in treatment-naive patients with genotype 1 chronic hepatitis C. *Hepatology* 2010;52(4):1208–15.

70. Schiff ER, Everson GT, Tsai N, *et al.* HCV-specific cellular immunity, RNA reductions, and normalization of ALT in chronic HCV subjects after treatment with GI-5005, a yeast-based immunotherapy targeting NS3 and core: a randomized, double-blind, placebo-controlled phase 1b study. *Hepatology* 2007;46(4 Suppl 1):816A.

71. Pockros P, Jacobson IM, Boyer TD, *et al.* GI-5005 therapeutic vaccine plus Peg-IFN/ribavirin improves sustained virologic response versus Peg-IFN/ribavirin in prior non-responders with genotype 1 chronic HCV infection. *Hepatology* 2010;52(Suppl 1):LB6.

72. Vierling JM, McHutchison JG, Jacobson IM, *et al.* GI-5005 therapeutic vaccine improves deficit in cellular immunity in IL28B genotype T/T, treatment-naive patients with chronic hepatitis C genotype 1 when added to standard of care (SOC) Peg-IFN-alfa-2A/ribavirin. *Hepatology* 2010;52(Suppl 1):1973A.

73. Kuzushita N, Gregory SH, Monti NA, *et al.* Vaccination with protein-transduced dendritic cells elicits a sustained response to hepatitis C viral antigens. *Gastroenterology* 2006;130(2):453–64.

74. Jones KL, Brown LE, Eriksson EM, *et al.* Human dendritic cells pulsed with specific lipopeptides stimulate autologous antigen-specific T cells without the addition of exogenous maturation factors. *J Viral Hepatitis* 2008;15(10):761–72.

75. Kuntzen T, Timm J, Berical A, *et al.* Naturally occurring dominant resistance mutations to hepatitis C virus protease and polymerase inhibitors in treatment-naive patients. *Hepatology* 2008;48(6):1769–78.

76. Bartels DJ, Zhou Y, Zhang EZ, *et al.* Natural prevalence of hepatitis C virus variants with decreased sensitivity to NS3.4A protease inhibitors in treatment-naive subjects. *J Infect Dis* 2008;198(6):800–807.

77. Sarrazin C, Zeuzem S. Resistance to direct antiviral agents in patients with hepatitis C virus infection. *Gastroenterology* 2010;138(2):447–62.

78. Thompson AJ, McHutchison JG. Antiviral resistance and specifically targeted therapy for HCV (STAT-C). *J Viral Hepatitis* 2009;16(6):377–87.

79. Forestier N, Susser S, Welker, MW *et al.* Long term follow up of patients previously treated with telaprevir *Hepatology* 2008;48(4 Suppl 1):760A.

80. Puyang X, Poulin DL, Mathy JE, *et al.* Mechanism of resistance of hepatitis C virus replicons to structurally distinct cyclophilin inhibitors. *Antimicrob Agents Chemother* 2010;54(5):1981–7.

81. Zeuzem S, Buggisch P, Agarwal K, *et al.* Dual, triple, and quadruple combination treatment with a protease inhibitor (GS-9256) and a polymerase inhibitor (GS-9190) alone and in combination with ribavirin (RBV) or PegIFN/RBV for

up to 28 days in treatment-naive, genotype 1 HCV subjects. *Hepatology* 2010;52(Suppl 1):LB1.

82. Rong L, Dahari H, Ribeiro RM, Perelson AS Rapid emergence of protease inhibitor resistance in hepatitis C virus. *Sci Transl Med* 2010;2(30):30ra32.

83. Ge D, Fellay J, Thompson AJ, *et al.* Genetic variation in IL28B predicts hepatitis C treatment-induced viral clearance. *Nature* 2009;461(7262):399–401.

84. Tanaka Y, Nishida N, Sugiyama M, *et al.* Genome-wide association of IL28B with response to pegylated interferon-alpha and ribavirin therapy for chronic hepatitis C. *Nat Genet* 2009;41(10):1105–9.

85. Suppiah V, Moldovan M, Ahlenstiel G, *et al.* IL28B is associated with response to chronic hepatitis C interferon-alpha and ribavirin therapy. *Nat Genet* 2009;41(10):1100–1104.

86. Thompson AJ, Muir AJ, Sulkowski MS, *et al.* Interleukin-28B polymorphism improves viral kinetics and is the strongest pretreatment predictor of sustained virologic response in genotype 1 hepatitis C virus. *Gastroenterology* 2010;139(1):120–29.e18.

87. Thompson AJ, Muir AJ, Sulkowski MS, *et al.* Hepatitis C trials that combine investigational agents with pegylated interferon should be stratified by interleukin-28B genotype. *Hepatology* 2010;52(6):2243–4.

Index

Page numbers in *italics* denote figures, those in **bold** denote tables.

Advanced Therapy for Hepatitis C, First Edition. Edited by Geoffrey W. McCaughan, John G. McHutchison and Jean-Michel Pawlotsky.
© 2012 Blackwell Publishing Ltd. Published 2012 by Blackwell Publishing Ltd.